Recent Results in Cancer Research

118

Recent Results in Cancer Research

L.Beck E.Grundmann R.Ackermann
H.-D. Röher (Eds.)

Hormone-Related
Malignant Tumors

With 83 Figures and 91 Tables

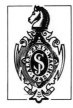

Springer-Verlag Berlin Heidelberg New York
London Paris Tokyo Hong Kong

Professor Dr. Lutwin Beck
Frauenklinik, Medizinische Einrichtungen
Universität Düsseldorf
Moorenstraße 5, 4000 Düsseldorf, FRG

Professor Dr. Ekkehard Grundmann
Gerhard Domagk-Institut für Pathologie
Westfälische Wilhelms-Universität Münster
Domagkstraße 17, 4400 Münster, FRG

Professor Dr. Rolf Ackermann
Urologische Klinik, Universität Düsseldorf
Moorenstraße 5, 4000 Düsseldorf, FRG

Professor Dr. Hans-Dietrich Röher
Chirurgische Klinik und Poliklinik I
Universität Düsseldorf
Moorenstraße 5, 4000 Düsseldorf, FRG

ISBN 3-540-51258-6 Springer-Verlag Berlin Heidelberg New York
ISBN 0-387-51258-6 Springer-Verlag New York Berlin Heidelberg

Library of Congress Cataloging-in-Publication Data
Hormone-related malignant tumors/L. Beck . . . (eds.).
p.cm.-(Recent results in cancer research; 118)
ISBN 0-387-51258-6: (U.S.: alk. paper)
1. Endocrine glands-Tumors. 2. Cancer-Endocrine aspects. I. Beck, Lutwin.
II. Series.
[DNLM: 1. Endocrine Diseases. 2. Hormones-adverse effects. 3. Hormones-
therapeutic use. 4. Neoplasms-drug therapy. 5. Neoplasms-etiology.
W1 RE106p v. 118/QZ 200 H8117] RC261.R35 vol. 118
[RC280.E55] 616.99'4 s-dc20 [616.99'44] DNLM/DLC
89-26231

Typesetting: Macmillan India Ltd., Bangalore-25, India
Printing: Druckhaus Beltz, Hemsbach/Bergstr.
Binding: J. Schäffer OHG, Grünstadt
2125/3140-543210-Printed on acid-free paper.

Preface

The growth and function of many tissues are influenced by hormones. Therefore it is quite understandable that hormones play a role in the development and treatment of malignant tumors. Numerous publications address this topic; however, the results of many studies are controversial and have not been unequivocally accepted. For nearly 50 years the carcinogenic effect of steroid hormones has been under debate, and their therapeutic value a matter of discussion for equally as long.

The present volume concentrates on substantiated data first obtained from the study of tumors developing from hormone-regulated or hormone-producing tissue, e.g., the thyroid, adrenal glands, prostate, and the female genital tract. Through a joint approach from the field of molecular biology, biochemistry, and histopathology, advances in the management of these tumors have been elaborated. Another exciting example is the endo-nuclear diagnosis of adrenal tumors. Antihormones, i.e. antian-drogens or GnRH analogues have proved to be important indeed since they exhibit a destructive effect on prostate carcinomas and breast cancer. Further improvements can be expected in the localization of hormones in tumor tissue by specific antibodies.

A special chapter is dedicated to the diffuse endocrine cell system (DECS), the clinical significance of which has mainly become obvious in the gastroenteropancreatic tract.

Doubtlessly we are on the threshold of a development which already affects medical oncology and may extend into the prevention of malignancies. This volume, bridging the gap between molecular biology and endocrine therapy, covers many aspects of hormone-related malignant tumors and offers both a survey of present knowledge and a basis for further research in this promising field.

Düsseldorf/Münster,　　　　　　　　　　L. Beck E. Grundmann
November 1989　　　　　　　　　　　R. Ackermann H.-D. Röher

Contents

VIII   Contents

List of Contributors*

Beck, T. *196*[1]
Bender, H. G. *260*
Berg, N.J. *233*
Böcker, W. *41*
Colvard, D.S. *233*
Dietel, M. *1*
Distler, W. *190*
Eidtmann, H. *225*
Fig. L.M. *113*
Friesen, S.R. *37*
Frilling, A. *48*
Goretzki, P.E. *48*
Graham, M.L. *233*
Grill, H.-J. *196*
Gross, M.D. *113*
Heitz, P.U. *19, 27*
Hoffmann, G. *196*
Ingle, J.N. *233*
Isaacs, J.T. *153*
Jacobi, G.H. *174*
Jonat, W. *225*
Käser, H. *97*
Khafagi, F. *113*
Klöppel, G. *27*
Kreienberg, R. *196*
Kügler, G. *225*

Kunz, T. *225*
Maass, H. *225*
Manz, B. *196*
Matthiessen, H. von *190*
Mosny, D.S. *260*
Müller, J. *106*
Niendorf, A. *1*
Pfleiderer, A. *252*
Podratz, K.C. *233, 242*
Pollow, K. *196*
Pontes, J.E. *186*
Raue, F. *64*
Roeher, H.-D. *48*
Saeger, W. *79*
Schaid, D.J. *233*
Schmidt-Gollwitzer, K. *196*
Schröder, F.H. *163*
Schröder, S. *41*
Schulze, H. *153*
Schweikert, H.-U. *145*
Shapiro, B. *113*
Simon, D. *48*
Spelsberg, T.C. *233*
Wells, S.A. Jr. *70*
Zingg, E.J. *139*

---

* The address of the principal author is given on the first page of each contribution.
[1] Page on which contribution begins.

Biological Basics

Cellular Receptors of Hormones and Nonhormone Ligands in Normal and Malignant Cells*

M. Dietel and A. Niendorf

Institut für Pathologie, Universitätskrankenhaus Eppendorf, Martinistraße 52, 2000 Hamburg 20, FRG

Introduction

The rate of cell division in multicellular organisms is controlled by humoral signals (e.g., hormones, growth factors, transport proteins or low-density lipoproteins), cell – to – cell interactions (e.g., contact inhibition), and cell-inherent factors such as certain genes and the associated gene products. Under physiological conditions there is a balance between creation and death of cells in response to requirement. For example, in case of local cell destruction fibroblasts, endothelia, pericytes, possibly keratinocytes, osteocytes, and other cell populations start to divide. Subsequent to repairment the cells stop growing. This process of growth regulation is under the control of various local signals. It is unclear up to now whether similar, but pathological, mechanisms also play a role in cell transformation with uncontrolled proliferation. Besides such local growth control many humoral factors are known to regulate cell proliferation. A prerequisite for the effectiveness of such growth-regulating substances are cellular receptors of the target cells through which the signals are transmitted into the cells to switch on and off the corresponding genes.

One of the characteristic features of cancer cells is the abnormal ability for unlimited and relatively uncontrolled growth. This has been assigned variously to changes of cyclic nucleotide levels, plasma membrane fluidity, signal proteins, cytoskeleton, ion fluxes, gene abnormalities, and cell receptor properties (for reviews see Alberts et al. 1983; Berridge 1981; Bishop 1985; Cooper and Hunter 1983; Horwitz and McGuire 1978; Hynes 1985; Paul 1984; Varmus 1985; Vasilev 1985; Weinberg 1983). There is some evidence that the cancer cells are less sensitive to most feedback mechanisms that control cell division. This can be demonstrated in vitro when the malignant cells pile up forming multilayered clusters, or

---

* This work was supported by the Deutsche Forschungsgemeinschaft, SFB 232 (Hamburg) and grant Di 276/1–2, as well as by the Hamburger Krebsgesellschaft, the Hamburger Stiftung zur Förderung der Krebsbekämpfung and the Erich und Gertrud Roggenbruck-Stiftung.

"domes," while normal cells grow only until confluent. There is a second control mechanism that has been lost in cancer cells; limitation of the number of cell divisions in a cell's life span, referred to as genetically programmed cell death (Alberts et al. 1983).

Most growth-control mechanisms are associated with cell receptors (Rc), which play a key role in signal transmission and thus in regulation of cell growth. This paper focuses on the function of membrane-bound and nuclear/cytosolic receptors in controlling proliferation of eukaryotic cells.

Types of Cell Receptors

The great variety of signaling substances (ligands) are identified by specialized Rc proteins located in the cell membrane, cytosol, or nucleus. In general, hydrophilic, mostly large ligands (peptides, glycoproteins, lipoproteins, viruses, many pharmacological agents) are recognized by cell surface Rc, while lipophilic, mostly small ligands (steroid hormones, thyroid hormones, certain amino acids, small artificial molecules) are recognized predominantly by cytosolic/nuclear Rc. An exception to the latter is the binding of small neurotransmitter molecules to surface Rc of the postsynaptic cell of nerve terminals.

Structure and Function of Surface Receptors

Cell surface Rc consist of extracellular, intramembrane, and intracytosolic domains (Figs. 1, 2). The receptor protein can perforate the membrane once or four– or sevenfold. The extracellular domain accounts for ligand binding. Signal transmission involves the activation of the intramembrane regulatory subunit (G-protein) including cleavage of the energy-rich guanosine triphosphate and subsequent activation of Rc-associated enzymes (adenylate cyclase, protein kinase, or phosphoesterase). The enzyme activation is performed by the intracellular domain and results in phosphorylation with activation of target proteins (Catt et al. 1979; Goldstein et al. 1979; Pastan and Willinghan 1981) which in response are able to trigger DNA activation. Concerning cell proliferation, possible steps of cellular signal transmission are the increase in intracellular calcium and cytosolic pH (Fig. 2, p. 4). Both events can stimulate cell division (Catt et al. 1979; Helmreich 1986).

Alternatively, calcium ions are involved in signal mediation, for example, of acetylcholin Rc (Carafoli and Peneston 1986). After ligand-Rc binding the gated calcium channels open followed by an increase in the cytosolic calcium concentration which activates mitogenic enzymes (Berridge 1981; Berridge and Irvine 1984). Several calcium binding proteins (calmodulin, troponin, vitamin D_3-dependent calcium binding protein) are involved in this mode of signal transmission.

Pathway and Sorting of the Ligand-Receptor Complex

Most ligands bind relatively tightly to their Rc (e.g., binding constant for several peptide hormones, $K_b = 1.9 \times 10^{-9}$), forming the ligand-receptor complex (LRC). As demonstrated morphologically, several LRC are concentrated by lateral movement (Fig. 3, p. 4) at certain areas on the cell surface (clustering) with subsequent membrane invagination (Fig. 4, p. 5). These structures are termed coated pits (CP). They dissociate from the membrane and form coated vesicles (CV) which are surrounded by a characteristic bristlelike coat of clathrin, a 180-kDa protein (Brown et al. 1983). The CV migrate to the inner part of the cell. The total process has been termed receptor-mediated endocytosis (Pastan and Willingham 1981) and is an energy-consuming process. Then, the CV looses the clathrin coat and fuses with the Golgi apparatus forming the compartment of uncoupling of receptor and ligand, (CURL). Most ligands are destroyed in lysosomes. Rc proteins, however, in general are recycled and reintegrated in the plasmalemma. Thus, the cell possesses an economical way for the redisposition of Rc avoiding repeated Rc synthesis.

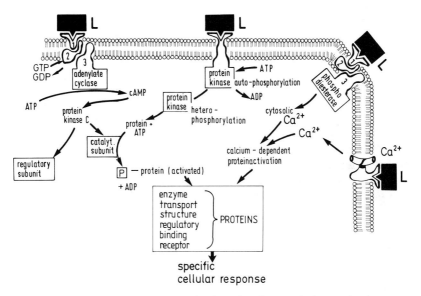

Fig. 1. Mechanisms of cell surface receptor activation, signal transmission, and subsequent intracellular processing. *Left*, ligand binding to an adenylate cyclase associated Rc: *1*, Extracellular domain; *2*, intramembranous regulatory protein (G-protein); *3*, intracellular enzymatically active domain. Production of cAMP and phosphorylation of cellular effector proteins. *Center*, ligand binding to a protein kinase associated Rc with autophosphorylation and heterophosphorylation. *Right*, ligand-receptor complex acting via a phophodiesterase with elevation of cytosolic calcium concentration. *Right lateral*, ligand binding to a calcium-associated Rc with activation of gated calcium channels, elevation of intracellular calcium levels, and stimulation of calcium-dependent cellular events, e.g., activation of enzymes. (From Dietel 1987)

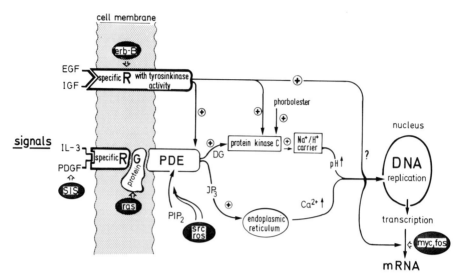

Fig. 2. Suggested interactions of growth factors, cell surface receptors, and subsequent signal transmission. At several steps oncogenes or oncogene products can interfere. Two mechanisms are demonstrated: (a) Activation of the phosphodiesterase (*PDE*) associated Rc converts phosphatidylinositol bisphosphonate (*PIP$_2$*) to diacylglycerol (*DG*) elevating cytoplasmic pH or to inositol triphosphonate (*IP$_3$*) elevating cytosolic Ca^{2+} concentration. Both events are suspected to stimulate cell growth. (b) Activation of the tyrosine kinase containing Rc appears to stimulate PDE, the cytoplasmic protein kinase C, and possibly directly the DNA replication. (From Dietel 1987)

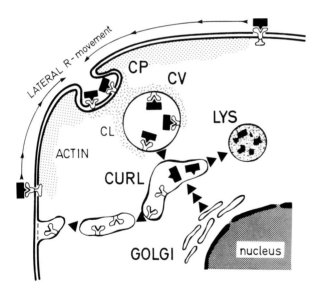

Fig. 3. Processing of the ligand–Rc complex during Rc-mediated endocytosis: ligand binding to a surface Rc, lateral Rc movement, internalization by clathrin (*CL*), coated pits (*CP*), transport to the compartment of uncoupling of Rc and ligand (*CURL*), lysosomal degradation (*LYS*) of the ligand, and reintegration of the Rc protein into the plasmalemma. (From Dietel 1987)

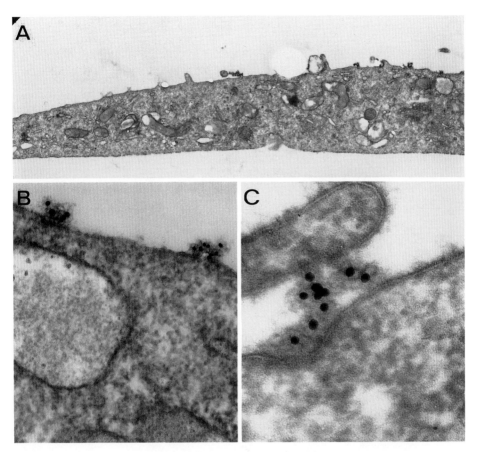

Fig. 4 A–J. Ultrastructural demonstration of Rc-mediated endocytosis. **A** Top to bottom section of the colon carcinoma cell line EPC 84–193 incubated with the ligand, i.e., gold–labeled LDL, for different time periods (10–120 min; × 3000). **B** The LDL binds to the surface Rc of LDL (× 85 000). **C** First step of internalization with ligand clustering and membrane indention (× 125 000). **D, E** Condensation of the cytoplasmic protein clathrin forming coated pits (× 125 000). **F, G** Subsequent constriction of coated vesicles (× 125 000, 85 000). **H** Tubuli-associated transport (× 50 000). **I, J** Lysosomal degradation (× 50 000). (Methods see Dietel 1987; Dietel et al. 1979). **D–F** see pp. 6,7

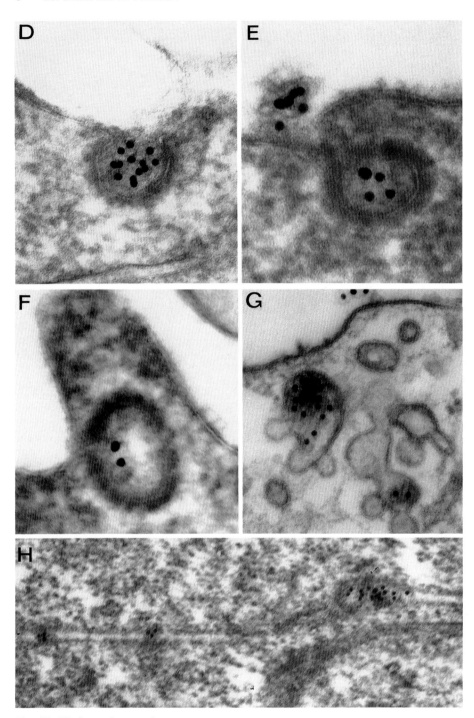

Fig. 4 D–H. Legend see p. 5

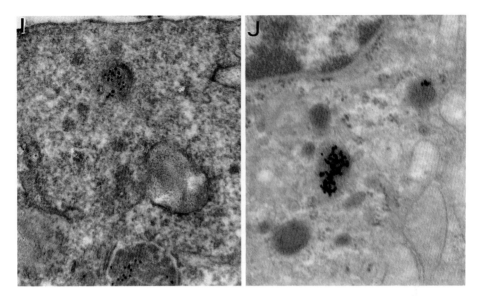

Fig. 4 I,J. Legend see p. 5

Cell Surface Receptors, Oncogenes, and Growth Promotion

The intention of a cell to divide is dependent in part upon environmental signals which are detected and transduced via surface Rc. Classic peptide hormones (growth hormone, somatostatin, somatomedins), hormone-like growth factors (GF), transport proteins (transferrin), and lipoproteins are groups of such signaling substances that participate in the Rc-mediated regulation of growth and differentiation of embryonic, mature, and tumorous tissue.

Peptide Hormones. Trophic hormones, such as growth hormone (GH), prolactin (PRL), somatostatin, somatomedin, and adrenocorticotrophic hormone (ACTH) contribute to regulate the proportional growth of mammalian tissues in development, childhood, and adolescence, as well as in physiological renewal of mature tissues. GH, for example, stimulates peripheral cells to divide either by binding directly to specific Rc or by inducing the liver to secret certain peptides (somatomedins) with growth-modulating activity. PRL and other mammotrophic hormones are found to influence maturation of the mammary tree and the surrounding mesenchymal tissue. Similar mechanisms are known for the promotion of tumor cells. Pituitary and hypothalamic hormones, insulin, gastrointestinal hormones, calcitonin, parathyroid hormone, and others stimulate or inhibit tumor growth (Emerman et al. 1985; Imagawa et al. 1985; Kinoshita et al. 1985; Lee et al 1986; Willingham et al. 1983; Rose 1979; Redding and Schally 1984). A prerequisite for these processes is that the target cells express the appropriate Rc. The initiation for growing cells (normal as well as malignant) to transcribe specific DNA regions which encode the specific Rc protein is not understood in detail. The regulation of

the various steps of Rc integration into the cell membrane is even more complicated.

Growth Factors. The family of GF were found to be important for growth control
of normal and transformed cells. One example is the epidermal growth factor
(EGF), which acts through a membrane-bound Rc. The EGF Rc, like other GF
Rc, exhibits tyrosine-specific protein kinase activity (Ushiro and Cohen 1980;
Hunter 1984) which can induce cell division (Fig. 2). EGF is involved in physiological development of many normal tissues as well as in atypical growth stimulation of malignant tumors (Carpenter and Cohen 1979; Hunter 1984; Sporn and
Roberts 1985; Willingham et al. 1983). In a number of tumors amplified EGF Rc
genes were found, e.g., primary brain tumors (glioblastomas) (Liberman et al.
1985), gastric carcinoma (Yamamoto et al. 1986), several cell lines of squamous
cell carcinomas (Kamata et al. 1986) and the intensively studied human epidermoid carcinoma cell line A 431. Transcription of these genes results in abnormally high number of the EGF Rc molecule which becomes integrated into the
cell surface. The Rc protein of A 431 cells is encoded by the activated *erb*B oncogen
(Ullrich et al. 1984). A correlation between growth rate, depth of invasion, and
density of EGF Rc has been demonstrated for malignant tumors (Neal et al. 1985;
Sainsbury et al. 1985) and may be of prognostic significance for patients.

The role of GF in maturation and differentiation of blood cells is extremely
complex. Many interactions are known between the blood cell associated GF
(interleukin, 1 and 2, T-cell GF, B-cell GF, macrophage GF, platelet-derived
GF, etc.) and their specific Rc (reviews see Alberts et al. 1983. Cantrell and Smith
1984; Hood et al. 1982; Waterfield et al. 1983). Other GF, e.g., patelet–derived
GF, fibroblast GF, transforming GF, colony–stimulating factor, angiogenesis
factor (Gullino 1981, Metcalf 1981) are also involved in the control mechanisms of
normal development, balanced growth, and tumorous overgrowth.

Other cellular oncogenes (c-*onc*) are known to code for several Rc proteins that
specifically recognize GF, e.g., the *ras* oncogene, which codes for the intramembrane G-protein and G-like proteins of the Rc complex (see Fig. 1). Activation of the c-*ras* oncogene results in an overproduction of the protein kinase C
triggering cell proliferation (Helmreich 1986). A strong candidate for the expression of a modified GF Rc is the c-*fms* oncogen. Its product is a transmembrane
glycoprotein with tyrosine kinase activity exposed on the cell surface which
probably is related to the Rc protein for a hematopoietic GF (CSF-1) acting on the
monocyte-macrophage lineage (Sherr et al. 1985).

Auto/Paracrine Growth Modulation and Transforming Growth Factors. Recently
oncogenes were discovered coding for transforming proteins that need to be
continuously present to preserve cellular transformation. The proposed mechanism describes an autocrine–induced transformation of tumor cells, i.e., some
tumor cells secret GF which stimulate their own cell growth by their action on
specific cell surface Rc. This has been demonstrated for the transforming growth
factor (TGF-α). In addition, a human small-cell lung cancer cell line was shown to
secret a bombesin-like peptide (Cuttitta et al. 1985) which was shown to activate

protein kinase C in the lung cancer cells from which it was secreted (Zachary et al. 1986).

Simultaneous activation of two or more oncogenes appears to enhance the transforming potency of the oncogene products (Rapp et al. 1985). The combination of *ras* and *myc* transforms fibroblasts and bone marrow cells with a higher activity than either alone. This is followed by different GF requirements for in vitro growth. Obviously the oncogene products are involved in different steps of Rc-mediated signal recognition and signal transmission to the nucleus to induce DNA replication.

A so-called negative, i.e., cell proliferation inhibiting, growth factor has been described by Knabbe and coworkers (1987). The TGF-β was shown to be secreted by the mammary carcinoma cells MCF-7 which simultaneously express TGF-β Rc in vitro suggesting an auto/paracrine mechanism. In these cells the production of TGF-β is stimulated by the application of antiestrogens. Thus, the growth-impairing effects of antiestrogens appear at least to be mediated by this negative growth factor. Further evidence for an antiproliferative potency of TGF-β was obtained by experiments which disclose a growth inhibitory effect of TGF-β also in nonhormonal dependent mammary carcinoma cells.

The mechanisms so far described offer possible explanations of how the activation of oncogenes can result in the uncontrolled growth of tumor cells. At the level of growth factors and their Rc, physiological development and malignant transformation may be closely related. Since the Rc are located in the cell membrane, they can easily be effected by intravenously applied substances. This may result in new therapeutic strategies, e.g., use of GF antagonists, Rc-blocking drugs, Rc antibodies etc. The regulation of oncogene activity may be influenced by regulatory genes, so-called antioncogenes (Green and Wyke 1985), which are involved in the switch on/switch off process of oncogenes.

Low-density Lipoproteins and Transferrin. Rapidly growing tumor cells synthesize relatively large amounts of membranes which requires cholesterol usually taken up by the cells as LDL. Consequently tumors cells carry a high density of LDL Rc (Dietel 1986; Lindguist et al. 1985; Vermeer et al. 1985). In own experiments, sufficient LDL supplement of the culture medium was found to be a prerequisite for optimal growth of tumor cells in vitro (Dietel 1986). Thus, LDL-linked antineoplastic compounds may be concentrated by tumor cells leading to selective cell death. This could become a new concept in cancer therapy (Vitols et al. 1984).

Proliferating cells require large amounts of iron as cofactor for the ribonucleotide reductase. For transport and internalization the iron molecule is coupled to the transport protein transferrin forming di – ferro – transferrin. This complex is internalized via Rc (Hannover and Dickson 1985). To satisfy the iron requirement of growing cells large amounts of the transferrin Rc must be expressed in malignant cells (Musgrove et al. 1984).

Viruses and Cell Transformation

Many viruses enter cells by Rc-mediated endocytosis (Dales 1973; March 1984; Pastan and Willingham 1985). The pathogenic effect manifests itself as simple infection or in some cases as malignant transformation (Table 1). Usually the viral genome is integrated into the DNA of the host cell. This requires some additional steps which are promoted by so-called cofactors: carcinogens, radiation, second virus, etc. (Fig. 5). The first virus with proven tumor-inducing potency was the Rous sarcoma virus that produces malignant mesenchymal tumors in chicken. Its tumor-promoting potency was found to be based on the binding of the virus to a surface Rc with subsequent endocytosis, followed by the transcription of the viral RNA to DNA by means of the reverse transcriptase and the integration of the oncogenic virus-DNA region (v-*src* oncogen) into host cell DNA. The *src* oncogen product is a protein kinase which activation results in mitosis (Hunter and Sefton 1980). The human T-cell leukemia virus III (HTLV-III) has been reported

Table 1. Viruses, oncogenes, and receptor-related oncogene products involved in cancero-genesis. (From Dietel 1987)

Oncog-enes	Virus	Species of origin	Rc-related oncogene proteins	Type of tumor
*erb*B	Avian erythroblast	Fowl		Leukemia, sarcoma
src	Rous sarcoma	Fowl		Sarcoma
yes	Yamaguchi sarcoma	Fowl	Membrane or	Sarcoma
fps	Fujinama sarcoma	Fowl	cytoplasmic,	Sarcoma
fgr	Pasheed feline sarcoma	Cat	tyrosine-specific	Sarcoma
fms	McDonough feline sarcoma	Cat	protein kinase	Sarcoma
fes	Feline sarcoma	Cat		Sarcoma
ros	Rochester-2 sarcoma	Fowl		Sarcoma
abl	Abelson murine leukemia	Mouse		Leukemia
sis	Simian sarcoma	Monkey	PDGF homologues	Sarcoma
mos	Moloney nurine sarcoma	Mouse	Phosphoprotein	Sarcoma
Ha-*ras*	Harvey murine sarcoma	Rat		Sarcoma
Ki-*ras*	Kirsten murine sarcoma	Rat	G Rc protein	Sarcoma
N-*ras*	??			Human carcinoma leukemia
myc	Myelocytomatosis MC 29	Fowl	Nuclear DNA Rc	Sarcoma, human carcinoma, leukemia
B-*lym*	??	Fowl	Nuclear DNA Rc	Malignant lymphoma

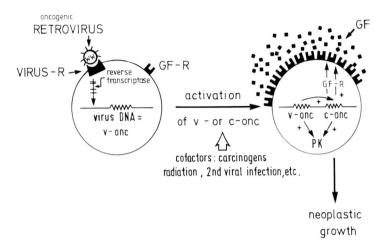

Fig. 5. Possible mechanisms of virus-induced cell transformation with involvement of cell surface receptors at two different sites. Viruses enter the cell by binding to special receptors (*R*); the virus (*v*) RNA is transcribed to v-DNA. Oncogenic v-DNA (*v-onc*) is integrated into cellular DNA (*left cell*). After activation by cofactors *v-onc* may activate cellular oncogenes (*c-onc*) that code for growth factor (*GF*) receptors (*right cell*). The elevated expression of growth factor receptors may be responsible for neoplastic growth. (From Dietel 1987)

to enter T4–lymphocytes via Rc–mediated endocytosis (McDouglas et al. 1986). The HTLV-III Rc can partly be blocked by an anti-Rc antibody reducing HTLV-III binding and thus internalization. Malignant transformation was shown for HTLV-I which can initiate leukemia (review, Sugamura et al. 1986). The HTLV-I proviral genome is integrated into the T-cell DNA inducing an activation of the gene that codes for the IL-2 Rc protein in T cells. Then, the IL-2 Rc is expressed at the surface of the infected cell in relatively large amounts. This was demonstrated in an HTLV-I transformed T-cell line (Poiesz et al. 1980) with enhanced transduction of the growth signal of IL-2. It is not clear whether the IL-2 Rc mediated signal is transduced by activating the protein kinase C, or whether other mechanisms are involved. In addition, an autointernalization of the IL-2 Rc with induction of cell growth in HTLV-1 transformed T-cell lines has been discussed (Sugamura et al. 1986). The general mechanisms of viral tumor induction and promotion have been reviewed recently (Bishop 1985; Varmus 1985).

Cytosolic/Nuclear Receptors and Growth Promotion

Cytosolic/nuclear Rc bind predominantly small lipophilic ligands such as steroid and thyroid hormones. After a ligand has entered a cell it couples to a specific cytosolic protein which moves toward the nucleus. There, the ligand binds to the specific DNA-associated Rc, a protein of the nonhistone class (Fig. 6). The

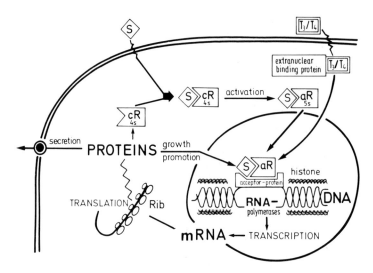

Fig. 6. Mechanisms of signal recognition, transmission, and growth promotion by cytosolic/nuclear receptors binding steroid or thyroid hormones (details, see text), *S*, Steroid hormone; T_3/T_4, Thyroid hormone; *cR*, cytosolic Rc protein; *aR*, activated Rc protein; *Rib*, ribosomes. (From Dietel 1987)

structure of the chromosomal steroid hormone (StH) receptor is known to consist of a steroid binding domain, a regulatory region, and a DNA binding domain. Receptor activation leads to the stimulation of transcriptorily active DNA regions.

The Steroid Hormones. The stimulating activity of estrogen (E) and progesterone (P) in estrogen receptor positive mammary and endometrium carcinomas, as well as in benign and malignant hepatic neoplasias (Nagasue et al. 1986; Wanless Medline 1982) is generally accepted. In addition, other StH are discussed as modulating cell activities and division in other types of tumors: androgens in prostate carcinomas (Geller and Albert 1984; Markland et al. 1978; Neumann et al. 1977) and glucocorticosteroids in leukemia. Recently, E Rc have also been demonstrated in gastric cancer of the diffuse type (Tokunaga et al. 1986), other gastrointestinal tumors (Sica et al. 1984), and several carcinomas of diverse types (Kamata et al. 1986; Kobayashi et al. 1982; Greenway et al. 1981). However, in these cases the growth-promoting potency of E has not yet been evidenced. To slow down the proliferation rate of StH Rc expressing tumors antagonists of StH are used. For treatment of mammary carcinoma one of the antagonists applied is the antiestrogen tamoxifen, and more recently 3-hydroxytamoxifen (Löser et al. 1985). They interfere with the E Rc in the nucleus of cancer cells (Horwitz and McGuire 1978; Rochefort and Bogna 1981); however, exact knowledge on the blocking action is lacking. One prerequisite for a successful therapy with StH antagonists is the presence of the appropriate Rc, which should be demonstrated morphologically and biochemically. The dual evidence is important, since an antiproliferative effect of StH antagonists on tumor cell growth depends on (a) the

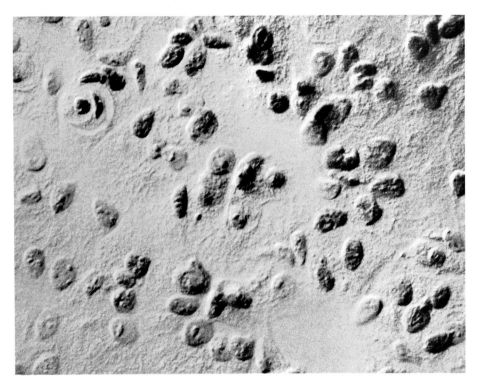

Fig. 7. Immunocytochemical visualization of the estrogen receptor in the mammary cancer cell line MCF-7 M1 cells (a cloned variant of the MCF-7 cell line). The receptor protein is located exclusively in the nuclei. The vast majority of the cells contain the estrogen receptor. However, some cells did not show an immunoreaction indicative for the cellular heterogeneity even of cell lines in vitro (× 40)

number of Rc molecules per tissue weight (determinable biochemically) and (b) the number Rc positive cells per tumor (determinable morphologically). Immunocytochemical studies using monoclonal antibodies specific for the nuclear Rc protein of estrogen demonstrated that even tumors with high amounts of E Rc (Fig. 7) often contain Rc-negative cell clones (Greene et al. 1980; King and Greene 1985). This explains experimentally obtained data confirming the lack of the expected inhibitory effect of StH antagonists in some StH Rc positive tumor cell lines (Dietel et al. 1985; Simon et al. 1984)

The StH-induced Rc activation stimulates synthesis of several gene products which enhance cell division. To obtain further insight into this problem Green and coworkers (1986) cloned and sequenced the complementary DNA (cDNA) of the E Rc in the E Rc positive breast cancer cell line MCF-7. Subsequently it was possible to express the cDNA in HeLa cells. The cDNA was found to code for a protein with the same molecular mass and same E binding capacity as the E Rc of MCF-7 cells. It is of great interest that the cDNA sequence of the E Rc shares strong sequence homology with the *erb*A gene of the oncogenic avian erythroblastosis virus (Green et al. 1986). Although the *erb*A oncogene is not itself carcinogenic, the *erb*A product may be involved in the Rc-mediated growth-promoting effect of E in breast cancer.

1,25 (OH)$_2$ Vitamin D$_3$. Another group of StH with growth-modulating potency are the calciferols (vitamin D). Most attention has been paid to the activated form of vitamin D$_3$, the 1,25 (OH)$_2$D$_3$. In several cancer cells lines and primary tumors 1,25 (OH)$_2$D$_3$ Rc have been found: melanoma, leukemia, osteosarcoma, breast, bronchic, and colonic carcinoma, parathyroid tumors, etc. (Colston et al. 1982; Dietel 1982; Dietel et al. 1979; Eisman et al. 1983; Pike 1984). The effects on cell replication are predominantly inhibitory. However, own experiments disclosed a decrease in cell growth only in two out of six cell lines from gastrointestinal tumors (Niendorf et al 1987).

Conclusions

There is general agreement that at least two, and presumably several events are required to transform normal cells into malignant ones (Land et al. 1983; Paul 1984). One step is immortalization and another is acquisition of the capability for invasive growth. Although this may be an oversimplification, we have learned that cell surface Rc as well as cytosolic/nuclear Rc are involved at multiple sites of oncogenesis, and that they may play a key role in induction and promotion of the cancer disease.

The multiple interactions between peptide hormones, steroid hormones, growth factors, viruses, and related Rc as well as the associated genes demonstrate the complex network in the regulation of tumor cell growth. Rc molecules can be reached relatively easy using the corresponding ligand. Thus, specific ligands, i.e., agents directly interfering with special Rc (modulating binding capacity, destroying, blocking etc.) or antihormones (preventing Rc activation), may prove a useful tool in cancer treatment. However, therapy of malignant tumors is complicated by the enormous heterogeneity of tumor cell populations within a given tumor (Dietel et al. 1986; Schnipper 1986). This means that one growth-modulating substance may be relevant only for a certain cell population of a given tumor. This unfortunately is also the case for Rc-mediated therapeutic approaches.

References

Alberts B, Bray D, Lewis J, Raff M, Roberts K, Watson JD (1983) Molecular biology of the cell. Garland, New York, pp 951–1012

Berridge MJ (1981) Receptor and calcium signalling. In: Lamble JW (ed) Towards understanding of receptors. Elsevier North Holland, New York, pp 122–131

Berridge MJ, Irvine RF (1984) Inositol triphosphate a novel second messenger in cellular signal transduction. Nature 312: 315–321

Bishop JM (1985) Viruses, genes and cancer II. Retrovirus and cancer genes. Cancer 55: 2329–2333

Brown MS, Anderson RGW, Goldstein JL (1983) Recycling receptors: the round trip itinerary of migrant membrane proteins. Cell 32: 663–667

Cantrell DA, Smith KA (1984) The interleukin 2–T-cell system: a new cell growth model. Science 224: 1316–1316

Carafoli E, Peneston JT (1986) The calcium signal. Sci Am (Germ edn) Jan 1: 76–85

Carpenter G, Cohen S (1979) Epidermal growth factor. Annu Rev Biochem 48: 193–216

Catt KJ, Harwood JP, Aguilera G, Dufau ML (1979) Hormonal regulation of peptide receptors and target cell responses. Nature 280: 109–116

Colston K, Colston MJ, Fieldsteel AH, Feldman D (1982) 1,25-dihydroxyvitamin D3 receptors in human epithelial cancer cell lines. Cancer Res 42: 856-859

Cooper JA, Hunter T (1983) Regulation of cell growth and transformation by tyrosine-specific protein kinase: the search for important cellular substrate proteins. In: Vogt PK, Kiprowski H (eds) Retroviruses 2. Current Topic Microbiology and Immunology, vol 107. Springer, Berlin Heidelberg New York, pp 125–161

Cuttitta F, Carney DN, Mulshine J, Moody TW, Fedorko J, Fischler A, Minna JD (1985) Bombesin-like peptides can function as autocrine growth factors in human small-cell lung cancer. Nature 316: 823–826

Dales S (1973) Early events in cell-animal virus interaction. Bacteriol Rev 37: 103–135

Dietel M (1982) Functional morphology and pathology of parathyroid glands. Fischer, Stuttgart

Dietel M (1986) Cell receptors – functions and deficiencies. Verh Dtsch Ges Pathol 70: 4–17

Dietel M (1987) What's new in receptor mediated growth promotion of normal and malignant cells? Pathol Res Pract 182: 431–442

Dietel M, Dorn G, Montz R, Altenähr E (1979) Influence of vitamin D3, 1,25-dihydroxyvitamin D3, and 24,25-dihydroxyvitamin D3 on parathyroid hormone secretion, adenosine 3′, 5′-monophosphate release, and ultrastructure of parathyroid glands in organ culture. Endocrinology 105: 237–245

Dietel M, Hölzel F, Arps H, Simon WE, Albrecht M (1985) Mamma carcinomas in vitro: cytoskeleton, tumor makers, nuclear DNA, and rate of proliferation in relation to hormones and cytostatics. Verh Dtsch Ges Pathol 69: 212–217

Dietel M, Arps H, Klapdor R, Müller-Hagen S, Sieck M, Hoffmann L (1986) Antigen detection by the monoclonal antibodies CA 19–9 and CA 125 in normal and tumor tissue and patients' sera. Cancer Res Clin Oncol 111: 257–265

Eisman JA, Frampton RJ, Sher E, Suva LJ, Martin TJ (1983) Presence and role of 1,25-dihydroxyvitamin D receptors in human cancer cells. In: Meyskens FL, Prasad KN (eds) Modulation and mediation of cancer by vitamins, 282–286. Karger, Basel

Emerman JT, Leathy M, Gout PW, Brucjovsky N (1985) Elevated growth hormone levels in sera from breast cancer patients. Horm Metab Res 17: 421–424

Geller J, Albert JD (1984) Antiandrogen and small dose of estrogen therapy as preferred treatment for prostate carcinoma. In: Hormones and cancer. Raven, New York

Goldstein JL, Anderson RGW, Brown MS (1979) Coated pits, coated vesicles and receptor-mediated endocytosis. Nature 279: 679–685

Green AR, Wyke JA (1985) Anti-oncogenes. A subset of regulatory genes involved in carcinogenesis. Lancet II (8453): 475–477

Green S, Walter P, Kumar V, Krust A, Bornert JM, Argos P, Chambon P (1986) Human oestrogen receptor cDNA: sequence, expression and homology to v-erb-A. Nature 320: 134–139

Green GL, Nolan C, Engler JP, Jensen EV (1980) Monoclonal antibodies to human estrogen receptor. Proc Natl Acad Sci USA 77: 5115–5119

Greenway B, Iqbal MJ, Johnson PJ, Williams R (1981) Oestrogen receptor proteins in malignant and fetal pancreas. Br Med J 283: 751–753

Gullino PM (1981) Angiogenesis factor(s). In: Baserga R (ed) Tissue growth factors. Springer, Berlin Heidelberg New York, pp 427–450 (Handbook of experimental pharmacology, vol 57)

Hannover JA, Dickson RB (1985) Transferrin: receptor mediated endocytosis and iron delivery. In: Pastan I, Willingham MC, (eds.) Endocytosis. Plenum, New York, pp 131–162

Helmreich EJM (1986) Fortschritte der molekularen Endokrinologie. Klin Wochenschr 64: 669–681

Hood LE, Weissman IL, Wood WB (1982) Immunology, 2nd edn. Benjamin Cummings Menlo Park, Ca

Horwitz KG, McGuire WL (1978) Nuclear mechanisms of estrogen action: effects of estradiol and anti-estrogens on estrogen receptors and nuclear receptor processing. J Biol Chem 253: 8185–8191

Hunter T, (1984) The proteins of oncogenes. Sci Am 251: 70–79

Hunter T, Sefton BM (1980) Transforming gene product of Rous sarcoma Virus phosphorylates tyrosine. Proc Natl Acad Sci USA 77: 1311–1315

Hynes RO (1985) Molecular biology of fibronectin. Annu Rev Cell Biol 1: 67–91

Imagawa W, Tomooka Y, Hamamoto S, Nandi S (1985) Stimulation of mammary epithelial cell gowth in vitro: interaction of epidermal growth factor and mammogenic hormones. Endocrinology 116: 1514–1524

Kamata N, Chida K, Rikimaru K, Horikoshi M, Enomoto S, Kuroki T (1986) Growth-inhibitory effects of epidermal growth factor and over expression of its receptors on human squamous cell carcinomas in culture. Cancer Res 46: 1648–1653

King WJ, Greene GL (1985) Monoclonal antibodies localize oestrogen receptor in the nuclei of target cells. Nature 307: 745–747

Kinoshita Y, Fukase M, Takenaka M, Nakada M, Miyauchi A, Fujita T (1985) Calcitonin stimulation of cyclic adenosine 3':5'-monophosphate production with growth inhibition in human renal adenocarcinoma cell lines. Cancer Res 45: 4890–4894

Knabbe C, Lippman ME, Wakefield LM, Flanders KC, Kasid A, Derynck R, Dickson RB (1987) Evidence that transforming growth factor-β is a hormonally regulated negative growth factor in human breast cancer cells. Cell 48: 417–428

Kobayashi S, Mizuno T, Tobioka T (1982) Sex steroid receptors in diverse human tumors. Gann 73: 439–445

Land H, Prada LF, Weinberg RA (1983) Cellular oncogenes and multistep carcinogenesis. Science 222: 771–778

Lee PDK, Rosenfeld RG, Hintz RL, Smith SD (1986) Characterization of insulin, insulin-like growth factors I and II, and growth hormone receptors on human leukemic lymphoblasts. J Clin Endocrinol Metab 62: 28–35

Libermann TA, Nusbaum HR, Razon N, Kris R, Lax I, Soreq H, Whittle N, Waterfield MD, Ullrich A, Schlessinger J (1985) Amplification, enhances expression and possible rearrangement of EGF receptor gene in primary human brain tumors of glial origin. Nature 313: 144–147

Lindquist R, Vitols S, Gahrton G, Öst A, Peterson C (1985) Low density lipoprotein receptor activity in human leukemic cells—relation to chrmosome aberrations. Acta Med Scand 217: 553–558

Löser R, Seibel K, Roos W, Eppenberger U (1985) In vivo and In vitro antiestrogenic action of 3—hydroxytamoxifen, tamoxifen and 4-hydroxitamoxifen. Eur J Cancer Clin Oncol 21: 985–990

March M (1984) The entry of enveloped viruses into cells by endocytosis. Biochem J 218: 1–10

Markland FS, Chiopp RT, Cosgrove MD, Howard EB (1978) Characterization of steroid hormone receptors in the Dunning R-3327 rat prostatic adenocarcinoma. Cancer Res 38: 2818–2826

McDouglas JS, Kennedy MS, Sligh JM, Cort SP, Mawle A, Nicholson JKA (1986) Binding of HTLV-III/LAV to T4$^+$ T cells by a complex of the 110K viral protein and the T4 molecule. Science 231: 382–385

Metcalf D (1981) Hemopoietic colony stimulating factors. In: Baserga R (Ed) Tissue growth factors. Springer, Berlin Heidelberg New York, pp 343–384 (Handbook of experimental pharmacology, vol 57)

Musgrove E, Rugg C, Taylor I, Hedley D (1984) Transferrin receptor expression during exponential and plateau phase growth of human tumour cells in culture. J Cell Physiol 118: 6–12

Nagasue N, Ito A, Yukaya H, Ogawa Y (1986) Estrogen receptors in heptacellular carcinoma. Cancer 57: 87–91

Neal DE, Marsh C, Bennett MK, Abel PD, Hall RR, Sainsbury JRC, Harris Al (1985) Epidermal growth factor receptors in human bladder cancer: comparison of invasive and superficial tumors. Lancet: 366–368

Neumann F, Graf KJ, Hason SH, Schenche B, Steinbeck H (1977) Central actions of antiandrogens. In: Martini GA, Motta JB (eds) Androgens and antiandrogens. Raven, New York, pp 163–171

Niendorf A, Arps H, Dietel M (1987) Effect of 1,25-dihydroxyvitamin D$_3$ on human cancer cells in vitro. J Steroid Biochem 27: 825–828

Pastan I, Willingham MC (1981) Journey to the center of the cell: role of the receptorsome. Science 214: 504–509

Pastan I, Willingham MC (1985) Endocytosis. Plenum, New York, pp 1–40

Paul J (1984) Oncogenes. J. Pathol 143: 1–10

Pike JW (1984) Monoclonal antibodies to chick intestinal receptors for 1,25-dihydroxyvitamin D3. J Biol Chem 259: 1167–1173

Poiesz BJ, Ruscetti FW, Mier JW, Woods AM, Gallo RC (1980) T-cell lines established from human T-lymphocytic neoplasias by direct response to T-cell growth factors. Proc Natl Acad Sci USA 77: 6815–6819

Rapp UR, Bonner TI, Moelling K, Jansen HW, Bister K, Ihle J (1985) Genes and gene products involved in growth regulation of tumor cells. In: Havemann K, Sorenson G, Gropp C (eds) Peptide hormones in lung cancer. Springer, Berlin Heidelberg New York, pp 221–236 (Recent results in cancer research, vol 99)

Redding TW, Schally AV (1984) Inhibition of growth of pancreatic carcinoma in animal models by analogs of hypothalamic hormones. Proc Natl Acad Sci USA 81: 248–256

Rochefort H, Bogna JL (1981) Differences between estrogen receptor and nuclear receptor processing. Nature 292: 257–259

Rose DP (1979) Endogenous hormones in the etiology and clinical course of breast cancer. In: Rose DP (ed) Endocrinology of cancer, vol 1. CRC, Boca Raton, pp 21–59

Sainsbury JRC, Farndon JR, Sherbet GV, Harris Al (1985) Epidermal growth factor receptors and estrogen receptors in human breast cancer. Lancet: 364–366

Schnipper LE (1986) Clinical implications of tumor-cell heterogeneity. N Engl J Med 314: 1423–1431

Sherr CJ, Rettenmier CW, Sacca R, Roussel MF, Look AT, Stanley ER (1985) The c-*fms* protooncogene product is related to the receptor for the mononuclear phagocyte growth factor, CSF-1. Cell 41: 665–676

Sica V, Nora E, Contieri E (1984) Estradiol and progesterone receptors in malignant gastrointestinal tumors. Cancer Res 44: 4670–4674

Simon WE, Albrect M, Tram G, Dietel M, Hölzel F (1984) In vitro growth promotion of human mammary carcinoma cells by steroid hormones, tamoxifen and prolactin. J Natl Cancer Inst 73: 313–321

Sporn MB, Roberts AB (1985) Autocrine growth factor and cancer. Nature 313: 745–747

Sugamura K, Fuji M, Ishii T, Hinuma Y (1986) Possible role of interelukin 2 receptor in oncogenesis of HTLV-I/ATLV. Cancer Rev 1: 96–114

Tokunaga A, Nishi K, Matsukura N, Tanaka N, Onda M, Shirota A, Asano G, Hayashi K (1986) Estrogen and progesteron receptors in gastric cancer. 57: 1376–1379

Ullrich A, Coussens L, Hayflick JS, Dull TJ, Gray A, Tam AW, Lee J, Yarden Y, Liberman TA, Schlessinger J, Downward J, Mayes ELV, Whittle N, Waterfield MD, Seeburg PH (1984) Human epidermal growth factor receptor cDNA sequence and abberant expression of the amplified gene in A 431 epidermoid carcinoma cells. Nature 309: 418–425

Ushiro H, Cohen S (1980) Identification of phosphotyrosine as a product of epidermal growth factor activated protein kinase in A 431 cell membranes. J Biol Chem 255: 8263

Varmus HE (1985) Viruses, genes and cancer. I. The discovery of cellular oncogenes and their role in neoplasia. Cancer 55: 2324–2328

Vasilev JM (1985) Spreading of non-transformed and transformed cells. Biochim Biophys Acta 780: 21–65

Vermeer BJ, Wijsman MC, Mommaas-Kienhuis AM, Ponec M (1985) Modulation of low density lipoprotein receptor activity in squamous carcinoma cells by variation in cell density. Eur J Cell Biol 38: 353–360

Vitols S, Gahrton G, Peterson C (1984) Significance of the low density lipoprotein (LDL) receptor pathway for the in vitro accumulation of AD 32 incorporated into LDL in normal and leukemic white blood cells. Cancer Treat Rep 68: 515–520

Wanless IR, Medline A (1982) Role of estrogens as promotors of hepatic neoplasia. Lab Invest 46: 313–320

Waterfield MD, Scrace T, Whittle N (1983) Platelet-derived growth factor is structurally related to the putative transforming protein p28^{sis} of simian sarcoma virus. Nature 304: 35–39

Weinberg RA (1983) A molecular basis of cancer. Sci Am 249: 126–143

Willingham MC, Haigler HR, Fitzgerald DJR, Gallo MG, Rutherford AV, Paştan IH (1983) The morphological pathway of binding and internalization of epidermal growth factor in cultured cells. Exp Cell Res 146: 163–175

Yamamoto T, Kamata N, Kawano H, Shimitsu S, Kuroki T, Toyoshima K, Rikimaru K, Nomura N, Ishizaki R, Pastan I, Gamou S, Shimizu N (1986) High incidence of amplification of the EGF receptor gene in human squamous carcinoma cell lines. Cancer Res 46: 414–416

Zachary I, Sinnett-Smith JW, Rozengurt E (1986) Early events elicited by bombesin and structurally related peptides in quiescent Swiss 3T3 cells. I. Activation of protein kinase C and inhibition of epidermal growth factor binding. J Cell Biol 102: 2211–2222

Localization of Hormones by Antibodies

P.U. Heitz

Institut für Pathologie, Universität Zürich, Schmelzbergstraße 12,
8091 Zürich, Switzerland

Hormones are substances produced by endocrine cells which are carried by the blood from the site of their secretion to the receptors of their target cells. At present hormones, including paracrine and autocrine substances, and neural messengers form the group of regulatory substances. Chemically they are peptides, proteins, glycoproteins, steroid hormones, iodothyronines or biogenic amines. Antibodies can be raised against many, if not all hormones, but the immunogenicity of the different substances varies widely.

Under physiological steady-state conditions a high local concentration of peptide, proteo-, and glycoprotein hormones and biogenic amines is present in the Golgi apparatus and especially in the post-Golgi pool of cytoplasmic secretory granules (Fig. 1; Kelly 1985; Heitz 1986). By contrast, the intracellular concentration of steroid hormones or of iodothyronines, not stored in a pool of secretory granules, is much lower.

Immunological tracing of hormones in cells makes use of various tracers, fluorescent substances, enzymes (of which horseradish peroxidase and acid phosphatase are the most important), and heavy metals, i.e. colloidal gold. The techniques can be classified as direct (primary antibody labelled) and indirect. Among the latter the unlabelled antibody enzyme method (PAP technique) based exclusively on immunological binding of the antigen and the various reagents, and the avidin-biotin complex method (ABC technique), exploiting the high chemical affinity of avidin for biotin, and variations thereof, have been most widely used (Guesdon et al. 1979; Sternberger 1986). Immunofluorescence can be applied exclusively at the light microscopical level; the other techniques can be extended to electron microscopy. At present, techniques using colloidal gold bound to staphylococcal protein A (Fig. 2), streptococcal protein G or to immunoglobulins are increasingly used at the light and electron microscopical level (Roth et al. 1985; Taatjes et al. 1987). In light microscopy the signal can be enhanced by photochemical silver amplification (Danscher 1981; Danscher and Nörgaard 1983; Holgate et al. 1983). The localization of antigens is precise, and in electron microscopy the contrast of colloidal gold particles is excellent due to their high atomic weight. The identification of endocrine cells by tinctorial stains or con-

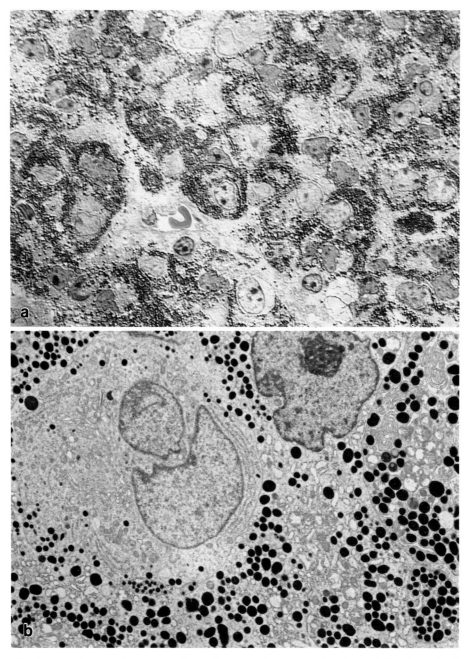

Fig. 1a, b. High local concentration of peptide hormones in the post-Golgi pool of cytoplasmic secretory granules. **a** Growth hormone producing pituitary adenoma. Semi-thin section of Epon embedded tissue (toluidin blue, original magnification × 800, differential interference contrast optics). **b** Thin section of the same tumour showing a large number of intracellular secretory granules of variable size and shape (uranyl-acetate and lead citrate, original magnification × 957)

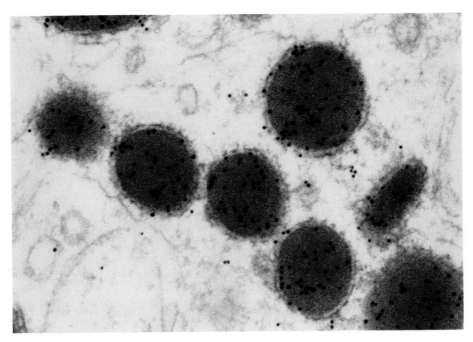

Fig. 2. Growth hormone producing pituitary adenoma inducing acromegaly. Growth hormone localized in secretory granules, using the protein A-gold technique. Diameter of the gold particles (*black dots*) 14 nm. (Original magnification ×20 300)

ventional electron microscopy is indirect. The morphology of the cells is rather typical, but in tumour cells it may be rather atypical and therefore difficult to recognize. Immunocytochemistry at the light and electron microscopical levels permits the direct identification and localization of post-translational products, including precursor molecules and subunits of hormones, and the final secretory products. In addition, post-transcriptional mRNA can now be visualized using *in situ* hybridization. The combination of these techniques has an enormous potential in future research.

The potential of immunocytochemical techniques lies in their specificity and sensitivity. The limitations of the methods are biological and technical. Biological limitations include hormones produced by tumours with a structure or conformation deviating from the normal and therefore no longer bearing the epitopes recognized by a given antibody, and a low concentration of secretory products in the post-Golgi pool of secretory granules is present in many tumour cells, especially in malignant tumours, because secretory products are by-passing the pool. A directed and regulated secretion may therefore become a constitutive secretion. The low intracellular concentration is one major difficulty in the visualization of steroid hormones and iodothyronines. In the thyroid the problem can be circumvented by visualizing thyroglobulin, the carrier protein of thyroid hormones (Fig. 3).

In addition to biological limitations a series of technical pitfalls must be realized and avoided.

Tissue processing is important for the successful use of immunocytochemical methods. At present many hormones can be reliably visualized in tissues fixed in liquid formaldehyde because the currently used immunocytochemical techniques are very sensitive. For work at the electron microscopical level monomeric glutaraldehyde may be added, and some antigens withstand a postfixation with osmium tetroxide. The type of fixation, its duration and the concentration of fixatives must be determined for every antigen and antibody. In general, a fixation without delay after excision of the tissue sample is essential for obtaining good results. Some antigens do not withstand a cross-linking or a precipitation by a fixative and must be localized in frozen or freeze-dried tissue. Their epitopes appear to be destroyed by fixation or to become inaccessible for the antibody due to a conformational change of the molecule. Every antibody must be tested in order to determine its possible use in immunocytochemistry. The determination of its optimal working concentration by titration is of paramount importance.

Technical pitfalls leading to non-specific reactions must be avoided by careful and extensive technical controls to be carried out for every incubation. Negative controls consist in the omission of reagents and their replacement by nonreactive control solutions in every step of a given reaction. The first step of the reaction (i.e. binding of the antibody to the antigen) must also be carried out using the antibody

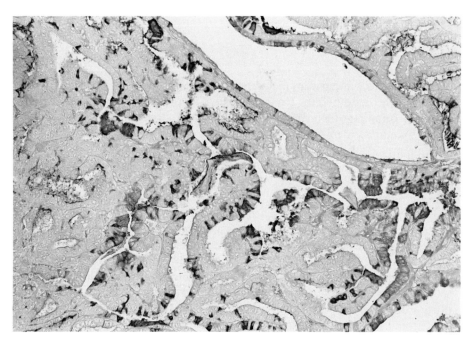

Fig. 3. Papillary carcinoma of the thyroid. Visualization of thyroglobulin production using the avidin-biotin complex technique. (Original magnification × 300)

absorbed with the appropriate (and possibly also inappropriate) antigens in an appropriate range of concentration, in order to block the reaction. Further controls include tissue not producing (negative control) and tissue known to produce the antigen (positive control).

The localization of a reaction in the tissue or cells can give important clues to the specificity or non-specificity of a reaction. The signal – to – noise ratio must be considered.

Additional controls using techniques based on other principles than immuno-cytochemistry should be carried out. Biochemical analysis of tissue extracts by radioimmunoassay or related techniques and, if possible, cell culture in which the secretion of a given antigen is demonstrated can confirm the validity of results obtained with immunocytochemical methods. A patient may be cured after excision of a hormone-producing tumour, and the concentrations of substances considered important in the pathogenesis of symptoms can be determined in the patients's serum.

The advances obtained in the knowledge of anatomy, biology and pathology of neuroendocrine cell systems due to the systematic combined application of the aforementioned techniques, including immunocytochemistry, are important (for reviews see Falkmer et al. 1984). Neuronal systems and pathways have been and are still being discovered. Endocrine, paracrine and autocrine cell systems and secretion have been discovered and/or "functionally dissected", i.e. the pituitary,

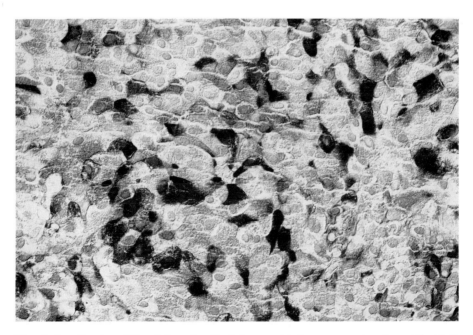

Fig. 4. Localization of the alpha-subunit of glycoprotein hormones using the avidin-biotin complex technique in an alpha-only pituitary adenoma. (Original magnification × 400, differential interference contrast optics)

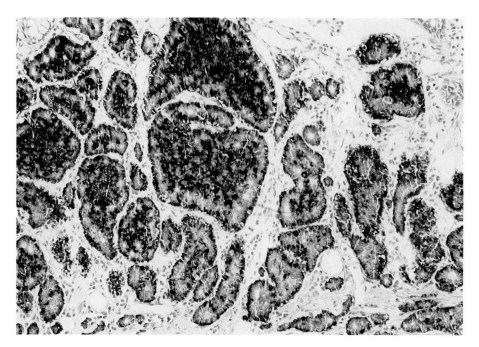

Fig. 5. Endocrine tumour of the ileum (carcinoid): large amount of substance P. Unlabelled antibody enzyme method. (Original magnification × 100)

the thyroid, the diffuse neuroendocrine system of the gastrointestinal tract, the pancreas, the bronchial tree, and the urogenital tract. Numerous previously unknown substances were found to be synthesized and secreted by endocrine cells. For the first time it is now possible to analyse precisely the aplasia, hypoplasia or the selective destruction of endocrine cells, i.e. in diabetes mellitus, or to define a hyperplasia of endocrine cells. Endocrine tumours can now be precisely defined, and new, previously unknown types of tumours have been detected, i.e. prolactinoma and alpha-only tumours of the pituitary (Fig. 4), medullary thyroid carcinoma producing calcitonin and related peptides, and CEA, pancreatic endocrine tumours, the classificiation of which has been revolutionized (Heitz and Klöppel 1987; Klöppel and Heitz 1988; similarly that of pituitary tumours, Heitz et al. 1987a), endocrine tumours (carcinoids) of the gastrointestinal tract (Chejfec et al. 1988) in which unexpected markers have been found (Fig. 5), and of the lung. In some groups of tumours the grade of functional differentiation can be determined by analysing their hormone production, i.e. in thyroid tumours by determining the production of thyroglobulin (Fig. 3; Ryff-de Léche et al. 1986), while in pancreatic endocrine tumours benign or malignant biological behaviour can be predicted with high sensitivity and specificity by determining their production of the alpha-chain of glycoprotein hormones (Heitz et al. 1983; 1987b). By using hormonal markers, in combination with broad-spectrum markers for neuroendocrine differentiation (Fig. 6) and antibodies directed against intermediate filament proteins metastases

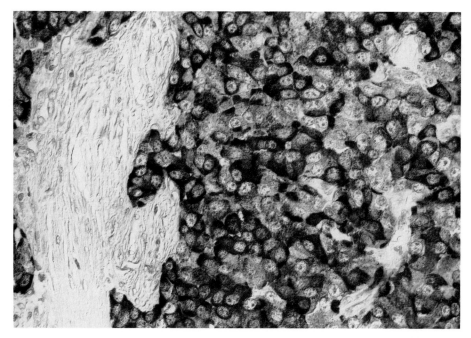

Fig. 6. Glucagonoma of the pancreas. Presence of chromogranin A in many but not all tumour cells. Avidin-biotin complex method. (Original magnification × 400, differential interference contrast optics)

of neuroendocrine tumours can be precisely defined or at least much better analysed than previously, and the primary may be localized subsequently, i.e. melanoma, Merkel cell tumour, carcinoids, etc. (Heitz 1987; Bishop et al. 1988). In addition "ectopic hormone secretion" can often be shown as well as the presence of neuroendocrine cells in many nonendocrine tumours.

One of the most important advances has been the detection of the phenotypic heterogeneity of cells in endocrine tumours (Heitz et al. 1971; Polak et al. 1976; Klöppel and Heitz 1988), a phenomenon which is apparently not restricted to endocrine tumours but is a general problem in tumour biology.

References

Bishop AE, Power RF, Polak JM (1988) Markers for neuroendocrine differentiation. Pathol Res Pract 183: 119–128

Chejfec G, Falkmer S, Askensten U, Grimelius L, Gould VE (1988) Neuroendocrine tumors of the gastrointestinal trat. Pathol Res Pract 183: 143–154

Danscher G (1981) Localization of gold in biological tissue. A photochemical method for light and electron microscopy. Histochemistry 71: 81–88

Danscher G, Nörgaard JOR (1983) Light microscopic visualization of colloidal gold on resin-embedded tissue. J Histochem Cytochem 31: 1394–1398

Falkmer S, Hakanson R, Sundler F (eds) (1984) Evolution and tumour pathology of the neuroendocrine system. Elsevier, Amsterdam

Guesdon JL, Ternynck T, Avrameas S (1979) The use of avidin-biotin interaction in immunoenzymatic techniques. J Histochem Cytochem 27: 1131–1139

Heitz PU (1986) Hormonale Tumormarker. Verh Dtsch Ges Pathol 70: 64–81

Heitz PU (1987) Neuroendocrine tumor markers. In: Seifert G (ed) Morphological tumor markers. General aspects and diagnostic relevance. Springer, Berlin Heidelberg New York, pp 279–306 (Current topics in pathology vol 77)

Heitz PU, Klöppel G (1987) Endokrine Tumoren des Pankreas und des Duodenum. Verh Dtsch Ges Pathol 71: 202–221

Heitz PU, Steiner H, Halter F, Egli F, Kapp JP (1971) Multihormonal amyloid-producing tumour of the islets of Langerhans in a twelve year old boy. Virchows Arch [A] 353: 312–324

Heitz PU, Kasper M, Klöppel G, Polak JM, Vaitukaitis JL (1983) Glycoprotein-hormone alpha-chain production by pancreatic endocrine tumors: a specific marker for malignancy. Immunocytochemical analysis of tumors of 155 patients. Cancer 51: 277–282

Heitz PU, Landolt AM, Zenklusen HR, Kasper M, Reubi JC, Oberholzer M, Roth J (1987a) Immunocytochemistry of pituitary tumors. J Histochem Cytochem 35: 1005–1011

Heitz PU, von Herbay G, Klöppel G, Komminoth P, Kasper M, Höfler H, Müller KM, Oberholzer M (1987b) The expression of subunits of human chorionic gonadotropin (hCG) by nontrophoblastic, nonendocrine, and endocrine tumors. Am J Clin Pathol 88: 467–472

Holgate CS, Jackson P, Cowen PN, Bird CC (1983) Immunogold silver staining: new method of immunostaining with enhanced sensitivity. J Histochem Cytochem 31: 938–944

Kelly B (1985) Pathways of protein secretion in eukaryotes. Science 230: 25–32

Klöppel G, Heitz PU (1988) Pancreatic endocrine tumors. Pathol Res Pract 183: 155–168

Polak JM, Bloom SR, Adrian TE, Heitz PU, Bryant MG, Pearse AGE (1976) Pancreatic polypeptide in insulinomas, gastrinomas, vipomas, and glucagonomas. Lancet 1: 328–330

Roth J, Kasper M, Heitz PU, Labat F (1985) What's new in light and electron microscopic immunocytochemistry? Application of the protein A-gold technique to routinely processed tissue. Pathol Res Pract 180: 711–717

Ryff-de Lèche A, Staub JJ, Kohler-Faden R, Müller-Brand J, Heitz PU (1986) Thyroglobulin production by malignant thyroid tumors: an immunocytochemical and radioimmunoassay study. Cancer 57: 1045–1053

Sternberger LA (1986) Immunocytochemistry, 3rd edn. Wiley, New York

Taatjes DJ, Chen TH, Ackerström B, Björck L, Carlemalm E, Roth J (1987) Streptococcal protein G-gold complex: comparison with staphylococcal protein A-gold complex for spot blotting and immunolabeling. Eur J Cell Biol 45: 151–159

Diffuse Endocrine Cell System

Morphology and Functional Activity of Gastroenteropancreatic Neuroendocrine Tumours

G. Klöppel and P.U. Heitz

Department of Pathology, Academic Hospital, Free University of Brussels, Laarbeeklaan 101, 1090 Brussels, Belgium

As components of the neuroendocrine cell system the gastroenteropancreatic (GEP) endocrine cells have a number of varied proteins in common. The best known of these specific components are neuron-specific enolase (NSE), chromogranins A, B and C, protein gene product 9.5, synaptophysin and Leu 7 (Bishop et al. 1988; Martin and Maung 1987). These markers and the specific neuroendocrine cell products, i.e. regulatory peptides, can be immunostained to define the nature of the cells. The tumours originating from these cells are rare, but by reproducing many of the morphological and functional features of their cell(s) of origin they reveal a distinct morphology and may give rise to a number of well-defined syndromes.

This review provides a condensed overview on the pathology, immunocyto-chemistry and biology of GEP neuroendocrine tumours. For further reading we refer to recent reviews and the original articles cited therein (Dayal and Wolfe 1984; Heitz 1984; Polak and Bloom 1985; Klöppel and Heitz 1988; Chejfec et al. 1988).

Nomenclature and Classification

Endocrine tumours of the pancreas and gut have been variously named, i.e. islet cell tumours, insulinomas, nesidioblastomas, B-cell tumours, non – B-cell tumours, carcinoids, EC-cell tumours, argentaffinomas, and APUDomas of the pancreas and gut. For endocrine neoplasms of the pancreas we prefer the term pancreatic endocrine tumour, since it is noncommittal concerning the ontogenetic origin of the cells and the histogenetic origin of the tumours. The name carcinoid is given to all of the tumours derived from the diffuse neuroendocrine system (DeLellis et al. 1984), with the exception of the medullary thyroid carcinoma, the small-cell lung carcinoma and the Merkel cell tumour of the skin (Table 1). If criteria of malignancy are present, the labelling as malignant or metastasizing should be added. Tumours associated with hormonal symptoms are designated as functioning or active, while tumours without these signs are classified as nonfunctioning or inactive. Due to advances in identifying hormonal products of tumours in the

Table 1. Neuroendocrine cell system and tumour classifiation

Cell system	Tumour type
Gland forming	
Pituitary	Adenoma
Parathyroids	Adenoma
Paraganglia	Paraganglioma
Adrenal medulla	Phaeochromocytoma
Diffusely distributed	
Skin	Merkel cell tumour
Thyroid C cells	Medullary carcinoma
Endocrine pancreas	Pancreatic endocrine tumour
Respiratory tract	
Thymus	
Stomach	
Small and large bowel	Carcinoid
Liver and biliary tract	
Urogenital tract	

serum or at the cellular level by immunological methods, the morphological classification may be extended by functional labellings. Taking into account the hormone with the most elevated serum concentration, which is believed to give rise to the observed clinical syndrome, and/or the major product detected by immunocytochemistry the tumours are accordingly named insulinomas, gastrinomas, vipomas, glucagonomas, etc. In nonfunctioning tumours containing only a few hormone-positive cells the hormones identified should be tabulated.

Criteria of Malignancy

The majority of pancreatic endocrine tumours lack reliable histological or cytological criteria of malignancy. Exceptions are some rare, poorly differentiated and fast growing neoplasms whose endocrine nature is barely recognized by conventional histology. In all the other slowly growing tumours the only clear criterion of malignancy is massive infiltration of adjacent organs or metastases to regional lymph nodes or the liver. As, however, metastases may become apparent only years after the removal of the primary, a long clinical follow-up period is needed to establish the benign nature of a tumour.

Gut carcinoids reveal their malignant potential by invasion of the bowel wall. However, their rate of malignancy varies according to size, site and stage of invasion. Thus appendix carcinoids, as a rule, show a benign behaviour. The same is true for small gastric and rectal carcinoids which do not invade the muscularis propria and can thus be removed by the endoscopist. In contrast, most carcinoids of the small and large intestine have progressed, when detected, to a stage where they have already metastasized (Table 2). Recently the nuclear DNA content of carcinoids, as studied by flow cytometry, was correlated with the course of the

Table 2. Approximate frequency and malignancy rate of gastrointestinal carcinoids

Site	Frequency	Malignancy rate
Appendix	50%	2%
Rectum	25%	10%
Ileum	15%	80%
Stomach	4%	20%
Duodenum	4%	40%
Colon	2%	80%

disease (Kujari et al. 1988). It was found that six of seven patients with aneuploid tumour and three of five patients with diploid tumour, observed for at least 10 years, died of the disease. We investigated the DNA distribution profiles of 29 pancreatic endocrine tumours with static cytofluorometry (G. Klöppel, C. Donow and P. U. Heitz, unpublished observations). The correlation with the clinical outcome revealed that patients with diploid tumours had an average survival time of 6.5 years as contrasted with 2.6 years in patients with aneuploid tumours. In contrast to the carcinoids, gangliocytic paragangliomas of the duodenum, containing neural as well as epithelial cells, can be considered benign (Hamid et al. 1986).

Gross Pathology, Histology and Ultrastructure

The majority of GEP neuroendocrine tumours are well demarcated neoplasms with firm consistency. They are usually solitary, but multiplicity may be found, particularly in the gut. In the pancreas the presence of multiple tumours is often associated with the syndrome of multiple endocrine neoplasia type 1 (MEN 1). Gut carcinoids arise in the submucosa and, by becoming larger, invariably invade the muscularis propria. In contrast, pancreatic tumours may become huge without showing any invasion of the surrounding organs.

Table 3. Classifications of carcinoids according to their histological pattern

Williams and Sandler 1963		Soga and Tazawa 1971
Foregut	Argyrophil	Type B: trabecular E: mixed C: glandular D: atypical
Midgut	Argyrophil and argentaffin	Type A: insular E: mixed
Hindgut	Nonargyrophil	Type E: mixed D: atypical

Histologically, the GEP tumours produce very similar, if not identical, patterns. In principle, trabecular structures, sometimes combined with gland-like elements, can be distinguished from solid (insular) patterns. While in the pancreas there is no preference to either histological growth pattern, midgut carcinoids (ileum, appendix) preferably display solid structures, foregut and hindgut carcinoids trabecular or mixed structures (Table 3). No consistent histological differences exist between functioning and nonfunctioning tumours. Histochemical stains still used for diagnosing GEP tumours include aldehyde fuchsin (B cells) and silver impregnation techniques (argentaffin and argyrophil cells). Electron microscopy reveals the endocrine nature of the tumours by demonstrating membrane-bound, electron-dense secretory granules. In well-differentiated tumours such as insulinomas and midgut carcinoids secretory granule morphology is indicative of the hormone stored in the respective cell. In poorly differentiated tumours such as vipomas and most gastrinomas and glucagonomas, morphology of the granules is not diagnostic.

Immunocytochemistry and Multihormonality

Precise classification of GEP neuroendocrine tumours requires immunocytochemical analysis. NSE, the chromogranins and the other aforementioned proteins serve as general markers for neuroendocrine tumours. Usually the hormone inducing the clinical syndrome can be localized. In pancreatic tumours without a syndrome pancreatic polypeptide is frequently found. When using a battery of antisera against hormones many tumours turn out to be multihormonal (Heitz et al. 1982; Klöppel and Heitz 1988; Chejfec et al. 1988). Multihormonality may vary from one area to another, and metastases may produce hormones not found in the primary. Some of the tumour hormones are ectopic with respect to the site of tumour origin (Heitz et al. 1981). These properties of the neuroendocrine tumours are best explained by a common gene expression which becomes apparent during neoplastic transformation of neuroendocrine cells.

Immunocytochemical Profile, Tumour Localization and Biological Behaviour

The immunocytochemical profile of GEP tumours reveals characteristic constellations, depending on whether they have arisen in the pancreas, stomach, duodenum, distal small bowel and appendix or in the colon and rectum (Fig. 1). Thus, the hormonal spectrum of the tumours usually reflects the normal distribution of their cell of origin. The typical carcinoid of the ileum and appendix, for instance, usually shows a pattern comprising only serotonin and substance P. However, there are a number of noteworthy exceptions such as the pancreatic gastrinomas, vipomas, and GHRF- and ACTH-producing neoplasms (Heitz et al. 1981). Tumours with ectopic hormone production and hormonal syndromes are greater in size and more often malignant than those producing orthotopic hormones. In pancreatic endocrine tumours, alpha-HCG seems to be an indicator of

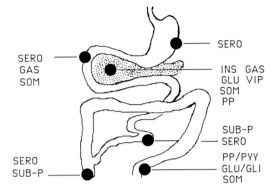

Fig. 1. Preferential hormone constellations in gastroenteropancreatic neuroendocrine tumours. *SERO*, serotonin: *SUB-P*, substance P; *INS*, insulin; *GLU/GLI*, glucagon/glicentin; *SOM*, somatostatin; *PP/PYY*, pancreatic polypeptide; *GAS*, gastrin; *VIP*, vasoactive intestinal peptide

malignancy. We found it in high prevalence in functioning malignant neoplasms, while it was virtually lacking in those with a benign behaviour (Heitz et al. 1983). In carcinoids, alpha-HCG expression appears to have no indicator function for predicting the likelihood of metastases (Heitz et al. 1987).

Functioning Tumours of the Pancreas

Insulinomas make up more than 70% of the functioning pancreatic endocrine tumours. Between 80% and 90% of insulinomas are benign and less than 2.5 cm in diameter when detected (Table 4). Virtually all of the insulinomas occur in the pancreas or attached to the pancreas. Inappropriate insulin secretion is the functional finding common to all types of insulinomas. However, insulinomas differ in the amount of proinsulin in the tumour tissue and released into the circulation, the insulin concentration in tumour extracts and the ability of insulinomas to respond to the inhibitory action of diazoxide and somatostatin. Insulinomas are followed in order of frequency by gastrinomas (Table 5), vipomas (Table 6), glucagonomas (Table 7) and tumours producing ACTH, GHRF, serotonin or PTH. The majority of these tumours are larger than insulinomas and show a malignant behaviour. The hormonal syndromes caused by these tumours are: Zollinger-Ellison syndrome (gastrin), Verner-Morrison syndrome (VIP), glucagonoma syndrome (glucagon), Cushing's syndrome(ACTH), acromegaly

Table 4. Characteristics of insulinomas associated with hypoglycaemic syndrome

Site	Intrapancreatic 99%
Size	<2.5 cm
Single	90%
Malignant	10%
Immunocytochemistry	100% positive for insulin; <50% multihormonal

Table 5. Characteristics of gastrinomas associated with Zollinger-Ellison syndrome

Site	Intrapancreatic <70%; extra-pancreatic (duodenal) >30%
Size	>2.5 cm intrapancreatic; <2.0 cm duodenal
Single	20%–50%
Malignant	60%–90%
Immunocytochemistry	80%–90% positive for gastrin; >50% multihormonal

Table 6. Characteristics of vipomas associated with Verner-
Morrison-syndrome

Site	Intrapancreatic 95%; Extra-pancreatic 5%; ganglioneuro-blastomas in children
Size	<4 cm
Single	99%
Malignant	69%–90%
Immunocytochemistry	80%–90% positive for VIP; commonly associated with PP

Table 7. Characteristics of glucagonomas associated with glucagonoma syndrome

Site	Intrapancreatic 99%
Size	>4 cm
Single	95%
Malignant	60%–90%
Immunocytochemistry	100% positive for glucagon; >50% multihormonal

(GHRF), carcinoid syndrome (serotonin and substance P), and hypercalcaemia
syndrome (PTH-like substance). The somatostatinoma syndrome is at present not
well defined (Vinik et al. 1987), and there are some doubts whether its symptomes
can be specifically ascribed to the effects of somatostatin.

Functioning Tumours of the Gut

Serotonin and substance P producing gut carcinoids which have metastasized to
the liver cause the well-known 'carcinoid-syndrome' (Dayal and Wolfe 1984).

Table 8. Hormonal syndromes associated with gastrointestinal carcinoids

Syndrome	Tumour site	Frequency
Carcinoid Syndrome	Ileum	70%
	Stomach	6%
	Duodenum	3%
	Colon	5%
Zollinger-Ellison syndrome	Duodenum	>95%
	Stomach	> 1%
Cushing's syndrome	Stomach	very rare

Virtually all of these carcinoids arise from the ileum (Table 8). According to their ultrastructural features and their strong reactivity with silver impregnation stains they are often called EC-cell carcinoids or argentaffin carcinoids. Gastrin-secreting carcinoids associated with the Zollinger-Ellison syndrome are preferentially located in the duodenum and are only rarely found at other sites such as the stomach antrum or the biliary tract (Bhagavan et al. 1986). The duodenal gastrinomas, which may be very small, show a malignancy rate of about 40%.

Nonfunctioning Tumours of the Pancreas and Gut

In pancreatic tumours not associated with a clinically recognizable syndrome the PP cell is often the prevailing cell type (Table 9). Less frequent are tumours rich in cells producing somatostatin, neurotensin or calcitonin (Klöppel and Heitz 1988). Tumours remaining nonreactive to a battery of antisera to various known hormones may nevertheless contain secretory granules by electron microscopy and stain for NSE and chromogranin. Nonfunctioning tumours may be small and found by chance during an operation or at autopsy. Others are large malignant tumours which cause nonspecific symptoms by invasion of organs adjacent to the pancreas or by metastasis. In the vast majority of carcinoids residing in the stomach, appendix, colon and rectum hormone production is not clinically evident (Chejfec et al. 1988). This is also true for some duodenal carcinoids which

Table 9. Characteristics of nonfunctioning pancreatic endocrine tumours presenting with symptoms related to mass effect and invasion of surrounding structures

Site	Intrapancreatic or adjacent to the pancreas
Size	Large (4–20 cm)
Single	95%
Malignant	60%–90%
Immunocytochemistry	Multihormonal but sparsely granulated; PP, somatostatin, neurotensin, calcitonin or no currently known hormone demonstrable

immunocytochemically display gastrin cells. Duodenal carcinoids with predominant somatostatin immunoreactivity frequently contain psammoma bodies and are associated with neurofibromatosis (Dayal et al. 1986; Stamm et al. 1986). In patients with chronic atrophic gastritis type A and pernicious anaemia multiple gastric carcinoids composed of ECL cells are observed in increasing frequency (Solcia et al. 1986).

Multiple Endocrine Neoplasia Type 1

The MEN-1 syndrome affects mainly the parathyroids, the endocrine pancreas and the adenohypophysis. The outstanding features of the pancreatic lesions are diffuse microadenomatosis combined with a few larger tumours showing a diameter greater than 0.5 cm (Klöppel et al. 1986). The rate of malignancy is low. Many of the microadenomas are rich in PP cells, glucagon cells or insulin cells. The high incidence of PPomas in these pancreases probably accounts for the elevated serum PP levels found in many MEN-1 patients (Friesen et al. 1983). Multihormonality is a consistent finding. When large insulinomas are present they may cause a hypoglycaemic syndrome. Despite the frequent occurrence of Zollinger-Ellison syndrome in MEN-1 patients, pancreatic gastrinomas are surprisingly uncommon, although the pancreas of these patients may be studded with tumours of varying size producing other hormones. In these cases a duodenal gastrinoma, which may be very small and therefore easily overlooked at operation, must be considered (Fig. 2) (Stamm et al. 1986). Rarely, a Werner-Morrison syndrome or a glucagon-oma syndrome has been reported in MEN-1 patients. In a few patients, pancreatic endocrine tumours have been observed in combination with von Hippel-Lindau disease or phaeochromocytoma (often bilateral; Klöppel and Heitz 1988;).

Mixed Endocrine-Exocrine Tumours

In the pancreas true endocrine-exocrine tumours are extremely rare. In the gut these neoplasms may be detected in higher frequency. Best known are the goblet cell carcinoids of the appendix (Höfler et al. 1984).

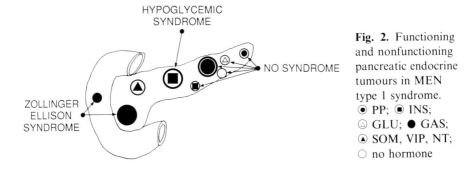

Fig. 2. Functioning and nonfunctioning pancreatic endocrine tumours in MEN type 1 syndrome. ⦿ PP; ◉ INS; ⊕ GLU; ● GAS; ▲ SOM, VIP, NT; ○ no hormone

References

Bhagavan BS, Slavin RE, Goldberg J, Rao RN (1986) Ectopic gastrinoma and Zollinger – Ellison – syndrome. Hum Pathol 17: 584–592

Bishop AE, Power RF, Polak JM (1988) Markers for neuroendocrine differentiation. Pathol Res Pract 183: 119–128

Chejfec G, Falkmer S, Askensten U, Grimelius L, Gould VE (1988) Neuroendocrine tumors of the gastrointestinal tract. Pathol Res Pract 183: 143–154

Dayal Y, Wolfe HJ (1984) Regulatory substances in clinically nonfunctioning gastrointestinal carcinoids. Evolution and tumour pathology of the neuroendocrine system. In: Falkmer S, Hakanson R, Sundler F (eds) Elsevier, Amsterdam, pp 497–517

Dayal Y, Kirsten K, Tallberg A, Nunnemacher G, DeLellis RA, Wolfe HJ (1986) Duodenal carcinoids in patients with and without neurofibromatosis. Am J Surg Pathol 10: 348–357

DeLellis RA, Dayal Y, Wolfe HJ (1984) Carcinoid tumors. Changing concepts and new perspectives. Am J Surg Pathol 8: 295–300

Friesen SR, Tomita T, Kimmel JR (1983) Pancreatic polypeptide update: its roles in detection of the trait for multiple endocrine adenopathy syndrome, type 1 and pancreatic polypeptide-secreting tumours. Surgery 94: 1028–1037

Hamid QA, Bishop AE, Rode J, Dhillon AP, Rosenberg BF, Reed JR, Sibley RK, Polak JM (1986) Duodenal gangliocytic paragangliomas: a study of 10 cases with immunocytochemical neuroendocrine markers. Hum Pathol 17: 1151–1157

Heitz PU (1984) Pancreatic endocrine tumours. In: Klöppel G, Heitz PU (eds) Pancreatic pathology. Churchill Livingstone, Edinburgh, pp 206–232

Heitz PU, Klöppel G, Polak JM, Staub J-J (1981) Ectopic hormone production by endocrine tumors: localization of hormones at the cellular level by immunocytochemistry. Cancer 48: 2029–2037

Heitz PU, Kasper M, Polak JM, Klöppel G (1982) Pancreatic endocrine tumors: immunocytochemical analysis of 125 tumors. Hum Pathol 13: 263–270

Heitz PU, Kasper M, Klöppel G, Polak JM, Vaitukaitis JL (1983) Glycoprotein-hormone alpha-chain production by pancreatic endocrine tumors: a specific marker of malignancy. Immunocytochemical analysis of tumors of 155 patients. Cancer 51: 277–282

Heitz PU, von Herbay G, Klöppel G, Komminoth P, Kaspar M, Höfler H, Müller KM, Oberholzer M (1987) The expression of subunits of human chorionic gonadotropin by non-trophoblastic, non-endocrine, and endocrine tumors. Am J Clin Pathol 88: 467–472

Höfler H, Klöppel G, Heitz PU (1984) Combined production of mucus, amines and peptides by goblet-cell carcinoids of the appendix and ileum. Pathol Res Pract 178: 555–561

Klöppel G, Willemer S, Stamm B, Hacki WH, Heitz PU (1986) Pancreatic lesions and hormonal profile of pancreatic tumors in multiple endocrine neoplasia type 1: an immunocytochemical study of nine patients. Cancer 57: 1824–1832

Klöppel G, Heitz PU (1988) Pancreatic endocrine tumors. Pathol Res Pract 183: 155–168

Kujari H, Joensuu H, Klemi P, Asola R, Nordman E (1988) A flow cytometric analysis of 23 carcinoid tumors. Cancer 61: 2517–2520

Martin JME, Maung RT (1987) Differential immunohistochemical reactions of carcinoid tumors. Hum Pathol 18: 941–954

Polak JM, Bloom SR (1985) Endocrine tumours. Churchill Livingstone, Edinburgh

Soga J, Tazawa K (1971) Pathologic analysis of carcinoids. Histologic reevaluation of 62 cases. Cancer 28: 990–998

Solcia E, Capella C, Sessa F, Rindi G, Cornaggia M, Riva C, Villani L (1986) Gastric carcinoids and related endocrine growths. Digestion 35 (Suppl 1): 3–22

Stamm B, Hedinger CE, Saremaslani P (1986) Duodenal and ampullary carcinoid tumors. A report of 12 cases with pathological characterisitcs, polpeptide content are relation to the MEN-1 syndrome and von Recklinghausen's disease (neurofibromatosis). Virchows Arch [A] 408: 485–489

Vinik AI, Strodel WE, Eckhauser FE, Moattari AR, Lloyd R (1987) Somatostatinomas, PPomas, neurotensiomas. Semin Oncol 14: 263–281

Williams ED, Sandler M (1963): The classification of carcinoid tumors. Lancet 1: 238–239

Clinical Implications of the Diffuse Gastroenteropancreatic Endocrine System

S.R. Friesen

Department of Surgery, University of Kansas School of Medicine,
Kansas City, KS 66103, USA

Introduction

The diffuse neuroendocrine system is composed of numerous amine-and peptide-secreting cells interspersed among other kinds of cells in the mucosa and submucosa of the gut and the pancreatic islets. Basic scientific investigations of this diffuse system, as contrasted to the endocrine *glands*, was delayed because the usual experimental observations following extirpation or transplantation of the cells was not possible.

The gastroenteropancreatic collection of diffuse neuroendocrine cells is a large reservoir of cells that secrete amines and peptides for the purpose of regulating and modulating normal physiologic control of carbohydrate metabolism, the digestion of proteins and fats, and the provision of an acid or alkaline pH appropriate for assimilation of nutrients. These neuroendocrine cells influence physiologic control by means of paracrine activity on neighboring cells, by neurocrine activity as aminergic and peptidergic neurotransmitters, and by their traditional endocrine function. For instance, carcinoid tumors of the duodenum arise from submucosal neurocrine cells that liberate amines as neurotransmitters (carcinoid syndrome) and peptides as endocrine hormones (ectopic duodenal gastrinomas, for instance).

The neuroendocrine cells that have the common cytochemical characteristics (amine precursor uptake and decarboxylation; Pearse 1969) are susceptible to stimulation and suppression; this is an important conceptual quality to be noted clinically. For instance, the response of hyperplastic cells to stimulation is an exaggerated normal response; on the other hand, stimulation of neoplastic tumor cells often results in a paradoxical response.

The peptide hormones that are released into the circulation seek out their specific membrane receptors on the end-organ target cells. These receptors, in turn, activate the cAMP second messenger system to activate the specific biologic activity of the end organ. For instance, the parietal cell of the stomach has four membrane receptors: two for the amines, histamine and acetylcholine, one for the peptide gastrin (all of which stimulate acid, H^+, secretion), and one for the peptide somatostatin that inhibits acid secretion.

Recent Results in Cancer Research. Vol. 118
© Springer-Verlag Berlin·Heidelberg 1990

Hypersecretion of amines and peptides occurs when there are pathologic processes of adenoma, carcinoma, carcinoid, microadenoma, or hyperplasia (Kloppel and Heitz 1984). The syndrome is an entopic one if the hypersecretion of peptides occurs from an organ in which that peptide is normally present; the syndrome is an ectopic one if that peptide is not normally present in the organ in which the neoplasm occurs. Ectopic tumor syndromes are usually malignant with the elaboration of large molecular peptides in preponderance (Lips et al. 1978).

Clinical Features

The clinical diagnosis of an endocrine syndrome due to hypersecretion of peptides is made on the basis of the following: (a) clinical picture, (b) stimulation or suppression tests, (c) measurement of elevated circulating peptides, and (d) confirmation by immunocytochemistry of the tumor. Localization of the tumors is by: (a) computerized tomography, (b) angiography, (c) selective venous assays, and (d) surgical exploration (Friesen 1982).

The most recent clinical investigative developments have occurred in the endocrinopathies of the pancreatic islets. These relate to (a) the hypersecretion of pancreatic polypeptide in the syndrome of multiple endocrine adenopathy type I (MEA I) (Wermer 1954) and (b) the ulcerogenic syndromes of both ectopic Zollinger-Ellison syndrome (gastrinomas) (Zollinger and Ellison 1955) and the entopic pseudo-Zollinger-Ellison syndrome of antral G-cell hyperplasia (AGCH) (Friesen and Tomita 1981).

The MEA I syndrome is a genetic (familial) triad of multiple organs (pituitary, parathyroid, and pancreas) with multiple cells involved in multiple pathologic states in multiple members of the family. It is an autosomal dominant trait. The new peptide human pancreatic polypeptide (hPP), discovered by Kimmel, the late biochemist of Kansas (Kimmel et al. 1975), is extremely useful in the diagnosis of this syndrome. It can be used to detect the genetic trait in asymptomatic members of a suspect family if there is an exaggerated response of circulating hPP ($>5\times$ basal) after a protein meal. This response correlates with islet cell hyperplasia. If the fasting plasma level is elevated ($>3\times$ normal), it signifies the presence of an islet cell tumor, even in an asymptomatic member of the family. The correlation, to date, is 100% in genetic MEA I patients but only 50% in patients with sporadic islet cell tumors (Friesen et al. 1983).

The ulcerogenic syndrome may be either ectopic or entopic. The ectopic form is the classical Zollinger-Ellison syndrome of recurrent ulcer disease with marked hypersecretion of gastric acids due to tumor gastrinomas of the islets or submucosal duodenal gastrinomas. Only recently has it been appreciated that the duodenal lesions are small tumors of neurocrine gastrin (G-17 and G-34) in the submucosa, like carcinoid cells. They metastasize to regional lymph nodes, and it is these nodes that are usually discovered first during surgical exploration. The primary lesions are found by careful inspection of the opened duodenum or the resected gastroduodenal specimen of total gastrectomy or pancreaticoduodenectomy (Delcore et al. 1988). There are a few rare cases of "isolated" lymph node gastrinomas without another primary gastrinoma detected (Delcore et al. 1988). Primary pancreatic gastrinomas with lymph node metastases usually also have hepatic metastases.

The entopic variety of the ulcerogenic syndrome is clinically called the pseudo-Zollinger – Ellison syndrome due to AGCH. This antral form is clinically similar to the classical ectopic form except that no tumor is present; only AGCH produces the hypergastrinemia and the hyperchlorhydria with ulceration. This entity can be differentiated from the tumor variety by stimulation tests (Friesen and Tomita 1984). Both have fasting hypergastrinemia, but meal stimulation further increases the serum gastrin concentration in patients with AGCH, and intravenous secretin stimulation further elevates the serum gastrin only in patients with tumor gastrinomas, a paradoxical response. Patients with ordinary duodenal ulcer with hyperacidity of neurogenic (vagal) origin have normal fasting serum gastrin concentrations with only mild stimulation by a meal and none by secretin.

Treatment

The treatment of ulcerogenic syndromes is sometimes controversial but need not be confusing if a correct pre-operative diagnosis has been made. There are several medical and surgical options regarding the endocrine mechanisms. The instigating cause of the hypergastrinemia, of either tumor or hyperplasia origin, is best treated (a) by excision of the tumor gastrinomas whether in nodes, duodenum, or pancreas and (b) by surgical antrectomy for the entopic AGCH. Medically the release of gastrin from the gastrinomas can be inhibited by the administration of long-acting somatostatin analogues (Mulvihill et al. 1986). Treatment of the end-organ hypersecretion of gastric acids can be accomplished medically by the use of (a) histamine 2 receptor blockers, (b) antacids, (c) omeprazole blockade of the H^+ pump, and (d) somatostatin analogue receptor blockage on the parietal cell. Surgically a total gastrectomy is the only certain method of completely eliminating the marked hypersecretion of acid. This latter traditional operation has additional benefits in that the specimen has been demonstrated to have small occult primary gastrinomas of the stomach and duodenum and may, in unusual circumstances, lead to regression of metastatic tumors (Friesen 1968). Although parietal cell vagotomy has been advocated to decrease the dosage of receptor blockers, it is inferior to the use of antroduodenectomy, which may not only disclose an occult submucosal primary duodenal gastrinoma but in patients with AGCH restore normal serum gastrin values and gastric acidity leading to healing of the ulceration.

References

Delcore R, Cheung LY, Friesen SR (1988) Outcome of lymph node involvement without hepatic metastases in patients with Zollinger-Ellison syndrome. Ann Surg 208: 291–298
Friesen SR (1968) A gastric factor in the pathogenesis of the Zollinger-Ellison syndrome. Ann Surg 168: 483–501

Friesen SR (1982) Tumors of the endocrine pancreas. N Engl J Med. 306: 580–590

Friesen SR, Tomita T (1981) Pseudo – Zollinger – Ellison syndrome: hypergastrinemia, hyperchlorhydria without tumor. Ann Surg 194: 481

Friesen SR, Tomita T (1984) Further experience with Pseudo-Zollinger-Ellison syndrome: its place in the management of neuroendocrine duodenal ulceration. World J Surg 8: 552

Friesen SR, Tomita T, Kimmel JR (1983) Pancreatic polypeptide update: its roles in detection of the trait for multiple endocrine adenopathy syndrome type I and pancreatic polypeptide-secreting tumors. Surgery 94: 1028

Kimmel JR, Hayden LJ, Pollock HG (1975) Isolation and characterization of a new pancreatic polypeptide hormone. J Biol Chem 250: 9369

Klöppel G, Heitz PU (1984) Pancreatic pathology. Churchill Livingstone, New York

Lips CJM, van der Sluys Veer J, van der Bonk JA, van Dam RH, Hackeng WHI. (1978) Common precursor molecule as origin for the ectopic – hormone – producing-tumor syndrome. Lancet 1: 16–18

Mulvihill S, Pappas TN, Passaro E, Debas HT (1986). The use of somatostatin and its analogs in the treatment of surgical disorder. Surgery 100:467

Pearse AGE (1969). The cytochemistry and ultrastructure of polypetide hormone-producing cells of the APUD series and the embryologic, physiologic and pathologic implications of the concept. J Histochem Cytochem 17: 303

Wermer F. (1954) Genetic aspects of adenomatosis of endocrine glands. Am J Med. 16: 363

Zollinger RM, Ellison EH (1955) Primary peptic ulcerations of the jejunum associated with islet cell tumors of the pancreas. Ann Surg 142: 709

Thyroid Gland (C-Cell Tumours)

Medullary Carcinoma of the Thyroid

W. Böcker[1] and S. Schröder[2]

[1]Gerhard-Domagk-Institut für Pathologie, Universität Münster, Domagkstraße 17,
4400 Münster, FRG
[2]Institut für Pathologie, Universität Hamburg, Martinistraße 52, 2000 Hamburg 20, FRG

Introduction

Medullary carcinoma (MC) originates in the C cells of the thyroid gland. Among the epithelial malignancies of this organ it accounts for some 3%–12% (Deftos 1983). Hazard et al. (1959) were the first to define it as a separate entity on the basis of amyloid deposits in the stroma. MC occurs in familial or sporadic form and with an approximately balanced sex distribution (Williams 1979; Deftos 1983; Emmertsen 1985). Its clinical course is characterized by a marked variability in morphologic structure and duration of disease (between a few months and several decades; Deftos 1983). Neither histologic nor cellular variations of MC (Kakudo et al. 1979; Harach and Williams 1983; Landon and Ordonez 1985; Mendelsohn et al. 1980; Martinelli et al. 1983; Fernandes et al. 1982; Zaatari et al. 1983; Golouh et al. 1985; Marcus et al. 1982; Kracht 1977; Zeman et al. 1978) can be correlated with the prognostic outlook, but morphologic differences are of distinctive significance for separating MC from the other types of thyroid carcinoma.

Recent immunohistochemical and biochemical investigations have disclosed the role of certain neuroendocrine and regulatory peptides and other tumor markers (De Lellis et al. 1978; Talerman et al. 1979; Wolfe et al. 1980; Lloyd et al. 1983; Saad et al. 1984; Holm et al. 1985; Schröder and Klöppel 1987; Williams 1979; Uribe et al. 1985; Krisch et al. 1985). The histogenetic derivation of MC from C cells has recently been questioned by some authors who have observed a coproduction of thyreoglobulin (TG) and calcitonin in otherwise typical MCs (Holm et al. 1985; Uribe et al. 1985; Sobrinho-Simoes et al. 1985).

The present analysis is based on results from our Hamburg material (Schröder 1988; Schröder and Klöppel 1987). Our investigations comprise conventional light microscopy and immune histology correlated with the respective clinical data.

Materials and Methods

Formalin-fixed paraffin-embedded material obtained from 39 primary medullary carcinomas was analyzed. The tumors were classified according to histologic

Table 1. Source and dilution of the employed antibodies

Antigen	Species	Source	Dilution
Cytokeratin	Mouse	Dianova (Hamburg, FRG)	1:1000
Vimentin	Mouse	Boehringer (Mannheim, FRG)	1:20
Neurofilament	Mouse	Dianova (Hamburg, FRG)	1:200
Thyreoglobulin	Mouse	Dianova (Hamburg, FRG)	1:200
Calcitonin	Rabbit	IBL (Hamburg, FRG)	1:3000
NSE	Rabbit	Dakopatts (Hamburg, FRG)	1:3000
Chromogranin A	Mouse	Camon (Wiesbaden, FRG)	1:500
CEA	Mouse	Behringwerke (Marburg, FRG)	1:3
CGRP	Rabbit	Amersham Int. (Amersham, UK)	1c17:200
Bombesin	Rabbit	IBL (Hamburg, FRG)	1:1000
S-100 protein	Rabbit	Dakopatts (Hamburg, FRG)	1:500
Leu-M1	Mouse	Becton-Dickinson (Heidelberg, FRG)	1:30

features and the presence of stromal amyloid as verified by Congo red staining. All cases were analyzed immunohistochemically for reactivity to calcitonin, neuron-specific enolase, carcinoembryonic antigen (CEA), serotonin, α-hCG, bombesin, somatostatin, and neurotensin (Table 1), Additional immunohistochemical tests using the avidin-biotin complex method, were performed for Leu $-$ M $-$ 1 antigen (monoclonal antibody available from Becton-Dickinson, Heidelberg, FRG) in 1:30 dilution. This Leu $-$ M $-$ 1 is a myelomonocytic antigen found in Reed-Sternberg cells of Hodgkin patients and in a number of adenocarcinomas, among them some papillary thyroid carcinomas (Schröder 1988).

In our study, Leu $-$ M $-$ 1 positive cells were counted, and the mean immuno-reactivity was defined as the proportion of positively staining cells per 100 tumor cells. The medical records of all patients in our series were followed to the summer of 1985.

Results

Histologically, the majority of MCs showed solid or trabecular structures, but as many as 15% revealed partly follicular or papillary patterns. A more marked nuclear pleomorphism was found in about 10%. No amyloid was observed in 27%

Table 2. Immunoreactivity of MC

Antigen	Percentage of positive cases	Intensity of staining reaction
CK	100%	+ + + +
Vimentin	55%	+ +/+ + +
Neurofilament	13%	+/+ +
Chromogranin A	100%	+ + +/+ + + +
NSE	75%	+ +/+ + +
Calcitonin	100%	(+)/*+ + + +
CGRP	92%	+ +/+ + + +
CEA	77%	+ +/+ + + +
α-hCG	23%	
Bombesin	18%	
Somatostatin	12%	
Neurotensin	3%	
TG	0%	

upon Congo red staining with polarization microscopy. On the whole, tests for amyloid often yield discordant patterns in the primary and its metastases, i.e., positivity in the one and absence of amyloid in the other.

Immunohistochemical results are summarized in Table 2. Calcitonin was found in varying amounts in all MCs, whereas none of them manifested TG expression in its tumor cells. Activity of chromogranin A was demonstrable in 100%, of CGRP in 92%, and of NSE in 75% of our cases. CEA was present in 77% of MCs, whereas all other regulatory peptids were observed in only very small percentages. With regard to intermediate filaments, all MCs were CK positive; coexpression of CK and vimentin was found in 55%, and neurofilaments appeared in only 13% of all cases.

Epithelial Leu–M–1 immunoreactivity was marked (i.e., more than 15% positive tumor cells) in 41% of cases; it was slight (15% or fewer positive cells) or absent in 46%. Kaplan-Meier curves demonstrating the probability of postoperative recurrence or survival for the respective patients revealed significant differences in clinical course (Fig.1). A marked epithelial Leu–M–1 reactivity correlated significantly with an unfavorable course (death or persistent disease), whereas patients without evidence of disease showed only slight positive staining or none at all. Neither histologic features (structure and cell type) nor immunohistochemical results (positive or negative immunoreactivity for CEA, chromogranin, CGRP, etc.) werefound to correlate with clinical outcome.

Discussion

The present World Health Organization classification is based on the concept of primary thyroid carcinomas originating either in C cells or in follicle cells. The

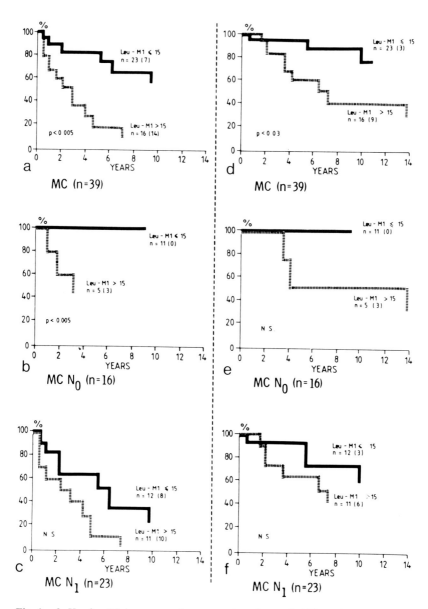

Fig. 1a–f. Kaplan-Meier curves demonstrating the probability of postoperative recurrent disease (**a-c**) and survival (**d-f**) of patients with MC, correlating the different degrees of epithelial Leu–M–1 immunoreactivity (<15% versus >15%) with tumor stages in the respective patients

hypothesis was founded for MC on the evidence of stromal amyloid deposits and other criteria such as calcitonin, CGRP, neuroendocrine markers and CEA, and for differentiated follicular carcinomas on the presence of TG, noted as a specific marker in a high percentage of cases. Reports on the coexistence of calcitonin and

TG in a number of otherwise typical MCs (Hales et al. 1982; Pfaltz et al. 1983; Ljungberg et al. 1984; Parker et al. 1985; Mills et al. 1986; Holm et al. 1986; Uribe et al. 1985; Sobrinho-Simoes et al. 1985) raised some doubts about the original concept of a basically differing carcinogenesis. Our own studies have shown that calcitonin antibodies may yield partly positive cross-reactions with normal thyroid parenchyma. This may be due to the preparation of calcitonin antibodies by immunization of rabbits with TG-conjugated calcitonin; consequently, we used only TG-absorbed calcitonin antisera in our assay. In our own material of 200 differentiated follicular cell carcinomas and medullary carcinomas, evidence of calcitonin was strictly limited to MCs, and that of thyreoglobulin to papillary and follicular thyroid carcinomas.

Morphologic diagnosis of MC may safely be based on the evidence of calcitonin in tumor cells. Additional immunohistochemical parameters may support it, although their diagnostic value is not as great. Considering the lack of evidence of amyloid in about 25% of all MCs, this parameter should be abandoned as a morphological criterion (Schröder 1988). The diagnostic value of CEA for MC has been well documented in the literature for many years (e.g., De Lellis et al. 1978; Talerman et al. 1979). Distinctly lower proportions of CEA-positive cases in our Hamburg series (75% versus 90% in the literature) may be due to our using a monoclonal antibody without NCA cross-reactivity (Schröder and Klöppel 1987).

Our investigations yielded additional evidence of certain hormonal and non-hormonal substances identified as secretion products of C cells or other neuroendocrine cells which may support the neuroendocrine differentiation of medullary carcinoma. However, no influence on the clinical course can be attributed to the varying histologic features nor to the immunohistologic criteria recorded in our study.

The observation of a prognostic impact of epithelial Leu–M–1 expression in MC is all the more surprising. This evidence may help to determine individual prognoses especially in carcinomas at the N_0 stage. Similar predictive properties of Leu–M–1 expression were also observed in papillary carcinomas but in no other type of thyroid carcinoma.

Summary

The results of our study may be summarized as follows:

1. Medullary carcinomas of the thyroid are derived from the C cells of the gland and are characterized by strong histologic and cytologic pleomorphism with inconstant stromal amyloid deposits.
2. The decisive morphodiagnostic criterion is immunohistochemical evidence of calcitonin coinciding with negative TG reactivity.
3. In addition to obligatory calcitonin expression, MCs may show variable synthesis of several polypeptids and biogenic (?) amines.
4. The varying immunoreactivity patterns are not related to the clinical behavior of the respective tumors.

5. Leu–M–1 antigen, a monocyte-granulocyte marker known to express in Reed-Sternberg cells and in certain nonhemopoietic neoplasms, can also be demonstrated in MCs. Leu–M–1 immunoreactivity was found to correlate significantly with an unfavorable course. Thus, the introduction of immunostaining for Leu–M–1 in cases of thyroid carcinoma may provide significant prognostic information for these patients.

References

Deftos LJ (1983) Medullary thyroid carcinoma. Karger, Basel

De Lellis RA, Rule AH, Spiler I, Nathanson L, Tashjian AT, Wolfe HJ (1978) Calcitonin and carcinoembryonic antigen as tumor markers in medullary thyroid carcinoma. Am J Clin Pathol 70: 587–594

Emmertsen K (1985) Medullary thyroid carcinoma and calcitonin. Dan Med Bull 32: 1–28

Fernandes BJ, Bedard YC, Rosen I (1982) Mucus-producing medullary cell carcinoma of the thyroid gland. Am J Clin Pathol 78: 536–540

Golouh R, US-Krasovec M, Auersperg M, Jancar J, Bondi A, Eusebi V (1985) Amphicrine-composite calcitonin and mucin-producing carcinoma of the thyroid. Ultrastruct Pathol 8: 197–206.

Hales M, Rosenau W, Okerlund MD, Gabanter M (1982) Carcinoma of the thyroid with a mixed medullary and follicular pattern. Morphologic, immunohistochemical and clinical laboratory study. Cancer 50: 1352–1359

Harach HR, Williams ED (1983) Glandular (tubular and follicular) variants of medullary carcinoma of the thyroid. Histopathology 7: 83–97

Hazard JB, Hawk WA, Crile G (1959) Medullary (solid) carcinoma of the thyroid–a clinicopathologic entity. J Clin Endocrinol Metab 19: 152–161

Holm R, Sobrinho–Simoes M, Nesland JM, Gould VE, Johannessen JV (1985) Medullary carcinoma of the thyroid gland: and immunocytochemical study. Ultrastruct Pathol 8: 25–41

Holm R, Sobrinho–Simoes M, Nesland JM, Johannessen JV (1986) Concurrent production of calcitonin and thyreoglobulin by the same neoplastic cells. Ultrastruct Pathol 10: 241–248

Kakudo K, Miyauchi A, Takai S, Katayama S, Kuma K, Kitamura H (1979) C-cell carcinoma of the thyroid–papillary type. Acta Pathol Jpn 29:653–659

Kracht JC (1977) C-Zellen und C-Zellengeschwülste. Verh Dtsch Ges Pathol 61: 235–264

Krisch K, Krisch I. Horvat G, Neuhold N, Ulrich W (1985) the value of immunohistochemistry in medullary thyroid carcinoma: a systematic study of 30 cases. Histopathology 9: 1077–1089

Landon G, Ordonez NG (1985) Clear cell variant of medullary carcinoma of the thyroid. Hum Pathol 16: 844–847

Ljungberg O, Bondeson L, Bondeson AG (1984) Differentiated thyroid carcinoma, intermediate type: a new tumor entity with features of follicular and parafollicular cell carcinoma. Hum Pathol 15: 218–228

Lloyd RV, Sisson JC, Marangos PJ (1983) Calcitonin, carcinoembryonic antigen and neuron-specific enolase in medullary thyroid carcinoma. An immunohistochemical study. Cancer 51: 2234–2239

Marcus JN, Dise CA, LI Volsi VA (1982) Melanin production in a medullary thyroid carcinoma. Cancer 49: 2518–2526

Martinelli G, Bazzocchi F, Govoni E, Santini D (1983) Anaplastic type of medullary thyroid carcinoma. An ultrastructural and immunohistochemical study. Virchows Arch [A] 400: 61–67

Mendelsohn G, Bigner SH, Egleston JC, Baylin SB, Wells SA (1980) Anaplastic variants of medullary thyroid carcinoma. Am J Surg Pathol 4: 333–341

Mills SE, Stallings RG, Austin MB (1986) Angiomatoid carcinoma of the thyroid gland. Anaplastic carcinoma with follicular and medullary features mimicking angiosarcoma. Am J Clin Pathol 86: 674–578

Parker LN, Kollin J, WU SY, Rypins EB, Juler GL (1985) Carcinoma of the thyroid with a mixed medullary, papillary, follicular and undifferentiated pattern. Arch Intern Med 145: 1507–1509

Pfaltz M, Hedinger CE, Muhlethaler JP (1983) Mixed medullary and follicular carcinoma of the thyroid. Virchows Arch [A] 400: 53–59

Saad MF, Ordonez NG, Guido JJ, Samaan NA (1984) The prognostic value of calcitonin immunostaining in medullary carcinoma of the thyroid. J Clin Endocrinol Metab 59: 850–856

Schröder S (1988) Pathologie und Klinik maligner Schilddrüsentumoren. Fischer, Stuttgart

Schröder S, Klöppel G (1987) Carcinoembryonic antigen and nonspecific cross-reacting antigen in thyroid cancer. An immunocytochemical study using polyclonal and mono-clonal antibodies. Am J Surg Pathol 11: 100–108

Schröder S, Baisch H, Rehpenning W, Müller–Gärtner HW, Schulzbischof K, Sablotny B, Meiners I, Böcker W, Schreiber HW (1987) Morphologie und Prognose des follikulären Schilddrüsencarcinoms. Eine klinisch–pathologische und DNS–zytome–Langenbecks Arch Chir 370: 3–24

Sobrinho-Simoes M, Nesland JM, Johannessen JV (1985) Farewell to the dual histogenesis of thyroid tumors? Ultrastruct Pathol 8: III–IV

Talerman A, Lindeman J, Kievit–Tyson PA, Dröge-Droppert C (1979) Demonstration of calcitonin and carcinoembryonic antigen (CEA) in medullary carcinoma of the thyroid (MCT) by immunoperoxidase technique Histopathology 3: 503–510

Uribe M, Fenolgio-Preiser CM, Grimes M, Feind C (1985) Medullary carcinoma of the thyroid gland. Clinical, pathological, and immunohistochemical features with review of the literature. Am J Surg Pathol 9: 577–594

Williams ED (1979) Medullary carcinoma of the thyroid. In: De Groot LJ (ed) Endocrinology, vol 2. Grune and Stratton, New York, pp 777–792

Wolfe HJ, De Lellis RA, Jackson CE, Greenwald KA, Block MA, Tashjian AH (1980) Immunocytochemical distinction of hereditary from sporadic medullary thyroid carcinoma. Lab Invest 42: 161–162

Zaatari GS, Saigo PE, Huvos AG (1983) Mucin production in medullary carcinoma of the thyroid.Arch Pathol Lab Med 107: 70–74

Zeman V, Nemec J. Platil A, Zamarazil V, Pohunkova D, Neradiolova M (1978) Anaplastic transformation of medullary thyroid cancer. Neoplasma 25: 249–255

Growth Regulation of Normal Thyroids and Thyroid Tumors in Man

P.E. Goretzki, A. Frilling, D. Simon, and H.-D. Roeher

Abteilung für Allgemeine- und Unfallchirurgie, Chirurgische Universitätsklinik Düsseldorf, Moorenstraße 5, 4000 Düsseldorf, FRG

Introduction

The biological importance of endocrine and paracrine growth stimulation of human thyroid gland and human thyroid tumors is still debated controversially. Most clinical data indicate a mitotic effect of thyrotropin (TSH) on thyrocyte growth in man (Abe et al. 1981; Clark et al. 1983; Goretzki and Clark 1988), whereas investigators using porcine follicles in culture question the direct effect of TSH on thyrocyte growth (Gaertner et al. 1985; Wanabe et al. 1985; Westermark et al. 1983, 1986). In these cells local active growth factors such as epidermal growth factor (EGF) stimulate cell proliferation (Westermark et al. 1986). In FRTL-5 cells, a permanent follicular thyroid cell clone from a rat thyroid tumor (Filetti et al. 1988; Jin et al. 1986; Tramontano et al. 1988), murine (Mothersill et al. 1984; Tamura et al. 1981) and canine thyrocytes (Roger et al. 1984; Roger and Dumont 1982) TSH proved to increase cell growth, which is at least partially related to TSH stimulation of adenylate cyclase (AC; Roger and Dumont 1982). Most of these studies, however, are of limited conclusiveness for humans. Thyrocytes demonstrate species-specific differences in growth regulation, and this requires the study of human thyrocytes. Additionally, using primary cell cultures these cells lack absolute purity because of fibroblast contamination, which can be excluded only by establishing defined permanent cell lines.

Assessing the biological importance of TSH and local active growth factors on growth regulation in human thyroids and in human thyroid tumors, we therefore used only human thyroid tissues. Our studies on cell membranes, primary cell cultures, and a defined human thyrocyte cell line have demonstrated, that both TSH and local active growth factors modulate human thyrocyte growth.

Material and Methods

Reagents. Bovine TSH was purchased from Armour (Chicago, USA). HAM F12 medium, MEM Dulbecco's medium, and forskolin were from Calbiochem (San

Diego, USA); creatine phosphokinase, phosphocreatine, bovine serum albumin, adenosine triphosphate, 3-isobutyl-1-methylxanthine (IBMX), bovine insulin, murine EGF, insulin-like growth factor (IGF), thymidine, dibutyryl cyclic adenosine monophosphate (dbcAMP), and cyclic adenosine monophosphate (cAMP) from Sigma (St. Louis, USA). Fetal calf serum (FCS) was obtained from Gibco (Paisley, UK). Collagenase (150 U/mg) and trypsin were from Boehringer (Mannheim, FRG). Neutral aluminum oxide, Sephadex G100, and Dowex AG were purchased from Merck (Darmstadt, FRG) and Ficoll from Pharmacia (Freiburg, FRG). Plastic material for culture technique was from Nunc (Roskilde, Denmark). Adenosine 5'-[α^{36}P]triphosphate (300 Ci/mmol), [^{3}H]thymidine (25 Ci/mmol), [^{3}H] adenosine 3'5'-cyclic monophosphate (30–50 ci/mmol) and cAMP RIA were obtained from Amersham (Braunschweig, FRG).

Thyroid Membrane Preparation. Human thyroid tissue was obtained at surgery, separated into tissue from differentiated thyroid cancer ($n=5$), follicular thyroid adenoma ($n=30$), and adjacent normal thyroid ($n=30$) in cases of a uninodular thyroid disease. In cases of multinodular thyroid disease ($n=12$) at least three aliquots from different localizations of the thyroid gland were pooled. Tissues were immediately placed on ice in sterile tubes, trimmed, minced, and homogenized in 4 ml buffer per gram tissue, containing 5 mM Tris-HCl (pH 7.5), 1 mM EDTA, and 0.25 M sucrose. After centrifugation at 1000 g and 4°C for 10 min the supernatant was aspirated and recentrifuged at 8000 g for 15 min. The pellet was extracted and resuspended in the same buffer to a total protein concentration of 1.5 mg/ml, measured by the method of Lowry et al.

Primary Thyrocyte Cultures. Normal human thyroid tissue was obtained at surgery, trimmed, and placed in PBS at room temperature. The tissue was minced, washed in PBS three times, and disintegrated with 1% collagenase for 5–45 min. After separating blood cells by centrifugation on a Ficoll layer thyrocytes were seeded in culture bottles containing minimal essential medium (MEM) and modified HAM F12 medium 1:1 with supplementation of 10% FCS, penicillin (50 IU/ml), streptomycin (50 μg/ml), and NaHCO$_3$ (36 mg/ml) for 24 h. Cells were then harvested using a rubber scaper, washed, and resuspended in medium without FCS. This was followed by a 24-h incubation of 20 000 cells per well in 24 well plates in medium with the tested substance, 2 μCi/ml [^{3}H]thymidine, but no FCS.

Short-Term Cultures. After seeding 500 000 cells per 80-cm^2 culture bottle in medium with 10% FCS for 3 days the supernatant was discarded. The cells were harvested using 0.5% trypsin in PBS and checked histologically and with trypan blue (85%–95% living cells). After one to three further propagations in 80-cm^2 culture bottles the cells were used when they had reached approximately 70% confluency. Checking for growth regulation, cells were seeded in 25-cm^2 culture bottles with medium, 10% FCS, and the tested substance (200 000 cells per bottle). Determining [^{3}H]thymidine incorporation into TCA-precipitable cell material, a 24-well plate (50 000 cells per well) and serum free medium was used.

Cell Line FTC-133. A 42 year old male patient was operated on for a metastatic follicular thyroid carcinoma in June 1987. Primary cell cultures from mediastinal lymph node metastases were passaged three times and cloned. One clone was further propagated 11 passages and was checked for thyroglobulin immunoreactivity. Cells from this clone were used, studying [³H]thymidine incorporation in serum free medium with TSH or local active growth factors added.

Proliferation Assay. In 25-cm² culture flasks 200 000 cells were seeded using 2 ml medium with 10% FCS. The medium was changed every 3rd day and cells were harvested at days 4, 8, 12, 16, and 20 with 0.5% trypsin and 0.01% EGTA in PBS. Viability was checked with 0.2% trypan blue. Cells were counted in a hemocytometer with 85%–95% viability. Experiments were performed in triplicates.

[³H]Thymidine Incorporation. In 400 μl 1:1 MEM Dulbecco's medium, HAM F12 medium 50 000 cells were seeded with 50 μl (1.0 μCi) [³H]thymidine and 50 μl tested substance for 24 h. Cells were centrifuged at 1000 g for 10 min, and the supernatant was aspirated. After washing cells with PBS twice 1 ml 10% TCA was added for 1 h. TCA was withdrawn and the pellet disolved in 500 μl 0.2 N NaOH at 4°C for 12 h. This solution was poured into 5 ml scintillation fluid and measured in a Beckman's beta counter.

cAMP Production in Thyrocytes. Cellular cAMP production was determined in 50 000 thyrocytes per well, kept in 400 μl salt-depleted Hank's medium (5.4 mol KCl, 1.3 mol $CaCl_2$, 0.8 mmol $MgSO_4$, 0.3 mmol HEPES and 0.5 IBMX) with the tested substance. After 90 min the medium was aspirated, lyophilized, and resuspended in 50 μl H_2O. Cells were covered with 400 μl 96% ethanol layer, stirred, and centrifuged at 10 000 g for 10 min. The supernatant was aspirated, evaporated, and resuspended in 50 μl H_2O. Both 50-μl H_2O extracts were poured together and determined for cAMP content following the RIA procedure.

Adenylate Cyclase Activity in Thyroid Membranes. The 8000 g particulate membrane fraction (100 μg) was incubated with increasing concentrations of bTSH (0.0003–0.1 IU/ml) or NaF (2 or 10 mmol/l) or forskolin (10^{-8}–10^{-4}mol/l) and adenosine 5'- [α^{32}P]triphosphate (20000 cpm) at 30°C for 30 min, as described previously. AC activity was determined by conversion of [α^{32}P]ATP to [^{32}P]cAMP, extracted by chromatography with an internal standard of [³H]cAMP (recovery of 75%–92%), as described previously (Clark et al. 1981).

Immunocytochemistry. For microscopic determination 100 000 cells were grown in culture flasks (16 ml) using medium with 10% FCS. After 3–5 days, when cells had reached confluency, the top was detached and the bottom washed in H_2O_2-enriched PBS three times to eliminate endogeneous peroxidase activity. After fixation in aceton at $-20°C$ for 10 min cells were left to dry at room temperature. Incubation with the primary antibody was carried out with a monoclonal antibody against thyroglobulin (Dakopatts) and a polyclonal antibody against EGF receptor (Amersham) for 18 h. Nonspecific background activity was suppressed using 1% horse serum. Thyroglobulin immunoreactivity was visualized by PAP technique, and EGF receptor immunoreactivity was visualized by ABC technique. For negative controls human fibroblasts were used.

Statistical Evaluations. For statistical evaluation of differences obtained in our assays we used distribution-free tests – the Wilcoxon rank test for unpaired or for paired samples, the Mann-Whitney test, and the χ^2 test.

Results

Studying AC activity in human thyroid tissues, we measured basal, TSH (0.1 IU/ml), NaF (2 mmol/1), Gpp(NH)p (0.1 mmol/1), and forskolin (0.1 mmol/1) stimulated AC. Tissues from thyroid adenomas demonstrated higher AC response to TSH than did tissues from normal thyroids, multinodular goiters, and differentiated thyroid cancers ($p < 0.05$; Table 1). TSH receptor unrelated AC stimulation by forskolin (2 mmol/1) gave comparable results in all four groups. Tissues from follicular thyroid adenomas showed the tendency for slightly higher AC responses to NaF (2 mmol/1) and Gpp(NH)p (0.1 mmol/1) when compared to normal and cancerous human thyroid tissues, but this was not statistically significant (Table 1).

In a prospective study we compared basal, TSH (0.1 IU/ml), and NaF (10 mmol/1) stimulated AC in normal and adenomatous human thyroid tissue from follicular adenomas with increased or decreased iodine uptake. Tissues from follicular thyroid adenoma with major degeneration (examined histologically), from thyroids with multinodular disease, and thyroid tissues from patients with preoperative antithyroid drug treatment were excluded from this study. The final 12 "cold" and 10 "hot" nodules with adjacent normal thyroid tissue demonstrated higher AC response to TSH (0.1 IU/ml) in tissues from follicular thyroid adenomas with increased and with decreased iodine uptake when compared to normal thyroid tissue of the same patient ($p < 0.005$ and 0.025; Table 2). AC stimulation by NaF (10 mmol/1), however, was increased only in tissue from "hot" follicular thyroid adenomas ($p < 0.005$) and not in tissue from "cold" adenomas when compared to normal thyroid tissue from the same patient (Table 2).

Table 1. Adenylate cyclase activity in the 8000 *g* particulate fraction of human thyroid tissues

Tissue	n	Basal[a]	TSH/b (0.1 IU/ml)	NaF/b (2 mmol)	Gpp (NH)p/b (0.1 mmol)	Forskolin/b (0.1 mmol)
Normal	8	74.5	3.11	6.64	10.26	7.95
Goiter	12	92.3	4.13	6.35	11.60	8.45
Adenoma	8	61.5	7.83	9.97	16.95	8.09
Cancer	5	92.4	3.07	4.71	10.88	7.26

[a] pmol cAMP/4 mg protein per 30 min.

Table 2. Adenylate cyclase activity of the 8000 g particulate fraction of normal and adenomatous human thyroid tissue with increased ("hot") or decreased ("cold") iodine uptake

Type of adenoma	n	Normal			Adenoma		
		Basal[a]	TSH/b (0.1 IU/ml)	NaF/b (10 mmol)	Basal	TSH/b (0.1 IU/ml)	NaF/b (10 mmol)
"Hot"	12	44	2.94	24.04	44	3.77[c]	35.71[c]
"Cold"	10	46	2.60	21.08	42	3.87[b]	21.96

[a] pmol cAMP/mg protein per 30 min.
[b] $p < 0.025$ (Wilcoxon rank test for unpaired samples).
[c] $p < 0.005$ (Wilcoxon rank test for unpaired samples).

TSH not only increased cAMP production in human thyrocytes (data not shown) but also caused increase [3H]thymidine incorporation in primary cell cultures from normal human thyroid tissues ($n = 7$), with maximal effectiveness at 0.1 mIU TSH/ml. EGF also stimulated [3H]-thymidine incorporation in these cells twofold, with maximal effectiveness at a concentration of 0.1 μg/ml (Fig. 1). Higher concentrations of TSH and EGF were less effective in stimulating [3H]thymidine incorporation in primary human thyrocyte cultures (Fig. 1).

Culturing human thyrocytes further, TSH sensitivity decreased, but maximal responsiveness to TSH (50–1000 mIU/ml) increased two to five fold when

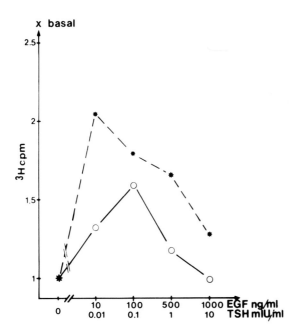

Fig. 1. [3H]Thymidine incorporation of human thyrocytes after incubation with EGF (*dotted line*) or TSH (*solid line*) for 24 h

Table 3. [³H]Thymidine incorporation into normal human thyrocytes after stimulation with dbcAMP or forskolin or dideoxyadenosine (ddA) in serum free medium for 24 h

Substance	n	Dose (mol/l)					
		0	10^{-8}	10^{-7}	10^{-6}	10^{-5}	10^{-4}
dbcAMP	3	$100+21$	$101+23$	$69+14$	$84+6$	$90+7$	$193+64$
Forskolin	3	$100+26$	$100+27$	$101+11$	$101+22$	$144+24$	$192+52$
ddA	8	$100+18$	—	$132+15$	$181+16$	$214+9$	$220+14$

[³H]thymidine incorporation was measured (Fig. 2). AC stimulation by forskolin (10^{-8}–10^{-4} mol/l) and the membranepermissable cAMP analogue dbcAMP (10^{-8}–10^{-4} mol/l) had no effect on [³H]thymidine incorporation in human thyrocytes up to a concentration of 10^{-5} mol/l. High concentrations of forskolin (10^{-4} mol/l) did increase [³H]thymidine incorporation in these cells twofold (Table 3). In contrast to AC stimulator forskolin dideoxyadenosine (ddA; 10^{-8}–10^{-4} mol/l), an inhibitor of AC, increased [³H]thymidine uptake in human thyrocytes up to tenfold (Table 3). TSH (100 mIU/ml) not only increased [³H]thymidine incorporation but also stimulated cell proliferation of human thyrocytes ($p < 0.001$; Fig. 3). The dbcAMP (10^{-4} mol/l) had no effect on thyrocyte proliferation (Fig. 3).

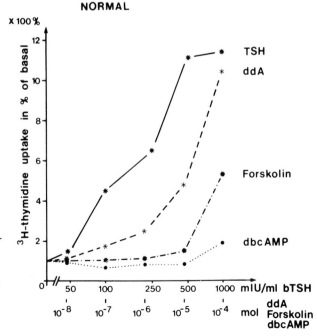

Fig. 2. [³H]Thymidine incorporation in short-term cultures of human thyrocytes after incubation with TSH, dideoxyadenosine (*ddA*), forskolin, or dbcAMP for 24 h

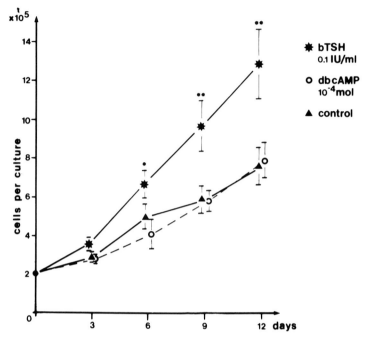

Fig. 3. Effect of TSH (0.1 IU/ml) and cAMP (10^{-4} mol/l) on cell growth of normal human thyrocytes growing in monolayer cultures ($n=9$). Values are means $+/-$ SD; $*p<0.05$; $**p<0.01$ (Wilcoxon rank test for unpaired samples)

Table 4. [^{3}H]Thymidine incorporation into human FTC-133 thyroid cells, rat FRTL-5 thyroid cells and human fibroblasts after incubation with TSH, EGF, IGF in serum free medium for 24 h ($n=4$)

Cells	Substance	Dose			
	TSH(mIU/ml)	0.1	1.0	10	100
FTC-133		$149 + 10$	$145 + 7$	$125 + 30$	$120 + 18$
FRTL-5		$123 + 19$	$154 + 16$	$229 + 67$	$302 + 37$
Fibroblast		——	$115 + 18$	$104 + 6$	$90 + 6$
	EGF(ng/ml)	1.0	10	100	1000
FTC-133		$181 + 19$	$187 + 27$	$185 + 39$	$203 + 37$
FRTL-5		$111 + 10$	$99 + 32$	$138 + 56$	$128 + 38$
Fibroblast		——	$115 + 18$	$105 + 6$	$90 + 6$
	IGF (ng/ml)	1.0	10		
FTC-133		$140 + 23$	$141 + 25$		
FRTL-5		$111 + 29$	$123 + 18$		
Fibroblast		$82 + 20$	$114 + 15$		

The permanent human cell line FTC-133 from a differentiated follicular thyroid cancer was positive in thyroglobulin immunoreactivity (Fig.4). There was no fibroblast contamination detectable in these cell cultures. Immunoreactivity was shown mainly cytoplasm near the nucleus (Fig. 4). The average production of TG was 9 ng per 48 h and 50 000 cells.

FTC-133 cells were also positive for EGF receptor immunoreactivity (Fig. 5). Distribution of EGF receptor, however, was different from thyroglobulin distribution. Major EGF receptor immunoreactivity was detectable at the cell membranes of cell surface and nucleus (Fig. 5).

In human FTC-133 cells TSH (0.1–100 mIU/ml), EGF (10^{-6}–10^{-3} g/l) and IGF (10^{-6}–10^{-5} g/l) stimulated [^{3}H]thymidine incorporation, with maximal effectiveness at 0.1 mIU TSH/ml and 10^{-3} g/l EGF (Table 4). In human fibroblasts TSH, EGF, and IGF had no effect on [^{3}H]thymidine incorporation. In rat FRTL-5 cell cultures TSH (0.1–100 mIU/ml) increased [^{3}H]thymidine incorporation in a dose-dependent manner. IGF had a questionable effect at 10^{-8} g/l

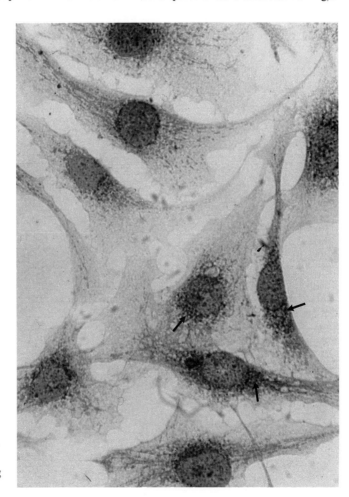

Fig. 4. Immunocyto-chemical staning of human FTC-133 cells, obtained from a differentiated folli-cular thyroid cancer for thyroglobulin. *Arrows* show the in-tracytoplasmatic dis-tribution of thyroglo-bulin in these cells (passage after cloning in passage three)

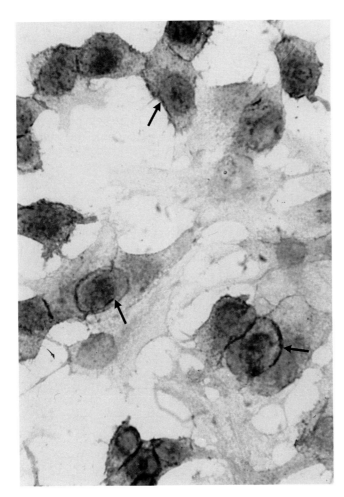

Fig. 5. Immunocytochemical determination of EGF receptors in FTC-133 cells. EGF receptor immunoreactivity is visualized mainly at the cell surface and the nucleus (*arrows*)

Table 5. [³H]Thymidine incorporation into FTC-133 human thyroid cells, primary cell cultures of normal thyrocytes, and short-term cultures of normal thyrocytes after incubation with TSH or TSH + IGF for 24 h

Cells	Dose (mIU/ml)			
	0	0.1	10	1000
FTC-133 (IGF 10ng/ml)	148 + 23	165 + 41	193 + 15	233 + 16
FTC-133	100 + 21	149 + 10	125 + 30	
Primary thyrocytes	100 + 16	163 + 23	98 + 14	
Short-term cultures	100 + 42	104 + 12	163 + 14	407 + 66

(not statistically significant) but was not tested over a wide range of IGF concentrations, EGF lacked any effect on [³H]thymidine incorporation in FRTL-5 cells (Table 4).

Adding IGF (10 ng/ml) and TSH (0.1–1000 ,mIU/ml) simultaneously to FTC-133 cells, TSH demonstrated a dose-dependent increase of [³H]thymidine incorporation. This is comparable to the TSH effect in short-term cultures of normal thyrocytes (Fig. 2). This is in contrast to the bell-shaped curve of [³H]thymidine incorporation in primary cell cultures of normal thyrocytes and in cell cultures of FTC-133 after TSH stimulation and without further addition of other stimulators (Table 5).

Discussion

The presented data indicated a stimulatory effect of TSH and local active growth factors, i.e., EGF and IGF, on DNA synthesis and cell growth in normal and pathological human thyrocytes. This growth effect of TSH in human thyrocytes was dependent neither on incubation of cells with serum nor on contamination of thyrocytes with fibroblasts, nor did it show a direct correlation to TSH-induced AC stimulation.

This stands in contrast to results obtained in bovine, (Eggo et al. 1984), canine (Roger and Dumont 1982), and porcine (Gaertner et al. 1985; Heldin et al. 1987; Heldin and Westermark 1988; Wanabe et al. 1985; Westermark et al. 1983, 1986) thyrocytes but partially parallels the results of other investigators using human thyrocytes (Ollis et al. 1986; Roger et al. 1988; Table 6).

Effect of TSH on cell growth. TSH stimulated DNA synthesis and cell growth in rat (Redmond and Tuffery 1981), sheep (Tamura et al. 1981), and dog (Roger et al. 1984) thyrocytes but lacked any effect on thyrocyte growth in porcine follicles in

Table 6. Present data on growth stimulation of canine, porcine, rat, and human thyrocytes

Authors	Investigated substance					Cell origin
	Iodine	TSH	cAMP	EGF	IGF	
Roger et al. (1982)		↑	↑			Canine
Heldin et al. (1987)	↑	O	↓	↑		Porcine
Gaertner et al. (1985)	↓	O	↓	↑		Porcine
Tramontano et al. (1988)		↑	↑	O	↑	Rat (FRTL-5)
Own experience		↑	O	↑	↑	Human (short-term culture, FTC-133)

culture (Gaertner et al. 1985; Heldin et al. 1987; Heldin and Westermark 1988; Wanabe et al. 1985; Westermark et al. 1983, 1986). Without addition of serum the effect of TSH on cell proliferation in human thyrocytes has been reported controversial (Eggo et al. 1984; Nitsch and Wollman 1980; Goretzki and Clark 1988; Goretzki et al. 1986, 1987 a, b). Recent results by Ollis et al. (1986) and our group (Goretzki and Clark 1988; Goretzki et al. 1986, 1987 a, b) demonstrated an TSH-induced increase of [³H]thymidine incorporation in human thyrocytes in monolayer culture, which has been confirmed by Roger et al. (1988). In all these cell cultures, however, fibroblast contamination was present, questioning the importance of these cells for thyrocyte growth (Wollman and Breitman 1970). The newly established permanent human thyrocyte cell line FTC-133, derived from a follicular thyroid cancer, is free of any fibroblast contamination. Studies with these cells confirmed our results obtained in fresh thyroid monolayer cultures, when [³H]thymidine incorporation was measured. Thus, TSH certainly stimulates [³H]thymidine incorporation in human thyrocytes seeded in serum free medium without fibroblast contamination. Studies by our group (Goretzki et al. 1987b) and by Roger et al. (1988) additionally show TSH-enhanced cell proliferation in human thyrocytes. These studies, however, are of questionable significance concerning the direct effects of growth stimulators on human thyrocytes because contamination with fibroblasts could not be eliminated totally. Fibroblasts accounted for at least 5% of all cells in these primary monolayer cultures (Roger et al. 1988). Further studies using human FTC-133 cells in serum free medium are in process, therefore, to elucidate the effect of TSH and local growth factors on human thyrocyte proliferation.

Importance of AC System. TSH was shown to stimulate AC activity in human thyroid tissues (Abe et al. 1981; Clark et al. 1981, 1983; Goretzki et al. 1987b; Roger et al. 1988, Trokoudes et al. 1981). Most studies additionally revealed an increased TSH response of AC in adenomatous human thyroid tissues (Burke and Szabo 1972; Clark et al. 1981, 1983; Goretzki and Clark 1988). Whether this increased AC response in functionally active as well as in functionally inactive follicular thyroid adenomas (estimated by amount of iodine trapping) may be related to an increase in growth stimulation of these cells remains questionable, however. Thus our studies using membrane-permissable cAMP (dbcAMP), forskolin, and the AC inhibitor ddA failed to show a direct correlation between AC activity and [³H]thymidine incorporation. But even in thyrocytes with elevated [³H]thymidine incorporation by ddA cell proliferation was unaffected (Fig. 6). Our results differ from those of other investigators using canine or rat thyrocyte cultures. (Filetti et al. 1988; Jin et al. 1986; Redmond and Tuffery 1981; Roger et al. 1984; Roger and Dumont 1982; Tramontano and Ingbar 1986; Tramontano et al. 1987, 1988). In these cultures cAMP was shown to stimulate cell proliferation. Some of these differences can be explained by differences in species-specific growth regulation of thyrocytes (Table 6), but even in primary human thyrocytes in monolayer culture Roger et al. (1988) demonstrated a growth stimulatory effect of cAMP. This contrasts not only with our findings but also with the clinical experience in patients with Graves disease. In these patients AC stimulation by

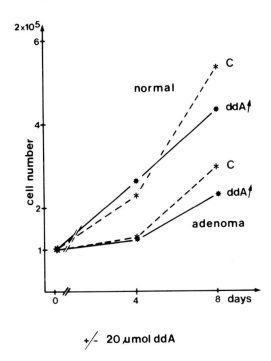

Fig. 6. Cell proliferation of human thyrocytes in dideoxyadenosine (ddA) enriched 2×10^{-5} mol/l medium with 10% FCS

+/- 20 μmol ddA

stimulating immunoglobulins does not always parallel thyroid growth, nor does every patient with hyperthyroidism due to cAMP stimulation develop thyroid gland enlargement (Harada et al. 1987; Wahl et al. 1982). Recently we could additionally demonstrate the independent effect of TSH on [³H]thymidine incorporation and AC stimulation in human thyrocytes from differentiated human thyroid cancers (Goretzki et al. 1986). These findings were confirmed by O.H. Clark (personal communication). TSH-induced cell growth stimulation in human thyrocytes is therefore not sufficiently explained only by the TSH stimulation of thyroidal AC but may be related to a number of other metabolic factors, such as phosphoinositol pathway, proto-oncogene expression, calcium, etc., (Sporn and Roberts 1987; Fig. 7).

Effect of Local Active Growth Factors. Our studies demonstrate the stimulatory effect of EGF and IGF on [³H]thymidine incorporation in human thyrocytes in culture. This is in accord with findings by Westermark et al. (1983, 1986) and Gaertner et al. (1985) who used porcine follicles. It partially confirms results obtained by Tramontano et al. (1987, 1988) on rat FRTL-5 cells, but these cells lack EGF receptors. FTC-133 cells demonstrate the first permanent human thyrocyte cell line, to our knowledge, which retains differentiated thyrocyte function. Thus, these cells can be propagated in serum free medium, demonstrate thryoglobulin immunoreactivity, and additionally show EGF receptor immunoreactivity (Damjanov et al. 1986). EGF- as well as IGF-stimulated [³H]thymidine uptake in these cells also confirms results reported by other investigators who

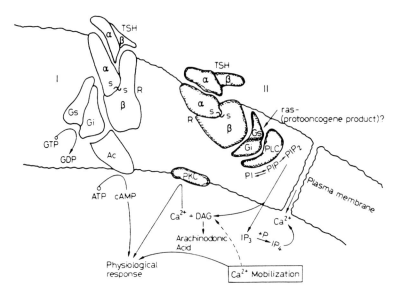

Fig. 7. Thyrocyte stimulation by TSH via a cAMP-dependent or a calcium and phosphoin-ositol mechanism?

could demonstrate EGF receptors in human thyroid tissues (Damjanov et al. 1986).

The effect of IGF on thyrocytes has been studied mainly in FRTL-5 cells, demonstrating a cAMP-independent proliferative effect of IGF on FRT-5 cells (Tramontano et al. 1987, 1988). In human FTC-133 cells IGF increased [^{3}H]thymidine incorporation, but this effect was small ($p > 0.05$; Table 4).

Synergism of TSH and Local Active Growth Factors. TSH has been shown to stimulate thyrocyte growth in different species but failed to increase cell pro-liferation in porcine follicles (Westermark et al. 1986). In these cells, however, TSH increased EGF receptor density probably due to an increase in cAMP levels. EGF secondarily stimulated cell growth in porcine follicles, which therefore can be augmented by TSH prestimulation (Westermark et al. 1986). In rat FRTL-5 cells IGF increased cell proliferation such as did TSH (Tramontano et al. 1988). By combining these substances a more than additive effect can be obtained (Tramon-tano et al. 1988). Comparable results could be demonstrated in human FTC-133 cells (Table 5), elucidating some of the more complex interactions of growth regulation in human thyrocytes and human thyroid cancer. Further studies will have to be performed in FTC-133 cells, however, to clarify some of the interactions between iodine, TSH, and local active growth factors in regulating the pro-liferation of human thyrocytes. Whether iodine decreases thyrocyte proliferation in human thyrocytes comparable to its effect on FRTL-5 cells (Becks et al. 1988) and porcine follicles in culture (Gaertner et al. 1985; Heldin et al. 1985) is also of socioeconomic interest in our iodine-deficient country. Additionally, we will have to investigate whether TSH primes human thyrocytes for other growth stimulators by cAMP or by phosphoinositol-dependent mechanisms (Fig. 7).

Summary

Our studies using thyrocyte membranes from different human thyroid tissues, monolayer cultures of human thyrocytes, and the permanant cell line FTC-133 demonstrate the stimulatory effect of TSH on metabolism, DNA synthesis, and cell growth in human thyrocytes. Up- and down- regulation of cAMP cell content fails to show direct effects on DNA synthesis and cell growth in primary thyrocyte cultures in man. Increased AC responsiveness to TSH in adenomatous human thyroid tissues, when compared to normal thyroids of the same patient ($p < 0.005$), is thus of only questionable importance for thyroid tumor growth.

The permanant cell line FTC-133 was established from differentiated follicular human thyroid cancer cells. FTC-133 cells proved to be of particular usefulness in assessing growth regulation of human thyroid tissue. These cells could be propagated in serum free medium, showed thyroglobulin immunoreactivity and EGF receptors, lacked any fibroblast contamination, and responded to TSH and local active growth factors such as EGF and IGF with a stimulated [³H]thymidine incorporation. The latter could be shown in primary cell cultures of normal and pathological human thyrocytes as well. Additional to the stimulatory effect of TSH and IGF on [³H]thymidine incorporation, these substances show an additive effect when incubated simultaneously.

Locally active growth factors and endocrine growth stimulation by TSH therefore act synergistically on thyrocyte growth in human thyrocyte cultures. Whether the TSH effect on cell growth is related to its stimulation of AC remains as yet questionable.

References

Abe Y, Ichikawa Y, Muraki T, Ito M, Homma T (1981) Thyrotropin (TSH) receptor and adenylate-cyclase activity in human thyroid tumors: absence of high affinity receptors and loss of TSH responsiveness in undifferentiated thyroid carcinoma. J Clin Endocrinol Metab 52: 23–28.

Becks GP, Eggo MC, Burrow GN (1988) Organic iodine inhibits deoxyribonucleic acid synthesis and growth in FRTL-5 thyroid cells. Endocrinology 123: 545–551

Burke G, Szabo M (1972) Dissociation of in vivo and in vitro autonomy in hyperfunctioning thyroid nodules. J Clin Endocrinol Metab 35: 199–202

Clark OH, Gerend PL, Core TC, Nissenson RA (1981) Thyrotropin binding and adenylate-cyclase stimulation in thyroid neoplasms. Surgery 90: 252–261

Clark OH, Gerend PL, Davis M, Goretzki PE, Nissenson RA (1983) Characterization of the thyrotropin receptor–adenylate cyclase system in neoplastic human thyroid tissue. J Clin Endocrinol Metab 57: 140–147

Damjanov I, Mildner B, Knowles BB (1986) Immunohistochemical localization of the epidermal growth factor receptor in normal human tissues. Lab Invest 55: 588–592

Eggo MC, Bachrach LK, Fayet G (1984) The effect of growth factors and serum on DNA synthesis and differentiation in thyroid cells in culture. Mol Cell Endocrinol 38: 141–150

Filetti S, Belfiore A, Amir SM, Daniels GH, Ippolito O, Vigneri R, Ingbar SH (1988) The role of thyroid-stimulating antibodies of Graves disease in differentiated thyroid cancer. N Engl J Med 318: 753–759

Gaertner R, Greil W, Demharter R, Horn K (1985) Bovine thyrotropin inhibits DNA synthesis inversely with stimulation of cyclic AMP production in cultured thyroid follicles. Moll Cell Endocrinol 42: 145–55

Goretzki PE, Wjst M, Koob R, Koller C, Simon R, Branscheid D. Clark OH, Roeher HD (1986) The effect of thyrotropin (TSH) and cAMP on DNA synthesis and cell growth of human thyrocytes in monolayer culture. Surgery 100: 1053–1061

Goretzki PE, Clark OH (1988) Thyroid stimulating hormone receptor studies. Prog Surg 19: 181–204

Goretzki PE, West M, Koob R, Koller C, Joseph K, Roeher HD (1987a) Adenylate cyclase stimulation and ^{3}H-thymidine incorporation in human thyroid tissues and thyrocyte cultures: the effect of IgG preparation from patients with different thyroid disorders. Acta Endocrinol [Suppl] (Copenh) 281: 281–287

Goretzki PE, Koob R, Koller C, Roeher HD (1987b) Thyrotropin (TSH) stimulates cell growth and DNA synthesis in monolayer cultures of human thyrocytes independent of the adenylatecyclase system. Acta Endocrinol [Suppl] (Copenh) 281: 273–280

Harada T, Shimaoka K, Mimura T, Ito K (1987) Current treatment Graves disease. Surg Clin North Am 67: 299–314

Heldin NE, Westermark B (1988) Epidermal growth factor, but not thyrotropin stimulates the expression of c-*fos* and n-*myc* messenger ribonucleic acid in porcine thyroid follicle cells in primary culture. Endocrinology 122: 1042–1046

Heldin NE, Karlsson FA, Westermark B (1987) A growth stimulatory effect of iodide is suggested by its effects on n-*myc* messenger ribonucleic acid levels, ^{3}H-thymidine incorporation and mitotic activity of porcine thyroid follicles in suspension culture. Endocrinology 121:757–764

Jin S, Hornicek FJ, Neylan D, Zakarija M, Mckenzie JM (1986) Evidence that adenosine 3′ 5′-monophosphate mediates stimulation of thyroid growth in FRTL-5 cells. Endocrinology 119: 802–810

Lowry OH, Rosebrough NJ, Farr AL, Randall RJ (1951) Protein measurement' with the Folin Phenol reagent. J Biol Chem 193: 265–269

Mothersill C, Seymour C, Malone JF (1984) Maintenance of differentiated sheep thyroid cells in primary culture for three months. Acta Endocrinol (Copenh) 107: 54–59

Nitsch L, Wollman SH (1980) Thyrotropin preparations are mitogenic for thyroid epithelial cells in follicles in suspension culture. Proc Natl Acad Sci USA 77: 2743–2747

Ollis CA, Davies R, Munro DS, Tomlinson S (1986) Relationship between growth and function of human thyroid cells in culture. J Endocrinol 108: 393–398

Redmond O, Tuffery AR (1981) Mitotic rate of rat thyroid follicular cells in vivo in response to a single injection of thyrotropin (TSH). Cell Tissue Kinet 14: 625–631

Roger PP, Dumont JE (1982) Thyrotropin and the differential expression of proliferation and differentiation in dog thyroid cells in primary culture. J Endocrinol 96: 241–249

Roger PP, Dumont JE, Boeynaems JM (1984) Lack of prostaglandin involvement in the mitogenic effect of TSH on canine cells in primary culture. FEBS Lett 166: 136–40

Roger P, Taton M, van Sande J, Dumont JE (1988) Mitogenic effect of thyrotropin and adenosine 3′ 5′-monophosphate in differentiated normal human thyroid cells in vitro. J Clin Endocrinol Metab 66: 1158–1165

Sporn MB, Roberts AB (1987) Peptide growth factors: current status and therapeutic opportunities. In: DeVita ST, Hellman S, Rosenberg SA (eds) Important advances in oncology 1987. Lippincott, Philadelphia, pp 75–86

Tamura K, Shimaoka K, Tsukada Y, Razack FA, Ericson LE (1981) Suppressive therapy for radiation-associated nodular thyroid disease. Jpn J Clin Oncol 11: 457–462

Tramontano D, Ingbar SH (1986) Properties and regulation of the thyrotropin receptor in the FRTL-5 rat thyroid cell line. Endocrinology 118: 1945–1951

Tramontano D, Moses AC, Picone R, Ingbar SH (1987) Characterization and regulation of the receptor for insulinlike growth factor-I in the FRTL-5 rat thyroid follicular cell line. Endocrinology 120: 785–790

Tramontano D, Moses Ac,Veneziani BM, Ingbar SH (1988) Adenosine 3',5'-monophosphate mediates both the mitogenic effect of thyrotropin and its ability to amplify the response to insulin-like growth factor I in FRTL-5 cells. Endocrinology 122: 127–132

Trokoudes KM, Michelsen H, Kidd A, Row VV, Volpe R (1981) Properties of human thyroidal and extrathyroidal TSH receptors. Acta Endocrinol (Copenh) 97: 473–479

Wahl RA, Goretzki P, Meybier H, Nitschke J, Linder MM, Roeher HD (1982) Coexistence of hyperthyroidism and thyroid cancer. World J Surg 6: 385–390

Wanabe Y, Amino N, Tamaki H, Iwatani Y, Miyai K (1985) Bovine thyrotropin inhibits DNA synthesis inversely with stimulation of cyclic AMP production in cultured porcine thyroid follicles. Endocrinol Jpn 32: 81–87

Westermark K, Westermark B, Karlsson FA, Ericson LE (1986) Location of epidermal growth factor receptors on porcine thyroid follicle cells and receptor regulation by thyrotropin. Endocrinology 118: 1040–1046

Westermark K, Karlsson FA, Westermark B (1983) Epidermal growth factor modulates thyroid growth and function in culture. Endocrinology 112: 71–79

Wollman SH, Breitman TR (1970) Changes in DNA and weight of thyroid glands hyperplasia and involution. Endocrinology 86: 322–327

Endocrine Aspects of Medullary Thyroid Carcinoma

F. Raue

Abteilung für Innere Medizin I, Endokrinologie und Stoffwechsel,
Medizinische Universitätsklinik, Bergheimer Straße 58, 6900 Heidelberg, FRG

Introduction

Medullary thyroid carcinoma (MTC) is a neoplasm of the calcitonin-secreting parafollicular, or C cells, of the thyroid gland; it comprises 5%–10% of all cases of thyroid cancer. In contrast to the follicular cells of the thyroid gland that metabolize iodine and produce the classical thyroid homones T_3 and T_4, the C cells produce and secrete calcitonin (CT) and related peptides. During embryogenesis the C cells migrate from the neural crest to the last branchial pouch and ultimately to the thyroid. The neural crest origin of the C cells is one explanation for the production of a wide variety of bioactive substances similar to other neuro-endocrine cells, but also for the association of MTC with other tumors of neural crest origin. Another important clinical feature of MTC is its familial occurrence with an autosomal dominant pattern, its multifocal development of C cell hyperplasia prior to malignant transformation, and its association with other endocrine tumors (e.g., bilateral pheochromocytoma).

Production of Bioactive Substances by MTC

MTC is characterized by the production of an abnormally high amount of CT, which is released into the peripheral blood (Raue et al. 1983). Although this CT is biologically active in other test systems, no definite long-term effect of chronic CT excess is observed in patients with MTC. Besides CT numerous other bioactive substances may be produced and secreted by MTC (Table 1). Katacalcin, the C-terminal flanking peptide of the CT precursor, is always cosecreted in equimolar quantities to CT. As a tumor marker katacalcin is likely to be as useful as CT in MTC. The presence of elevated CEA levels is generally associated with progression or recurrence of the disease. Although CEA measurement may serve as a useful prognostic indicator in follow-up of the disease, CEA determination lacks specificity for MTC. In rare cases of MTC ectopically produced ACTH leads to Cushing's syndrome. Immunohistochemical techniques have been used to demon-

Table 1. Bioactive substances produced or secreted by medullary thyroid carcinoma

Hormones
  Calcitonin
  Katacalcin
  Calcitonin gene related peptide
  β-Endorphin
  β-Melanocyte-stimulating hormone
  Substance P
  Somatostatin
  Neurotensin
  Prostaglandin
  Adrenocorticotropic hormone
  Serotonin
Enzymes
  Neuron-specific enolase
  Histaminase
  Dopadecarboxylase
Factors
  Carcinoembryonic antigen
  Nerve growth factor
  Synaptophysin

strate several additional markers in MTC tissue, including neuron-specific enolase and synaptophysin (Grauer et al. 1987; Wiedenmann et al. 1987).

Calcitonin as a Tumor Marker

In most patients with MTC, basal concentration of CT is sufficiently elevated to be diagnostic of tumor presence. There is a positive correlation between the tumor mass and the level of the tumor markers CT, katacalcin, and CEA (Raue et al. 1983, 1987); CT levels above 10 ng/ml and CEA levels above 100 ng/ml are found mostly in patients with distant metastases. Compared to other secretory products CT is of superior specificity for diagnosis of MTC; however, other diseases may also be accompanied by elevated levels of serum CT, i.e., renal failure (decreased renal clearance of CT) and other neoplasms (ectopic production by oat cell carcinoma of the lung). The frequency of hypercalcitoninemia in these conditions depends on the regional specificities of the CT antibodies used. Furthermore, none of the patients with lung cancer exhibits an exaggerated increase of serum CT in response to provocative testing (Samaan et al. 1980).

The sensitivity and diagnostic significance of CT determination is superior to the sensitivity of the other bioactive substances secreted by MTC. Patients with occult C-cell carcinoma may have normal or only slightly elevated CT levels. To identify these patients, provocation tests for CT secretion have been developed. These are highly specific and can differentiate between healthy persons and patients with C-cell hyperplasia or occult MTC. Pentagastrin (0.5 µg/kg body weight injected i.v. over 15 s) is a widely used provocative agent for CT secretion in patients with MTC (Sizemore and Go 1975). Within 2–5 min a prompt increase in serum CT is observed, even in patients who formerly had a normal basal CT level. The test often leads to unpleasant sensations, commonly described as burning or flushing. An alternative is the calcium infusion test (3 mg/kg body weight over 10 min i.v.), which produces an abnormal increase in serum CT in MTC patients within 10–20 min. This test is relatively well tolerated. Most C-cell tumors respond to either agent, and there are only rarely false-negative results. Both procedures should be carried out before the possibility of MTC is excluded. In addition, determination of katacalcin can be used as an independent marker (Raue et al. 1987). Monitoring of serum CT is an effective method for evaluating therapy in patients with MTC. Serum CT levels generally fall within days during the immediate postoperative period, whereas CEA declines only over weeks. Postoperative determination of CT is valuable to assess the radicality of surgery. Elevated basal and/or pentagastrin -stimulated CT levels are considered to indicate residual tumor and/or metastatic disease, even though this may not be demonstratable by other means. Localizing investigations may then be indicated. In the absence of inoperable metastases in the liver, bone, or lung, selective venous catheterization is used in order to localize tumor deposits by means of CT determination in the various venous blood samples. Further surgical efforts may then be directed to the appropriate area in the neck or mediastinum. Selective venous catheterization is comparable to other methods such as ultrasound, computerized tomography, and fine-needle biopsy (Table 2) with respect to diagnostic value.

Rapidly rising serum CT and CEA levels within months reflect serious and spreading disease. In disseminated progressive disease cytotoxic chemotherapy must be considered. The beneficial effect of adriamycin alone or in combination with *cis*-platinum has been confirmed. Measurement of the tumor markers CT and CEA seems to be useful in the assessment of chemotherapy (Raue et al. 1985); remission or progression can be confirmed by decrease or increase in serum levels of the tumor markers. CT serum levels seem to be a prognostic factor for MTC. Patients with normal CT levels after total thyroidectomy seem to be cured of MTC – the 5-year survival rate is 100% (Table 3) – while all patients who die from MTC show marked increases in CT and CEA levels prior to death.

Table 2. Comparison of different localization methods for local regional recurrences in MTC

Methods	% of positive findings[a]
Palpation	60
Ultrasound	79
Computerized tomography	72
Selective venous catherization	62

[a] Histologically confirmed recurrences in 48 reinterventions.

Table 3. Calcitonin levels in the follow-up and outcome of patients with MTC

Calcitonin (ng/ml)	Number of Patients	
	Alive	Dead
Normal (< 0.1–0.3)	15	0
Elevated (> 0.3)	32	12

Diagnosis of MTC

In the majority of patients with MTC the presenting symptoms and clinical findings are nonspecific and do not differ from those of other thyroid tumors (Saad et al. 1984). The diagnosis is often made by histopathological examination of surgically removed thyroid tissue. Thyroid enlargement (31%), thyroid nodule (30%), and cervical lymph nodes (15%) are the main clinical presentations of the disease in our series of 61 patients with MTC. In 5% watery diarrhea is the prominent feature. This diarrhea is humorally mediated and, as it is related to tumor mass, it often reflects metastatic disease. Prostaglandins or CT gene related peptide may be the possible humoral mediators.

During preoperative investigations the tumor was palpable in 73% of cases; it showed a cold nodule in the thyroid scintigram in 87% and a hypoechogenic area at ultrasound in 92% of cases; on further physical examination the cervical lymph nodes were involved in 38% and watery diarrhea was diagnosed in 18%. At the time of diagnosis our youngest patient was 9 years of age, the oldest 75 years, the average age being 44 years. The peak incidence was in the fifth decade. The male to female ratio was 1:1.26.

Familial Medullary Thyroid Carcinoma

The familial form of MTC may occur in association with multiple endocrine neoplasia (MEN) IIa (MTC, pheochromocytoma, primary hyperparathyroidism), MEN IIb (MTC, pheochromocytoma, multiple mucosal neuromas), and without accompaning endocrinopathies. The early diagnosis of familial MTC depends solely on the use of biochemical parameters to detect the tumor before any clinical signs have evolved (Gagel et al. 1988). In patients with very early tumor and absence of any clinical signs, the basal CT level may be normal; after a CT stimulation test with pentagastrin or calcium, however, a pathological increase is observed, and the presence of tumor can be detected. All patients genetically at risk for familial MTC, starting at about the age of 5, are followed up in our clinic by repeating provocative tests annually. In the literature, even younger patients have

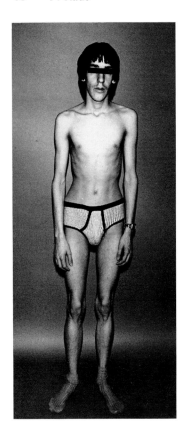

Fig. 1. Appearance of a patient with multiple endocrine neoplasia type IIb showing marfanoid habitus, thickening of the lips (neuromata), and elongated face

been reported. In addition, blood tests are carried out to screen for the presence of hyperparathyroidism and pheochromocytoma. Whenever a pheochromocytoma is suspected, it should be removed prior to surgery for the thyroid tumor. The MEN IIb syndrome is characterized by a typical phenotype, i.e., a marfanoid habitus with long, thin extremities, poor muscle development, a characteristic facies with bumpy lips caused by neuromas which can involve the tongue, eyelids, conjunctiva, and cornea. These are important clinical signs since children with familial MTC may be suspected of having MEN IIb by evaluating of their characteristic phenotype (Fig. 1; Frank et al. 1984).

The specific genetic defect in MEN is localized to chromosome 10. Hence it is likely that diagnosis in the neonate will be possible within the next few years when the specific nucleic acid abnormality in MEN is determined and a specific genetic marker becomes available (Mathew et al. 1987).

Acknowledgements. We wish to thank Mrs. M.C. Jockers-Scherübl, M.D., for helpful suggestions and Mrs. D. Skalecki for her help in the preparation of this manuscript.

References

Frank K, Raue F, Gottwinter J, Heinrich U, Meybier H, Ziegler R (1984) The importance of early diagnosis and follow up in sproadic MEN IIb. Eur J Pediatr 143: 112

Gagel RF, Tashijian AH, Cummings T, Papathanasopoulos N, Kaplan MM, DeLellis RA, Wolfe HJ, Reichlin S (1988) The clinical outcome of prospective screening for multiple endocrine neoplasia type 2a. N Engl J Med 318: 478

Grauer A, Raue F, Rix E, Tschahargane C, Ziegler R (1987) Neuron-specific enolase in medullary thyroid carcinoma: immunohistochemical demonstration, but no significance as serum tumor marker. J Cancer Res Clin Oncol 113: 599

Mathew GGP, Chin KS, Easton DF, Thorpe K, Carter C, Liou CI, Fong SL, Bridges CD, Haak H, Kruseman HC, Schifter S, Hansen HH, Telenius H, Telenius-Berg M, Ponder BAJ (1987) A linked genetic marker for multiple endocrine neoplasia type 2a on chromosome 10. Nature 328: 527

Raue F, Schmidt-Gayk H, Ziegler R (1983) Tumormarker beim C–Zell–Carcinom (medulläres Schilddrüsencarcinom). Dtsch Med Wochenschr 108: 283

Raue F, Minne H, Ziegler R (1985) Cisplatin, Adriamycin und Vindesin. Eine Kombinations-Chemotherapie beim differenzierten Schilddrüsencarcinom. Tumor Diag Ther 6: 134

Raue F, Boden M, Girigs S, Rix E, Ziegler R (1987) Katacalcin, ein neuer Tumormarker beim C–Zell–Carcinom der Schilddrüse. Klin Wochenschr 65: 82

Saad MF, Ordonez NG, Rashid RK, Guido JJ, Hill CS, Hickey RC, Saaman NA (1984) Medullary carcinoma of the thyroid, a study of the clinical features and prognostic factors in 161 patients. Medicine 63: 319

Samaan NA, Castillo S, Schultz PN, Khalil KG, Johnston DA (1980) Serum calcitonin after pentagastrin stimulation in patients with bronchogenic and breast cancer compared to that in patients with medullary thyroid carcinoma. J Clin Endocrinol Metab 51: 237

Sizemore GW, Go VLW (1975) Stimulation tests of diagnosis of medullary thyroid carcinoma. Mayo Clin Proc 50: 53

Wiedenmann B, Kuhn C, Schwechheimer K, Waldherr R, Raue R, Brandeis WE, Kommerell B, Franke WW (1987) Synaptophysin identified in metastases of neuroendocrine tumors by immunocytochemistry and immunoblotting. Am J Clin Pathol 88: 560

Multiple Endocrine Neoplasia Type II

S.A. Wells, Jr.

Department of Surgery, Washington University School of Medicine,
4960 Audubon Avenue, St. Louis, MO 63110, USA

Introduction

There are two general categories of multiple endocrine neoplasia (MEN) syndromes, types I and II; type II is further subdivided into subtypes a and b. MEN I (Wermer's syndrome) was described in 1954 (Wermer 1963) and is characterized by the concurrence of neoplasia of the parathyroid glands, pituitary gland, and pancreatic islet cells. Less commonly, adenomas of the adrenal cortex or the thyroid gland occur. Most often, the parathyroid glands are involved, and affected patients have hypercalcemia, although many are asymptomatic. Clinical syndromes or biochemical abnormalities associated with pituitary or pancreatic islet cell neoplasia occur much less commonly. Majewski and Wilson (1979) in a recent autopsy study noted evidence of pathologic changes in the pituitary gland, pancreatic islet cells, and parathyroid glands in virtually 100% of patients affected with MEN I even though many of the patients had no clinical or laboratory evidence of disease prior to death.

MEN IIa (Steiner et al. 1968) is characterized by medullary thyroid carcinoma (MTC), pheochromocytomas, and parathyroid hyperplasia. Patients with MEN IIb (Chong et al. 1975) have MTC and pheochromocytomas, but they do not have parathyroid hyperplasia. Additionally, these patients have multiple mucosal neuromas, ganglioneuromatosis, and a characteristic phenotypic appearance.

Both MEN I and MEN II are inherited as autosomal dominant traits, and genetically the diseases have complete penetrance but variable expressivity. Virtually all patients with MEN I develop hyperparathyroidism, however fewer than 50% have pituitary adenomas or pancreatic islet cell lesions. All patients with MEN IIa develop MTC, however approximately 50% develop pheochromocytomas, and approximately 50% develop hyperparathyroidism. Among patients with MEN IIa 25% develop clinical manifestations of all components of the disease. MTC is also uniformly present in patients with MEN IIb, as are the characteristic phenotypic appearance, mucosal neuromas, and ganglioneuromatosis. Approximately 60% of patients with MEN IIb develop pheochromocytomas.

Recent Results in Cancer Research. Vol. 118
© Springer-Verlag Berlin·Heidelberg 1990

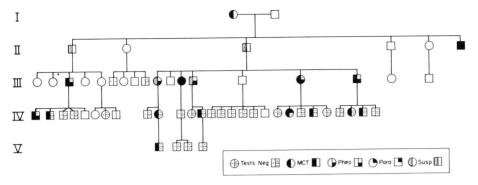

Fig. 1. Pedigree of a kindred with MEN IIa. (From Cance and Wells 1985)

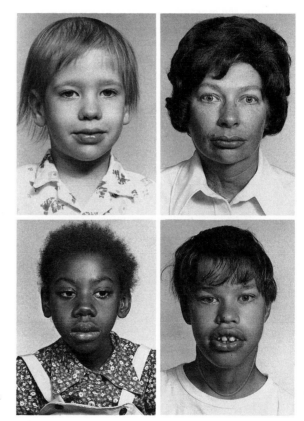

Fig. 2. Characteristic facial appearance of four patients with MEN IIb. (From Norton et al. 1979)

MEN IIa is much more common than MEN IIb. The disease has been described worldwide, and the clinical presentation is generally the same regardless of race. A typical pedigree from kindred with MEN IIa is shown in Fig. 1. The characteristic physical appearance of patients with MEN IIb is shown in Fig. 2.

Diagnosis

Shortly after MTC was discovered in 1959 (Hazard et al. 1959) Copp and associates (1962) discovered the polypeptide hormone calcitonin (CT). These investigators originally thought that the hormone arose from the parathyroid glands, but it was subsequently learned that it was secreted by the C cells of the thyroid gland. It is now known that MTC arises from the C cells, and that CT serves as a tumor marker for this neoplasm (Tashjian and Melvin 1968). Tashjian and associates (1970) demonstrated that intravenously administered calcium is a potent CT secretagogue. It has subsequently been shown by our group and others (Cooper et al. 1971; Rude and Singer 1977; Wells et al. 1978) that the rapid intravenous administration of pentagastrin (0.5 μg/kg in 5 s) or calcium gluconate (2 mg/kg in 1 min) or both stimulated higher peak calcitonin levels than a long calcium infusion (Fig. 3). The combined infusion of calcium and pentagastrin represents the most effective screening test for MTC since higher peak CT levels are achieved with a combined infusion than following the administration of either agent alone. Furthermore, some patients appear to respond to one of the two secretagogues but not the other (Fig. 4).

The importance of these provocative tests in screening kindred at risk for the development of MTC cannot be overemphasized since abnormal stimulated plasma CT levels are often the first indication of disease, and many patients are detected biochemically before clinical disease is evident. Generally, peak plasma

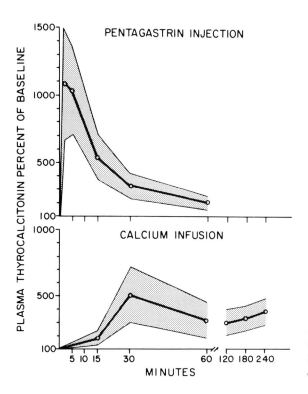

Fig. 3. Combined responses of seven patients with elevated baseline levels of plasma CT to pentagastrin injection and calcium infusion. Each patient underwent both tests on separate days. *Open circles and solid lines* indicate mean responses; *shaded areas* indicate SE range. (From Hennessey et al. 1974)

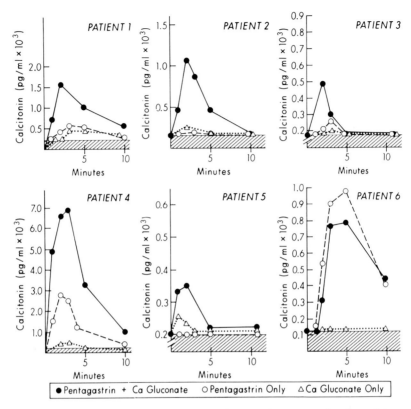

Fig. 4. Variable responses of plasma calcitonin to infusion of pentagastrin plus calcium gluconate, pentagastrin alone, and calcium gluconate alone in six patients with MTC. (From Wells et al. 1978)

CT levels in normal subjects are below 300 pg/ml. Individuals having levels in excess of 1000 pg/ml may be presumed to have MTC until proven otherwise. If such persons are kindred at risk for MTC, they should be subjected to thyroidectomy. Persons with intermediate plasma CT levels of 300–1000 pg/ml should be followed carefully and either tested again in 3–6 months, or they should have selective inferior thyroid vein (ITV) catheterization by way of a transfemoral approach and sampling during provocative testing with calcium and pentagastrin. Strikingly higher CT levels (usually five- to ten fold) are detected in ITV plasma compared to peripheral blood levels, whereas in normal subjects peripheral and central plasma CT levels are similar following provocative testing (Wells et al. 1982a).

Persons with either MEN IIa or MEN IIb who are diagnosed as having MTC should also be evaluated for the presence of hyperparathyroidism and pheochromocytomas. Hyperparathyroidism can be diagnosed by the presence of an elevated serum calcium concentration, usually associated with an increased serum parathyroid hormone level. The presence of a pheochromocytoma can be detected by identifying increased urinary excretion rates of catecholamines and metabolites. If a pheochromocytoma is present, this disease should be treated prior to thyroidectomy and/or parathyroidectomy.

Treatment

Medullary Thyroid Carcinoma. The treatment of MTC is total thyroidectomy. In patients with familial MTC the tumor is bilateral and affects both thyroid lobes (Fig. 5a). The tumors are usually located in the upper portion of the thyroid poles, and they are also frequently multicentric (Fig. 5b). It is also important to perform a modified neck dissection of lymph nodes in the central zone of the neck ranging from the thyroid notch superiorly to the sternal notch inferiorly and to the great vessels laterally. A standard radical neck dissection may be indicated in patients with extensive lateral neck disease.

Hyperparathyroidism. When parathyroid disease is present in patients with MEN IIa, it usually presents as a pseudonodular hyperplasia and affects all four glands. It has been our custom in such patients to perform a total parathyroidectomy with autotransplantation of tissue to the forearm muscle. If graft-dependent hypercalcemia develops, subsequently a portion of the transplanted parathyroid can be removed under local anesthesia.

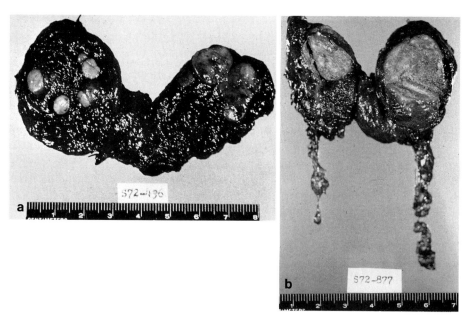

Fig. 5 a, b. Primary medullary thyroid carcinoma in total thyroidectomy specimens. The tumors exhibit a solid growth pattern, are multicentric, and are situated in the upper poles. (From Keiser et al. 1973)

Pheochromocytomas. After the diagnosis of pheochromocytoma has been determined biochemically, a computed tomographic scan of the abdomen is performed. Approximately 50%–75% of patients with MEN IIa or MEN IIb have bilateral pheochromocytomas (Fig. 6). Prior to exploring these patients transabdominally α-blockade is indicated, usually with the drug phenoxybenzamine. Such preparation takes 1–2 weeks, and patients should be essentially asymptomatic and normotensive with volume repletion prior to operation. β-Blockade is indicated only in patients who develop tachycardia with or without arrhythmias. There is some controversy regarding the management of pheochromocytomas in patients with MEN IIa or MEN IIb.

It is generally agreed that if both adrenal glands contain large pheochromocytomas, they should be removed. In patients, however, who have unilateral pheochromocytomas with a grossly normal-appearing contralateral gland, some investigators have elected to remove this gland also since adrenal medullary hyperplasia is usually present. Others, however, have felt that the adrenal gland should be left intact and the patient carefully followed. This conservative course is recommended because patients do not require glucocorticoid or mineralocorticoid replacement therapy, and they are not at risk for being addisonian and suffering increased morbidity or mortality if they sustain severe trauma, illness, or injury. Obviously, if the normally appearing adrenal gland is left intact, patients must be serially evaluated for the subsequent development of a pheochromocytoma.

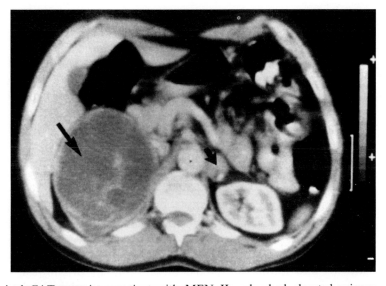

Fig. 6. Abdominal CAT scan in a patient with MEN IIa who had elevated urinary catecholamines. This scan (with contrast) demonstrates a large right adrenal pheochromocytoma (*large arrow*) and a smaller left adrenal pheochromocytoma (*small arrow*). (From Cance and Wells 1985)

Pathology

Medullary Thyroid Carcinoma. On gross section the tumors appear to be white or pale tan in color. Histologically, the neoplasms are composed of spindle cells and are highly vascular. There is a histologic finding associated with early MTC which is termed C-cell hyperplasia (CCH). This is a well-defined pathologic state which is considered a premalignant form of MTC. CCH is often associated with modest increases in calcitonin following provocative testing. Most patients with CCH have disease confined to the thyroid gland, and there is rarely involvement of regional lymph nodes. It is obviously important to diagnose MTC or CCH as early as possible since most patients who have only biochemical evidence of disease are cured by thyroidectomy. On special staining with Congo red or thioflavine T, the presence of amyloidlike material is evident in MTC. The material appears to be a prohormone of CT and is not a light-chain immunoglobulin as typical for amyloids.

Mucosal Neuromas and Ganglioneuromatosis. Patients with MEN IIb have neuromas present on the mucous membranes of the lips, mouth, and nasopharynx. They also have ganglioneuromatosis of the gastrointestinal tract. The ganglioneuromatosis appears to be associated with gastrointestinal disorders during early life since many children who present with this disease have constipation and bowel malfunction often leading to the erroneous diagnosis of (and their occasional treatment for) Hirschsprung's disease.

Prognosis

Patients with MEN IIa have a much better prognosis than do those with MEN IIb. This is due to the biologic character of the MTC, which grows much more rapidly and metastisizes earlier in patients with MEN IIb than in those with MEN IIa. Of our nine patients with MEN IIb none has been cured by thyroidectomy, even though some have been treated as early as age 3–4 years.

   The prognosis is relatively good in patients with MEN IIa especially if they are diagnosed early by biochemical testing while the disease is clinically occult. We evaluated a large number of patients with MEN IIa and determined evidence of lymph node metastases, residual MTC (as indicated by increased concentrations of plasma CT following stimulation in the postoperative period), distant metastases, and death. As can be seen in Table 1, there is an excellent correlation between the preoperative CT value and prognosis. Generally, patients presenting with stimulated CT levels lower than 1000 pg/ml rarely have evidence of lymph node metastases or residual MTC, and none of these patients developed distant metastases or died during the period of observation. In contrast, patients whose presenting CT levels were greater than 10 000 pg/ml had relatively advanced disease, and most had evidence of regional and distant metastases at the time of thyroidectomy. As one might expect, the prognosis is better in patients who are diagnosed biochemically compared to those who are diagnosed by clinical evaluation.

Table 1. Prognostic significance of preoperative stimulated plasma calcitonin (CT) levels. (From Wells et al. 1982b)

Group	Preoperative CT (pg/ml)	Regional lymph node meta-stases (%)	Postoperative CT (>300 pg/ml) (%)	Distant metastases (%)	Death (%)
1 ($n = 25$)	250–1000	1 (4)	1 (4)	0	0
2 ($n = 36$)	1000–5000	3 (8.3)	6 (16.7)	0	0
3 ($n = 8$)	5000–10 000	2 (25)	1 (12.5)	0	0
4 ($n = 23$)	> 10 000	13 (57)	14 (61)	4 (17)	2 (8.7)

Group 1 and group 2 versus group 4, $p < 0.001$.

The importance of biochemical testing and the early diagnosis and treatment of patients at risk for familial MTC can be appreciated when the alternative therapies for this disease are considered. MTC is relatively resistant to chemotherapeutic agents and even though we have employed a large number of chemotherapeutic regimens in patients with metastatic MTC, fewer than 10% of our patients have responded, and each of these responded only to the drug doxorubicin hydrochloride. Since these tumors do not arise from the thyroid follicles, they are not sensitive to radioactive iodine. Similarly, the tumor is relatively insensitive to external beam radiotherapy. At present the employment of biologic response modifiers or immunotherapeutic regimens have not been developed for MTC, and surgery is the only effective therapy.

Discussion

Even though MTC was described less than 30 years ago, the disease has attracted the interest of basic investigators and clinicians alike. Because it presents in the fascinating clinical syndromes of MEN IIa and MEN IIb, it is currently of great interest to geneticists who are using molecular biologic techniques to define the deranged gene which causes the disease. In all likelihood familial MTC will be diagnosed in the near future by DNA analysis rather than by biochemical testing. Nevertheless, clinicians who follow kindreds of patients with MEN IIa or MEN IIb must assume the responsibility not only for evaluating patients for the full expression of the disease but for evaluating the relatives of affected kindred as well.

References

Cance WG, Wells SA (1985) Multiple endocrine neoplasia type IIa. Curr Probl Surg 22: 1
Chong GC, Beahrs OH, Sizemore GW, Woolner LH (1975) Medullary carcinoma of the thyroid gland. Cancer 35: 695
Cooper CW, Schwesinger WH, Mahgoub AM, Ontjes DA (1971) Thyrocalcitonin: stimulation of secretion by pentagastrin. Science 172: 1238
Copp DH, Cameron EC, Cheney BA et al. (1962) Evidence for calcitonin – a new hormone from the parathyroid that lowers blood calcium. Endocrinology 70: 638
Hazard JB, Hawk WH, Crile G (1959) Medullary (solid) carcinoma of the thyroid: a clinico-pathologic entity. J Clin Endocrinol Metab 19: 152
Hennessey JF, Wells SA, Ontjes DA et al. (1974) A comparision of pentagastrin injection and calcium infusion as provocative agents for the detection of medullary carcinoma of the thyroid. J Clin Endocrinol Metab 39: 487
Keiser HR, Beaven MA, Doppman J et al. (1973) Medullary thyroid carcinoma, pheochromocytoma, and parathyroid disease. Ann Intern Med 78: 561
Majewski JT, Wilson SD (1979) The MEA syndrome: an all or none phenomenon? Surgery 86: 475
Norton JA et al. (1979) Multiple endocrine neoplasia type IIb: the most aggressive form of medullary thyroid carcinoma. Surg Clin North Am 59: 109
Rude RK, Singer FR (1977) Comparison of serum calcitonin levels after a 1-minute calcium injection and after pentagastin injection in the diagnosis of medullary thyroid carcinoma. J Clin Endocrinol Metab 44: 980
Steiner AL, Goodman AD, Powers SR (1968) Study of a kindred with pheochromocytoma, medullary thyroid carcinoma, hyperparathyroidism and Cushing's disease: multiple endocrine neoplasia, type 2. Medicine 47: 371
Tashjian AH, Howland BG, Melvin KEW, Hill CS (1970) Immunoassay of human calcitonin. Clinical management, relation to serum calcium in studies in patients with medullary carcinoma. N Engl J Med 283: 890
Tashjian AH, Melvin KEW (1968) Medullary carcinoma of the thyroid gland: studies of thyrocalcitonin in plasma and tumor extracts. N Engl J Med 279: 279
Wells SA, Baylin SB, Linehan WM et al. (1978) Provocative agents and the diagnosis of medullary carcinoma of the thyroid gland. Ann Surg 188: 139
Wells SA, Baylin SB, Johnsrude IS, Harrington DP, Mendelsohn G, Ontjes DJ, Cooper CW (1982a) Thyroid venous catheterization in the early diagnosis of familial medullary thyroid carcinoma. Ann Surg 196: 505
Wells SA, Baylin SB, Leight GS (1982b) The importance of early diagnosis in patients with hereditary medullary thyroid carcinoma. Ann Surg 195: 595
Wermer P (1963) Endocrine adenomatosis: peptic ulcer in a large kindred. Am J Med 35: 205

Adrenal Gland

Tumours of the Adrenal Gland

W. Saeger

Abteilung für Pathologie, Marienkrankenhaus, Alfredstraße 9, 2000 Hamburg 76, FRG

In the pathology of the adrenal gland, tumours of the adrenal cortex must be strictly separated from those of the adrenal medulla.

Adrenal Cortex

The World Health Organization (WHO) classification (Table 1; Williams et al. 1980) presents a very useful and relatively simple manual for the morphological diagnosis of tumours of the cortex. However, if morphological structures are to be correlated with clinical and functional data, conventional light microscopy on paraffin sections must be supplemented by further methods, in particular by electron microscopy.

Three main diagnoses must be differentiated in tumour pathology of the adrenal cortex: hyperplasia, adenoma and carcinoma.

Hyperplasia are generally bilateral. They may be diffuse, in which case we find enlarged adrenals with broadened cortex and rounded outlines. Their weight exceeds 6 g. They may be nodular; in these cases we see mostly yellow nodules measuring up to 2.5 cm and compressing the surrounding cortices. In most of those cases larger and smaller nodules are demonstrable.

Adenomas are well demarcated tumours consisting of cords and nests of cells resembling normal cortical cells but lacking the normal structural pattern. One differentiates clear-cell or spongiocytic adenomas with lipid-rich cells showing a vacuolated cytoplasm in paraffin sections from compact-cell adenomas with lipid-poor cells of the inner-cortex type containing a non-vacuolated eosinophilic cytoplasm often with lipofuscin. The rare third type is the adenoma of glomerulosa cells and consists almost entirely of small cells from round, dense and small to medium width clear cytoplasm. The fourth type is the mixed-cell adenoma containing clear cells and compact cells in varying proportions.

Differentiation between adenoma and nodular hyperplasia is the first clinically very important problem which cannot be solved without knowledge of the endocrinological data. Spongiocytic nodules of various sizes measuring up to 2.5 cm

Recent Results in Cancer Research. Vol. 118
© Springer-Verlag Berlin·Heidelberg 1990

Table 1. WHO histological classification of tumours of the adrenal cortex. (From Williams et al. 1980)

Epithelial tumours
  Benign
    Adenoma
      Clear cell (spongiocytic)
      Compact cell
      Glomerulosa cell
      Mixed cell
  Malignant
    Carcinoma (adenocarcinoma)
Epithelial tumour-like lesions
  Nodular hyperplasia
    Single nodule
    Multiple nodular hyperplasia
  Capsular extrusion
  Accessory adrenal cortex
  Others
Mesenchymal tumours and tumour-like lesions
  Benign
    Myelolipoma
    Lipoma
    Cysts
    Others
  Malignant
Secondary tumours
Unclassified tumours

usually in a slightly hyperplastic gland are very frequent in arterial hypertension. They seem to correlate with the likewise hyperplastic ACTH cells in the anterior pituitary. These never develop into an adenoma (Neville and O'Hare 1982). The hyperplastic gland in ACTH-dependent Cushing's disease is very similar to that in cases with arterial hypertension, but in hypercortisolism the intervening cortex between the nodules is diffusely hyperplastic. The bilateral hyperplasia causing a primary hyperaldosteronism is generally characterized by many small, only microscopically identifiable nodules and some lipid-rich yellow intraglandular nodules measuring up to 1.0 cm (Neville and O'Hare 1982). Non-functioning nodules as single localized overgrowth of adreno-cortical cells of 2–3 cm in diameter in the otherwise normal gland may be found in post-mortem series in up to 3% of normotensive subjects. Non-functioning adenomas probably do not exist. All larger inactive adrenocortical tumours are malignant (Neville and O'Hare 1982).

The third main diagnosis is adrenocortical carcinoma. This is usually much larger than an adenoma and usually shows a diffuse growth pattern, capsular and vascular invasions and areas of necroses. Cellular pleomorphism and nuclear atypia may be demonstrable but are not really reliable criteria of malignancy as pleomorphism may also be present in adenomas. Therefore, if invasive growth is

Table 2. Adrenal morphology in primary hyperaldosteronism. (From Neville and O'Hare 1982)

Adrenocortical tumour	125	81.7%
Adenoma with hyperplasia of zona glomerulosa	50	32.7%
Adenoma with hyperplasia of zona glomerulosa and with nodules	70	45.8%
Carcinoma	5	3.3%
No adrenocortical tumour	28	18.3%
Hyperplasia of zona glomerulosa	4	2.6%
Hyperplasia of zona glomerulosa with micronodules	14	9.1%
Hyperplasia of zona glomerulosa with micronodules and macro-nodules	5	3.3%
Normal zona glomerulosa with micronodules	5	3.3%
Total	153	100.0%

not demonstrable, tumour weight is the most reliable parameter, but the clinical hyperfunction must also be taken into account. All tumours weighing more than 200 g in hyperaldosteronism, more than 250 g in Cushing's syndrome, more than 400 g in adrenogenital syndrome and all really inactive adrenocortical tumours are malignant (Symington 1969; Neville and O'Hare 1982).

What do we find in surgical specimens of adrenal glands in various types of endocrine hyperfunction?

In hyperaldosteronism (Table 2) with low plasma renin we find in 18% of cases no tumour but a hyperplasia of the zona glomerulosa often with micronodules or macronodules. The zona glomerulosa is demonstrable around the entire periphery of the cortex and is increased in width (Neville and O'Hare 1982). The cells seem to be unchanged. In many cases, some nodules are not of the zona glomerulosa type but consist of fasciculata cells. Some authors (Neville and O'Hare 1982) therefore believe that they probably stem from, rather than cause, the hypertension. In 82% of cases adenomas are found in primary hyperaldosteronism; these are single in over 90% of cases. In women the left gland harbours the adenoma more often than does the right gland. They weigh less than 2 g in 34% of cases but may weigh up to 200 g. Histologically cells are arranged in cords and nests. They are similar to those of the zona fasciculata or of the intermediate cells but rarely similar to those of the zona glomerulosa. The nuclei are more vesicular and often contain inclusions. These nuclear structures – present only in adenomas – are very helpful in the often difficult differentiation between adenoma and macronodule.

The carcinomas causing hyperaldosteronism in 3.3% of cases weigh from 30 g to more than 2000 g, on average more than 500 g. They are very vascular and show haemorrhage, necroses, cystic changes and calcifications. Histologically different patterns of cell arrangements, mostly a trabecular type, can be found separated by prominent vascular sinusoids. The cellular pleomorphism is variable and is often but not necessarily increased in comparison with adenomas. Mitoses are very rare or lacking.

In Cushing's disease (Table 3) due to an ACTH-secreting lesion of the pituitary both adrenals are hyperplastic and weigh (as surgical specimens) more than 11 g.

Table 3. Adrenal morphology in Cushing's disease and Cushing's syndrome

	Children	Adults
ACTH-dependent types	42%[a]	78%[a]
Diffuse hyperplasia		22%[b]
Micronodular hyperplasia		22%[b]
Macronudular hyperplasia		33%[b]
Primary non–ACTH–dependent hyperadreno-corticism	58%[a]	22%[a]
Adenoma	12%[a]	13%[a]
Carcinoma	46%[a]	9%[a]
Primary nodular dysplasia (adenomatosis)	Very rare	Extremely rare

[a] From Neville and O'Hare (1982).
[b] From Smals et al. (1984).

The contours are rounded, and the cortex is broadened. Small nodules (micronodular hyperplasia) or larger nodules (macronodular hyperplasia) may be developed (Smals et al. 1984). These are mostly bilateral and multiple. They may be localized within the cortex, in the capsule or around the central vein. These nodules never transform into adenomas. In hyperadrenocorticism due to an ectopic ACTH syndrome the adrenals are more enlarged but nodules develop only rarely.

In non–ACTH–dependent primary hyperadrenocorticism (Table 3) adrenal tumours are found. The adenomas are sharply demarcated, having an elastic consistency and a yellow or brown cut surface. They usually weigh less than 50 g. Necroses or bleedings are very sparse. Microscopically (Fig. 1) one can differentiate compact-cell type or spongiocytic adenomas. In adenomas with high spongiocytic proportions cortisol secretion may frequently be stimulated by ACTH whereas this is not possible in most compact-cell adenomas (Mitschke et al. 1973). The carcinomas are softer and larger than the adenomas in Cushing's syndrome. They weigh more than 50–100 g. Their capsule is disrupted. The cut surface shows large areas of necroses and bleedings. The histological pattern (Fig. 2) is solid or medullary or–due to necroses–pseudopapillary. Generally the cells resemble neither typical compact cells nor spongiocytes, but in more differentiated tumours typical compact cells are present. The blood sinusoids reveal a frequently disrupted endothelium and may contain microthrombi. Carcinomas causing Cushing's syndrome have a very poor prognosis due to local recurrences and metastases mostly in liver and lung. Survival rates of 13% at 5 years are reported (Bradley 1975).

The rarest type of Cushing's syndrome (less than 1% of cases) is the primary nodular dysplasia or bilateral nodular adenomatosis occurring mostly in children. The adrenals are not enlarged. They may weigh less than normal (Iseli and Hedinger 1985). Cut surfaces reveal small nodules measuring between 2 and 5 mm. Light microscopy shows large cells with granular eosinophilic or vacuolated cytoplasm and occasional PAS-positive bodies. The nuclei are variously pleomor-

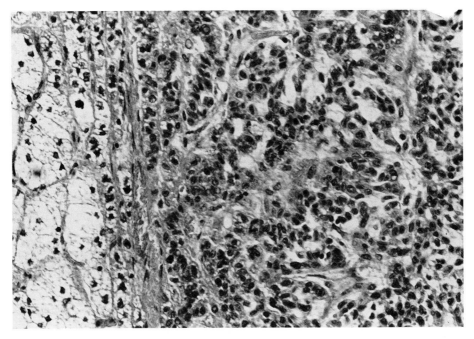

Fig. 1. Adrenal adenoma in Cushing's syndrome. Spongiocytes (*left side*) and smaller compact cells (*right side*), sparse connective tissue. Hematoxylin-eosin, magnification × 280

phic and are often very large, containing distinctly enlarged nucleoli. These small nodules are the cause of the hyperfunction. The surrounding cortex is atrophic.

A reliable morphological sign of glucocorticoid hyperfunction in Cushing's syndrome due to adrenal tumour is the atrophy of surrounding ipsilateral gland and the contralateral gland. In the pituitary, typical Crooke's cells are demonstrable. Cushing's syndrome is therefore one of the few endocrine hyperfunctions which can be identified by pathologists in post-mortem examinations without knowledge of the clinical data.

The third type of hyperfunction is the adrenogenital syndrome (Table 4), which is based on a congenital bilateral hyperplasia in children or an androgen-producing tumour in children or adults. Estrogen-secreting tumours also belong to the adrenogenital syndrome. These are very rare.

Virilizing adenomas weigh between 4 and 400 g and are encapsulated. The cut surface is uniformly brown or brown-red. Under the microscope the cells are seen to be arranged in short cords, acini or trabeculae. They are compact-type cells with vesicular nuclei and lipid-poor eosinophilic cytoplasm. Abundant lipofuscin is demonstrable. The cells often resemble regular cells of the zona reticularis, but spongiocytic cells of the fasciculata type may be present focally. The larger the tumour, the more developed are the thin-walled vascular sinusoids. Cellular and nuclear pleomorphism is often demonstrable in these larger tumours, which are difficult to classify as benign or malignant (Neville and O'Hare 1982; Saeger und

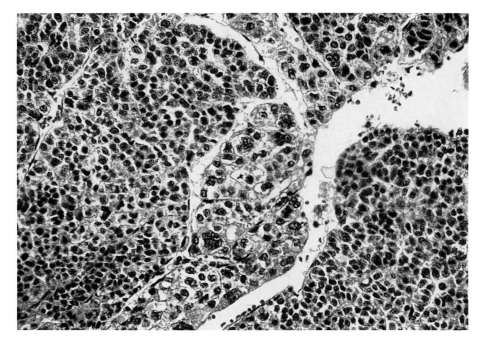

Fig. 2. Adrenal carcinoma in Cushing's syndrome. Medium-sized, partly very pleomorphic cells in medullary pattern, lacking connective tissue. Sinusoids with disrupted endothelium. Hematoxylin-eosin, magnification × 225

Table 4. Adrenal morphology of adrenogenital syndrome. (From Neville and O'Hare 1979, 1982)

Congenital bilateral adrenal hyperplasia[a]	
21-Hydroxylase deficiency	90%
11 β-Hydroxylase deficiency	5%
Δ^5-3β-Hydroxysteroid dehydrogenase-Isomerase deficiency	
Very rare other types	
Adrenal adenoma[b]	38%
Adrenal carcinoma[b]	62%

[a] 1 in 5000 births.
[b] Androgen-secreting tumours: 12% of adrenal specimens in hypercorticalism.

Mitschke 1989). We have encountered a small tumour weighing 20 g with distinct nuclear pleomorphism and defects of basal membrane and endothelial layer in the sinusoidal vessels, although the capsule was intact; we classified this as carcinoma. Otherwise, virilizing carcinomas weigh up to 2000 g and show defects of capsule and vessel walls and occasionally large areas of necroses. Their cells are of compact type or are uncharacteristic (Fig. 3). Spongiocytes are lacking. Nuclei are markedly

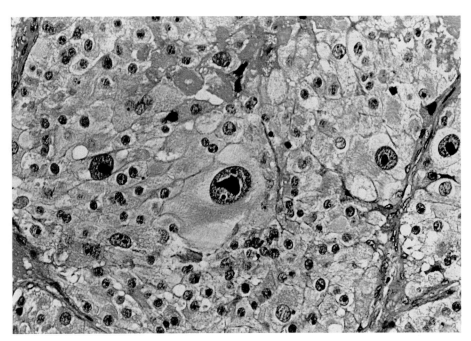

Fig. 3. Virilizing adrenal carcinoma. Partly very large cells with large nuclei and large nucleoli. Hematoxylin-eosin, magnification × 450

pleomorphic, harbouring large and occasionally double nucleoli. Mitoses are very rare. The adjacent and contralateral glands are normal. Atrophy does not develop.

Adrenal tumours causing feminization are the rarest type of active adrenalcortical tumours; 90% of these patients are male. These tumours are malignant in 84% of cases (Neville and O'Hare 1982). The adenomas are mostly small, measuring up to 5 cm and weighing up to 50 g. Histologically they are very similar to virilizing adenomas, showing compact cells in an often alveolar arrangement. The feminizing carcinomas generally weigh more than 200 g (up to 3500 g), but there is a marked overlap between benign and malignant tumours in size, weight and histological appearance (Fig. 4). The pleomorphism of cells varies. The nuclei may be more vesicular and have distinct, large nucleoli. Necroses and bleedings may be present especially in larger tumours (Mitschke et al. 1978).

Non-functioning adrenocortical tumours are exclusively malignant (non-hormonal carcinomas). In smaller lesions measuring less than 5 cm the differentiation between nodule and tumour is difficult (see above), but small inactive carcinomas are extremely rare. Most of these are larger than the active malignant tumours, measure more than 10 cm (up to 40 cm) in diameter and weigh more than 500–1000 g (up to 4.5 kg; Neville and O'Hare 1982). Benign, so-called myelolipomas as inactive tumours (Table 1) may be very large, but histologically they are easily differentiated from carcinomas by their typical arrangement of adipose cells and marrow elements. Histologically the carcinomas are similar to glucocorticoid- or androgen-secreting tumours, showing lipid-poor compact cells in diffuse

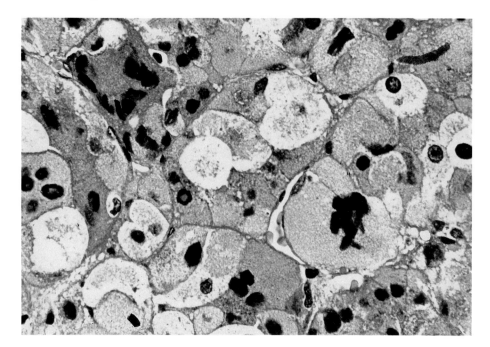

Fig. 4. Estrogen-secreting adrenal carcinoma. Pleomorphic cell, partly multinucleated. Giemsa stain, magnification × 750

or solid arrangement, but often many clear cells can be found which are not of spongiocytic type.

Without either distinct morphological criterion for the diagnosis of the non-functioning carcinoma, clinical data are mandatory. Any signs of adrenocortical hyperfunction must be absent. In patients suffering only from an arterial hypertension one can speculate as to whether hypertensiogenic steroids from the tumour are the cause of hypertension.

Morphological Methods for Identification of Cell Function. The immunohistochemistry for steroid hormones deals with many problems (Tayler 1986). The antibodies with specificity against one of the steroid hormones show measurable cross-reactivities against other steroid hormones or their precursors. It is astonishing that steroid hormones are demonstrable to any extent in paraffin-embedded tissues although such specimens have been processed extensively through organic solvents which might be expected to remove all of the steroids. On the other hand, one can find non-specific bindings of the reagents to charged components within tissue sections which may also cause many problems. Sex hormone positivity may be observed in other non-endocrine tumours such as hepatomas or breast carcinomas possibly due to absorption of the hormone by a specific receptor. Therefore, immunoperoxidase staining for steroid hormones may be of diagnostic value, but this method alone is not a reliable indicator of the type of hormone produced by any individual morphological type of tumour. Other immunohistological markers seem to be of minor importance. Intermediate filament proteins may be demonstrated in many adrenal cortical carcinomas and in some adenomas (Miettinen et al. 1985).

Electron microscopy is the method that we prefer for the more detailed scientific analysis of adrenocortical pathology and for clinical-pathological correlations. Features associated with steroid hormone synthesis are liposomes, extensive smooth endoplasmic reticulum, well-developed Golgi apparatus and mitochondria. Details of organelle distribution and their fine structures vary from zone to zone, but in contrast to the abrupt transitions seen by light microscopy, intermediate cell types can be seen with electron microscope (Neville and O'Hare 1979). The zona glomerulosa is characterized by small cytoplasmic volumes, scanty smooth endoplasmic reticulum, elongated mitochondria with small lamellar cristae, scanty osmiophilic liposomes and few lipofuscin granules. The outer zona fasciculata contains cells with very large cytoplasmic volume, scanty smooth endoplasmic reticulum, ovoid small mitochondria with few short tubules and vesicules, many osmiophilic free droplets or many empty membrane-bound vacuoles and few lipofuscin granules. The inner zona fasciculata shows large cells with increased smooth endoplasmic reticulum, spherical mitochondria of variable sizes and many internal vesicles, many osmiophilic free droplets or many empty membrane-bound vacuoles — like the outer zona fasciculata — and increased lipofuscin granules. The zona reticularis is composed of cells with intermediate cytoplasmic volume, densely packed smooth endoplasmic reticulum, ovoid medium-sized tubulovesicular cristae, very few vacuoles or osmiophilic droplets and many lipofuscin granules. Many adenomas and some carcinomas are similar to one (or occasionally two) zones of the normal adrenal cortex.

Many *aldosterone-secreting tumours* resemble partially the normal zona fasciculata and partially the zona glomerulosa, as they generally show a broad cytoplasm with many lipid vacuoles of fasciculata type but elongated small mitochondria with lamellar cristae of glomerulosa type (Tannenbaum 1973; Neville and Mackay 1972; Neville and O'Hare 1982; Shigematsu 1982). The ultrastructure of other adenomas is more similar to normal zona glomerulosa (Kano et al. 1979; Kuramoto und Kumazawa 1985), which is also demonstrable in hyperplastic nodules with primary hyperaldosteronism.

The tumours *in Cushing's syndrome* are ultrastructurally comparable with lipid-rich fasciculata cells (spongiocytic adenoma) or with compact fasciculata cells (compact-cell adenoma) showing varying levels of liposomes, more or less ovoid or spherical mitochondria with vesicles and less or more smooth endoplasmic reticulum. In contrast to normal zona fasciculata, organelles may be pleomorphic. Mitochondria may be bizarre and large; the endoplasmic reticulum may consist of distended vesicles (Mitschke et al. 1973; Neville and Mackay 1972; Tannenbaum 1973; Neville and O'Hare 1982). Most pleomorphic features are demonstrable in carcinomas (Fig. 5), but this is not proof of malignancy.

In *adrenogenital syndrome* the tumours frequently have a normal zona reticularis, showing densely packed smooth endoplasmic reticulum, round medium-sized mitochondria with tubulovesicular or partially lamellar cristae, sparse lipo-

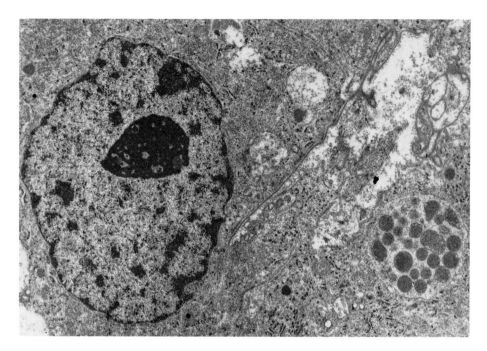

Fig. 5. Ultrastructure of adrenal carcinoma in Cushing's syndrome. Nucleus with large nucleolus, increased rough endoplasmic reticulum and increased numbers of ribosomes in the cytoplasm, decreased pleomorphic mitochondria. Uranyl acetate, lead citrate, magnification × 12 080

somes and many pigment granules (Fig. 6). The presence of intramitochondrial dense granules and/or lamellar cristae seems to be typical for this type of hyperfunction (Gorgas et al. 1976; Akhtar et al. 1984; Saeger and Mitschke 1989).

Estrogen-secreting tumours (Fig. 7) contain pleomorphic nuclei, various amounts of differently structured mitochondria and smooth endoplasmic reticulum, very sparse liposomes and many microbodies of unknown origin. Lipofuscin granules are rare. Intramitochondrial granules are frequent (Mitschke et al. 1978). These tumours may resemble androgen-secreting adenomas or carcinomas.

Non-hormonal adrenocortical carcinomas (Neville and O'Hare 1982) show relatively high amounts of rough endoplasmic reticulum, but the smooth endoplasmic reticulum is sparsely developed. Mitochondria vary in number and structure. Their cristae are mostly tubulovesicular or atypical. Liposomes vary widely in number, size and arrangement. Lipofuscin granules are sparse. The ultrastructure resembles that of active carcinomas, but morphometric analysis (Saeger et al. 1979) demonstrates a lesser content of organelles.

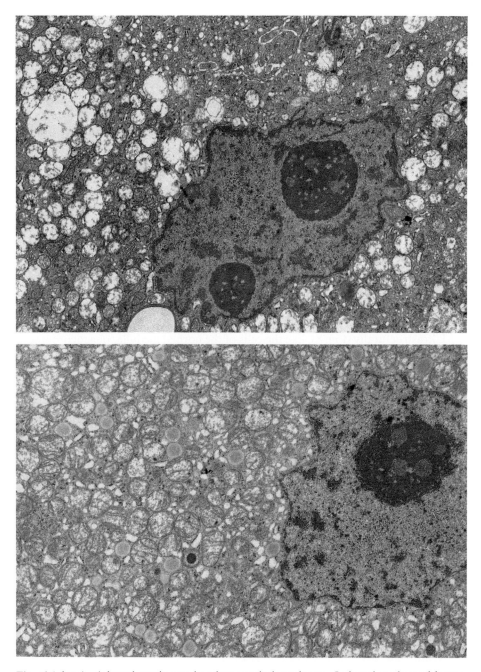

Fig. 6 (*above*). Adrenal carcinoma in adrenogenital syndrome. Lobated nucleus with two nucleoli, pleomorphic mitochondria, smooth surfaced and also rough endoplasmic reticulum. Uranyl acetate, lead citrate, magnification × 7970

Fig. 7 (*below*). Estrogen-secreting adrenal carcinoma. Lobated nucleus with large nucleolus, many mitochondria, some with intramitochondrial granules, some lipid bodies. Uranyl acetate, lead citrate, magnification × 9330

Adrenal Medulla

Tumours of the adrenal medulla are of neuroendocrine or neural type and are closely related to those of the extra-adrenal paraganglionic structures, including chemoreceptor organs which consist of very similar neuroendocrine tissue. The WHO classification (Table 5) differentiates between neuroendocrine, neural and mixed neuroendocrine-neural tumours (Williams et al. 1980). All types have a benign and a malignant variant, the differentiation of which may be very difficult or – with only morphological methods — impossible.

Phaeochromocytomas are round or ovoid tumours with a fibrous capsule over which the adrenal cortex may be stretched or which may even form a pseudocapsule. They weigh between 1.4 g and 3600 g with an average of 100 g (Neville and O'Hare 1979). The solid, partly lobulated cut surface is gray to brown. Areas of necroses and bleedings occur especially in larger tumours. Histologically, they are usually composed of polygonal, fusiform or pleomorphic cells in solid or alveolar arrangement with mostly sparse regular connective tissue. The abundant cytoplasm contains chromaffin granules. Immunohistological investigations (Table 6) demonstrate a long list of various hormonal or other neuroendocrine markers (Hacker et al. 1988). S-100 protein was found in satellite cells but not in tumour cells (Lauriola et al. 1985; Hacker et al. 1988).

Ultrastructurally (Fig. 8), like the cells of the normal medulla, phaeochromocytoma cells contain varying numbers of secretory granules of the norepinephrine or of the epinephrine type. Norepinephrine granules measuring between 75 and 250 nm have a dense core and a broad halo, epinephrine granules are less dense and have a slightly granular core (Tannenbaum 1970). The ratio of epinephrine to norepinephrine, 85:15 in normal medulla, is reversed in most adrenal phaeochromocytomas (Neville and O'Hare 1979). The mitochondria may be increased in size and number. The rough endoplasmic reticulum is well developed and focally dilated. Golgi fields may be doubled in some cells. Capillaries are fenestrated. Nerve fibres are lacking in phaeochromocytomas.

Probably 10% of all phaeochromocytomas are familial (Page et al. 1986). They are associated with various syndromes (Table 7) and are more often malignant than the sporadic tumours especially when associated with medullary thyroid carcinoma. About 10% of phaeochromocytomas are malignant, but differentiation between malignant and benign types is very difficult and often impossible in surgical specimens. Only metastases demonstrate malignancy (Table 8). Otherwise there do not exist reliable criteria to indicate malignancy. Therefore, in some cases the diagnosis of malignancy can be made only by their progress. Some unreliable indications of malignancy are increased mitoses and necroses, increased weight of the tumour, vascular invasions, and only few neuropeptides in immuno-histology.

Neural tumours (Table 5) of the adrenal medulla include the benign neurofibromas and ganglioneuromas and the malignant neuroblastomas and ganglioneuroblastomas. Benign tumours are about ten times less frequent than the malignant ones (Mitschke and Schäfer 1981).

Whereas *ganglioneuromas* have been reported to occur in all ages, with a tendency to older age groups, *neuroblastomas* are very frequent in infancy and

Table 5. WHO Histological classification of tumours of the adrenal medulla. (Without paragangliomas; from Williams et al. 1980)

Neuroendocrine tumours
  Benign
    Phaeochromocytoma
  Malignant
    Malignant phaeochromocytoma
Neural tumours
  Benign
    Neurofibroma
    Ganglioneuroma
  Malignant
    Ganglioneuroblastoma
    Neuroblastoma
Mixed neuroendocrine-neural tumours
  Benign
  Malignant
Miscellaneous
Secondary tumours
Unclassified tumours
Tumour-like lesions

Table 6. Immunhistological findings in phaeochromocytomas. (From Hacker et al. 1988)

Chromogranin	11/12	92%
Neuron-specific enolase	12/12	100%
Protein gene-product 9, 5	9/9	100%
Neurofilament protein	5/12	42%
Glial fibrillary acidic protein	0/12	0%
S-100 protein	0/12	0%
Tyrosine hydroxylase	6/12	50%
Dopamine β-hydroxylase	1/12	8%
Phenylethanolamine-N-methyltransferase	4/12	33%
Leucine enkephalin	7/12	58%
Methionine enkephalin	7/12	58%
Adrenocorticotropic hormone	2/12	17%
Bombesin	1/11	9%
Calcitonin	2/12	17%
Calcitonin gene-related peptide	2/12	17%
Somatostatin	5/12	42%
Neuropeptide tyrosine	10/12	83%
Vasoactive intestinal polypeptide	2/12	17%
Neurotensin	0/12	0%
Galanin	6/12	50%
Serotonin	3/12	40%

Table 7. Familial phaeochromocytoma syndromes. (From Heitz and Steiner 1981; Page et al. 1986)

Syndrome	Components of syndrome	Frequency of phaeochromocytoma
Multiple endocrine neo- plasia (type II, type IIa)	C-cell hyperplasia-medullary thy- roid carcinoma; adrenal medullary hyperplasia-phaeochromocytoma; parathyroid hyperplasia-adenoma	20%–40%
Multiple endocrine neo- plasia (type III, type IIb)	C-cell hyperplasia-medullary thy- roid carcinoma; adrenal medullary hyperplasia-phaeochromocytoma; corneal, mucocutaneous, and gas- trointestinal ganglioneuromatosis; marfanoid habitus	20%–40%
Lindau-von Hippel disease	Angiomatosis retinae; haeman- gioblastomas of central nervous system; renal, pancreatic hepatic, and epididymal cysts; renal carci- noma; phaeochromocytoma	5%–50%
von Recklinghausen's disease	Cutaneous or visceral neurofi- bromas; café au lait spots; benign and malignant schwannoma; men- ingioma; glioma; phaeochromocy- toma	0.5%–5%
Sturge-Weber syndrome	Cavernous haemangiomas invol- ving the first or all of the three divisions of the fifth cranial nerve; phaeochromocytoma	5%

childhood — the most common solid extracranial tumour of this age having an incidence of 9.6 cases per one million children (Young and Miller 1975) – and are very rare in adults. Familial neuroblastoma have been reported in rare cases.

The adrenal medulla is the most common site of origin (36% of neuro- blastomas; Page et al. 1986). Small incidental neuroblastomas are frequently found in routine microscopic sections of adrenal medulla from patients younger than 3 months of age (so-called in situ neuroblastomas). These generally show degenera- tive changes. Because of the high frequency of these tumours in neonatal autopsies and the relatively low incidence of clinically apparent neuroblastomas it has been concluded (Beckwith and Perrin 1963) that the vast majority of incidental neuro- blastomas must undergo spontaneous degeneration or maturation into neural or neuroendocrine tissue. The size of clinically apparent neuroblastomas ranges from relatively small lesions to those tumours which fill nearly the entire abdomen. The capsule is usually infiltrated. The tumours are soft. The gray to white cut surface often shows necroses and cystic degenerations. Microscopically, the neuroblas- tomas reveal a solid and sometimes lobular growth pattern. Pseudorosettes with a

Table 8. Differential diagnosis of benign and malignant phaeochromocytoma

	Benign	Malignant
Frequency[a]	90%	10%
Sex ratio[a]	55% females	70% females
Mean weight	150 g	760 g
Pleomorphism[b]	− to + + +	+ to + + +
Mitoses[b]	− to + +	+ to + + +
Necroses[b]	− to +	+ to + + +
Capsule invasion[c]	− to + (?)	− to + +
Vascular invasion[c]	− to + (?)	− to + +
Immunohistology[d]	Many neuropeptides	Few neuropeptides
Bilateral occurrence	Possible	Possible
Metastases	−	+

[a] Neville and O'Hare 1979.
[b] Williams et al. 1980.
[c] Mitschke and Schäfer 1981.
[d] Linnoila et al. 1988.

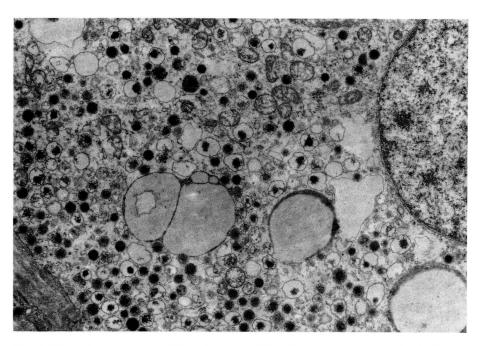

Fig. 8. Phaeochromocytoma of the adrenal medulla. Many secretory granules (with or without halo), some lysosomes with lipid bodies. Uranyl acetate, lead citrate, magnification × 10 700

central zone of nerve fibres may be present. Areas of haemorrhage, necroses, and calcifications are frequent. The round to ovoid nuclei are hyperchromatic. The nucleoli are inconspicuous. The scanty cytoplasm has poorly defined cell borders. Between the tumour cells a fibrillar eosinophilic matrix is demonstrable. By immunohistology, neuron-specific enolace and neurofilament are generally demonstrable whereas S-100, glial fibrillary acid protein, and myelin basic protein are negative.

The ultrastructure of neuroblastomas (Page et al. 1986) shows round nuclei with moderately condensed chromatin and small nucleoli and prominent process formation of the cytoplasm, which contains large numbers of mono- and polyribosomes, sparsely developed rough endoplasmic reticulum, inconspicuous Golgi fields and moderate amounts of mitochondria. Secretory granules measuring 50–200 nm are demonstrable in perinuclear cytoplasm and processes. Lysosomes measuring up to 900 nm may be present. Processes contain intermediate filaments and microtubules. Glycogen may be found. Schwann's cells may be included in the tumour and can be immunohistologically identified by demonstration of S-100 protein. Very rarely neuroblastomas show a focal or extensive maturation into mature ganglioneuromas (Page et al. 1986). Spontaneous regressions have also been reported (Evans et al. 1976). A histological grading (grades I–IV) based on the degree of differentiation (amount of neurofilaments, enlargement of cells and nuclei) has been proposed and seems to be correlated with prognosis (Beckwith and Martin 1968). Otherwise, the prognosis depends upon the age at diagnosis (the younger the better) and the stage.

Ganglioneuroblastomas are tumours composed of a mixture of neuroblasts and ganglion cells in various stages of differentiation (Williams et al. 1980) presenting neuroblastoma with partial differentiation and maturation. The mature areas can be immunostained by S-100 protein, neuron-specific enolase, myelin basic protein and neurofilament. If fibrous tissue is also developed (neurofibroma) vimentin is positive additionally (Taylor 1986). The prognosis of these tumours is unpredictable. Encapsulated ganglioneuroblastomas generally do not recur after complete surgical excision. Tumours showing extensive local invasion behave like neuroblastomas.

In rare cases, ganglioneuroblastomas and ganglioneuromas may be mixed with phaeochromocytomas (Table 5). The prognosis of the malignant type is unpredictable; that of the benign variant is excellent.

References

Akhtar M, Gosalbez T, Young I (1974) Ultrastructural study of androgen producing adrenocortical adenoma. Cancer 34: 322–327

Beckwith JB, Martin RF (1968) Observations of the histopathology of neuroblastomas. Pediatr Surg 3: 106–110

Beckwith JB, Perrin EV (1963) In situ neuroblastomas: a contribution to the natural history of neural crest tumors. Am J Pathol 43: 1089–1104

Bradley EL (1975) Primary and adjunctive therapy in carcinoma of the adrenal cortex. Surg Gynecol Obstet 141: 507–511

Evans AE, Gerson J, Schnaufer L (1976) Spontaneous regression of neuroblastoma. NCI
Monogr 44: 49–54

Gorgas K, Böck P, Wuketich S (1976) Fine structure of a virilizing adrenocortical adenoma.
Beitr Pathol 159: 371–397

Hacker GW, Bishop AE, Terenghi G, Varndell IM, Aghahowa J, Pollard K, Thurner J,
Polak JM (1988) Multiple peptide production and presence of general neuroendocrine
markers detected in 12 cases of human phaeochromocytoma and in mammalian adrenal
glands. Virchows Arch [A] 412: 399–441

Heitz PU, Steiner H (1981) Pluriglanduläre endokrine Regulations-störungen. In: Altenähr
E, Böcker W, Dhom G, Gusek W, Heitz PU, Klöppel G, Lietz H, Mitschke H, Saeger W,
Schäfer H, Staub J-J, Steiner H (eds) Pathologie der endokrinen Organe. Springer, Berlin
Heidelberg New York, pp 1137–1204 (Spezielle pathologische Anatomie, vol 14/II)

Iseli BE, Hedinger CE (1985) Histopathology and ultrastructure of primary adrenocortical
nodular dysplasia with Cushing's syndrome. Histopathology 9: 1171–1194

Kano K, Sato S, Hama H (1979) Adrenal adenomata causing primary aldosteronism – ultrastructural study of 25 cases. Virchows Arch [A] 384: 93–102

Kuramoto H, Kumazawa J (1985) Ultrastructural studies of adrenal adenoma causing
primary aldosteronism. Virchows Arch [A] 407: 271–278

Lauriola L, Maggiano N, Sentinelli S, Michetti F, Cocchia D (1985) Satellite cells in the
normal human adrenal gland and in phaeochromocytomas. An immunohistochemical
study. Virchows Arch [B] 49: 13–22

Linnoila RI, Lack EE, Steinberg SM, Keiser HR (1988) Decreased expression of neuropeptides in malignant paragangliomas: an immunohistochemical study. Hum Pathol 19:
41–50

Miettinen M, Lehto V-P, Virtanen I (1985) Immunofluorescence microscopic evaluation of
the intermediate filament expression of the adrenal cortex and medulla and their tumors.
Am J Pathol 188: 360–366

Mitschke H, Schäfer H (1981) Nebennierenmark. In: Altenähr E, Böcker W, Dohm G,
Gusek W, Heitz PU, Klöppel G, Lietz H, Mitschke H, Saeger W, Schäfer H, Staub JJ,
Steiner H (eds) Pathologie der endokrinen Organe. Springer, Berlin Heidelberg New
York, pp 971–1048 (Spezielle Pathologische Anatomie, vol 1412)

Mitschke H, Saeger W, Breustedt H-J (1973) Zur Ultrastruktur der Nebennierenrindentum-
oren beim Cushing-Syndrom. Virchows Arch [A] 360: 253–264

Mitschke H, Saeger W, Breustedt H-J (1978) Feminizing adrenocortical tumor. Histological
and ultrastructural study. Virchows Arch [A] 377: 301–309

Neville AM, Mackay AM (1972) The structure of the human adrenal cortex in health and
disease. In: Mason AS (ed) Diseases of the adrenal gland, vol 1. Saunders, London, pp
361–395

Neville AM, O'Hare MJ (1979) The human adrenal gland: aspects of structure, function
and pathology. In: James VHT (ed) The adrenal gland. Raven, New York, pp 1–66

Neville AM, O'Hare MJ (1982) The human adrenal cortex. Pathology and biology-an
integrated approach. Springer, Berlin Heidelberg New York

Page DL, DeLellis RA, Hough AJ (1986) Tumors of the adrenal. In: Hartmann WH, Sobin
LH (eds) Atlas of tumor pathology, sec series, fasc 23. Armed Forces Institute of
Pathology, Washington

Saeger W, Mitschke H (1989) Androgenbildende Prozesse der Nebennierenrinde. Aktuel
Endokrinol Stoffwechsel 10: 162–169

Saeger W, Saager G, Caselitz J (1979) Ultrastructural and morphometrical study of
endocrinologically active and of non-functioning adenomas of the human adrenal cortex.
Acta Endocrinol [Suppl] (Copenh) 225: 55

Shigematsu K (1982) Comparative studies between hormone contents and morphological appearances in human adrenal cortex – special reference to non-functioning tumors (adenoma and adenomatous nodule) and functioning adenoma. Acta Histochem Cytochem 15: 386–400

Smals AGH, Pieters GFF, Van Haelst UJG, Kloppenborg PWC (1984) Macronodular adrenocortical hyperplasia in long-standing Cushing's disease. J Clin Endocrinol Metab 58: 25–31

Symington T (1969) The adrenal cortex. In: Symington T (ed) The adrenal gland, vol 3. Livingstone, Edinbourgh, p 218

Tannenbaum M (1970) Ultrastructural pathology of adrenal medullary tumors: In: Sommers SC (ed) Pathology annual, vol 5 Appleton-Century Croft, New York, pp 145–171

Tannenbaum M (1973) Ultrastructural pathology of the adrenal cortex. In: Sommers SC (ed) Pathology annual, vol 8. Appleton-Century Croft, New York, pp 109–156

Taylor CR (1986) Immunomicroscopy: a diagnostic tool for the surgical pathologist. In: Bennington JL (ed) Major problems in pathology, vol 19. Saunders, Philadelphia, pp 1–452

Valente M, Penelli N, Segato P, Bevilacqua L, Thiene G (1978) Androgen producing andrenocortical carcinoma. A histological and ultrastructural study of two cases. Virchows Arch Path Anat 378: 91–103

Williams ED, Siebenmann RE, Sobin LH (1980) Histological typing of endocrine tumours. International histological classification of tomours, No. 23 World Health Organization, Geneva

Young JL, Miller RW (1975) Incidence of malignant tumors in children. J Pediatr 86: 254–260

Clinical and Diagnostic Findings in Patients with Chromaffin Tumors: Pheochromocytomas, Pheochromoblastomas

H. Käser

Institut für klinische und experimentelle Tumorforschung, Universität Bern, Tiefenaustraße 120, 3004 Bern, Switzerland

Chromaffin tumors are defined as neoplasias composed of catecholamine-producing, -storing, and -secreting cells. They therefore develop not only in the adrenal medulla but also in sympathetic paraganglia. Regardless of their intra- or extra-adrenal localization, we shall use the term pheochromocytoma for all expansive growing forms of these tumors and the term pheochromoblastoma for all infiltrating and metastasizing forms (Table 1; Käser 1985). However, it must be emphasized that even the nonmalignant pheochromocytoma must be considered as lifethreatening disease. In fact, its endocrine activity may lead to death if the tumor remains unrecognized and untreated. However, if correctly diagnosed, this neural crest tumor can be removed by surgery, and most patients can thus be cured.

A thorough knowledge of the clinical symptoms and the availability of specific chemical methods are a prerequisite to diagnose these neoplasias. Furthermore, the methods used should allow discrimination between pheochromocytoma and pheochromoblastoma. I will therefore, review briefly the current knowledge regarding these tumors, taking into consideration our own experience with 177 patients.

Chromaffin tumors are very rare and only one or two new cases per million people are reported every year (Gifford et al. 1985; Käser 1985; Stenström and Svärdsudd 1986). In the past few years, we have examined only 19 patients with pheochromoblastoma but 158 patients with pheochromocytoma. For this reason I will first discuss the latter form of these tumors.

Pheochromocytoma

Contrary to general belief, this neoplasia is not found predominantly in adults but occurs in individuals at any age (Fig. 1; Käser and Wagner 1982; Sutton et al. 1981). Our youngest patient was 5 months old at the time of diagnosis. In fact, the morbidity in childhood is not significantly lower than in the overall population (Niklaus 1986) The sexes are equally represented.

Pheochromocytoma cells are genetically derived from primitive neuroectodermal elements, the so-called sympathogonia. These cells migrate during embryonic

Recent Results in Cancer Research. Vol. 118
© Springer-Verlag Berlin·Heidelberg 1990

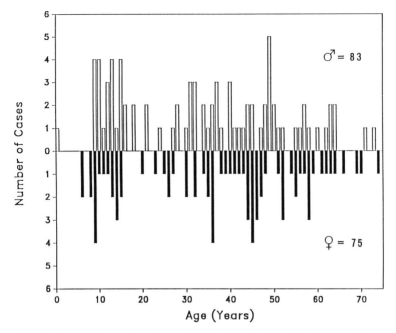

Fig. 1. Age at diagnosis and sex of 158 patients with pheochromocytoma

Table 1. Nomenclature of chromaffin neoplasias

Benign (pheochromocytoma)
  Intra–adrenal: pheochromocytoma
  Extra–adrenal: sympathetic paraganglioma
Malignant (pheochromoblastoma)
  Intra–adrenal: malignant pheochromocytoma
  Extra–adrenal: malignant sympathetic paraganglioma

development from the neural crest in a caudal direction dorsolaterally and anterior to the aorta. Some of the cells accumulate at the site of originating sympathetic ganglia, but the majority of them finally enter the developing fetal adrenal cortex. Following this migration they start to differentiate first to pheochromoblasts and then to the mature chromaffin cells of the adrenal medulla and the extra-adrenal sympathetic paraganglia. The latter process extends to childhood and is accompanied by a regression of the extra-adrenal chromaffin cells (Fig. 2) so that the adrenal medulla remains virtually the only chromaffin organ after puberty (Coupland 1965, 1981; Langmann 1970).

Considering the ontogenesis of the adrenomedullary system, it is not surprising that 90% of pheochromocytomas are found in the medulla in adults but only 50% in children (Table 2). Most of the extra-adrenal tumors are likewise located in the retroperitoneal region, but they may develop anywhere along the sympathetic

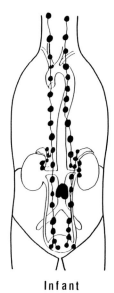 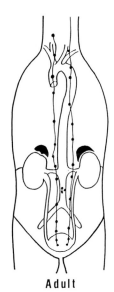

Fig. 2. Distribution of chromaffin tissue in the infant and the adult

Infant   Adult

Table 2. Location pattern of pheochromocytoma

Occurence/site	Adults (n = 114)		Children (n = 44)	
Single tumors				
Adrenal [a]	84% ⎱		30% ⎱	
		90%		55%
Extra-adrenal	6% ⎰		25% ⎰	
Multiple tumors				
Biadrenal	6% ⎱		20% ⎱	
Extra-adrenal	3%	10%	10%	45%
Adrenal/extra-adrenal	1% ⎰		15% ⎰	

[a] Right 55%, left 45%.

trunk from the cervical ganglion down to the pelvis (Gauer et al. 1988; Manger and Gifford 1977). Pheochromocytomas occur as a single tumor in most adults but as multiple tumors in some 50% of children. In the case of multiple tumors both adrenals are generally involved. However, especially in children, multifocal tumors of very different locations may be expected (Fries and Chambertin 1968; Käser 1987).

Since the cells of this neoplasia produce catecholamines, as do the chromaffin cells of the sympathetic paraganglia and the adrenal medulla, a plethora of symptoms may occur depending on the quantity of norepinephrine and/or epinephrine that the tumor produces. The most common symptoms are headaches, sweating with or without paleness of the face, palpitations, nervousness or anxiety, nausea, and also tremulousness, weakness and fatigue (Table 3). Less frequent are visual disturbances, tinnitus, dizziness, constipation or pain in chest and abdomen. In some very rare instances patients also complain of polyuria, polydipsia or polyphagia, depression and Raynaud's phenomenon, or other symptoms. These clinical manifestations may occur as single symptoms or in combination. They may be permanently present in the patients or occur as paroxysmal attacks. These attacks may occur frequently or only every few months, and their duration varies considerably, lasting from minutes to hours. The causes of these attacks are usually unclear. Nevertheless, it is known that changes in body position, coughing, laughing, or even defecation may lead to such attacks in some patients. Also, seizures may be caused by drugs such as sympathomimetics and β-adrenergic blockers, by certain foods and beverages which contain histamine, tyramine, or related biogenic amines (e.g., oranges, tangerines, mustard, several wines and cheeses), and even by chocolate. Finally, affective reactions such as anger or fear are also known to provoke paroxysms (Käser 1987; Labhart 1971; Manger and Gifford 1977).

Because of the rarity of this tumor and the great variety of its associated symptoms, pheochromocytoma is often not considered. But if the above-mentioned manifestations are further accompanied by persistent or paroxysmal hypertension, tachycardia, and/or hypermetabolism, the presence of a pheochromocytoma must be suspected. This is especially true if the observed symptoms cannot be associated with any other disease. In all these patients the presence of a chromaffin tumor must be confirmed or rejected.

In the past, provocative and blocking tests were used to diagnose pheochromocytoma. Today, the chemical quantitation of catecholamines and their metabolites (Fig. 3) has established itself as the method of choice (Plouin et al. 1981; Ziegler 1985). Even the simple determination of the vanilmandelic acid (VMA), the common breakdown product of epinephrine and norepinephrine, has proven very

Table 3. Incidence of symptoms resulting from elevated catecholamine levels

Subjective symptoms	Incidence (%)
Headache	70–90
Sweating	60–70
Pallor	40–60
Palpitations	40–60
Nervousness, anxiety	30–60
Nausea, vomiting	30–40
Tremulousness	25–30
Weakness, fatigue	20–30
Abdominal pain	15–25
Visual disturbances, tinnitus, vertigo	10–15
Chest pain, backache	10–15
Obstipation	10–15

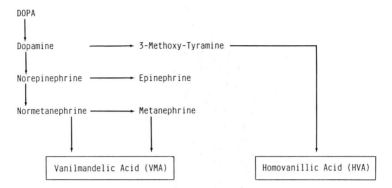

Fig. 3. Main metabolic pathways of catecholamines

valuable as an indicator. In about half of our patients we observed excretion of this metabolite exceeding five times the limit of normal. These observations have provided us conclusive evidence of a chromaffin tumor. Additionally, in 40% of our patients VMA was clearly elevated, although not as much as in the first group, and in only 5% was the VMA value at the upper normal range. Therefore, to ensure a clear diagnosis in the last two groups additional tests are required. Principally the quantitation of methoxyamines has proven very valuable. We have been able to show that all patients with a pheochromocytoma excrete high levels of normetanephrine and/or metanephrine, even though VMA excretion was not significantly elevated (Gauer et al. 1988).

Quantitative determinations of the catecholamines and of their metabolites represent the method of choice in confirming or rejecting the presence of a pheochromocytoma.

Nevertheless, the following conditions must be fulfilled:

– The urine specimen must have been collected according to a precise protocol.
– The total amount of metabolites must be quantitated in pooled 24-h urine and not in a single sample.
– Specific methods must be used which avoid errors due to the intake of drugs or to nutritional factors.
– The values must be interpreted taking into account the strongly age-dependent variation of the normal range.

As a result, one must be cautious in interpreting the values given by so-called quick tests used to determine an elevated VMA excretion or the total catecholamine and total metanephrine levels.

Abnormally high concentrations of norepinephrine, epinephrine, and their metabolites are also found in the blood of pheochromocytoma patients. However, since several factors unrelated to the tumor, such as stress, cause an elevation of the catecholamine level, blood collection must be performed under standardized conditions in order to yield conclusive results (Bravo et al. 1979; Cordes 1985; Ziegler 1985).

Table 4. Relationship between pattern of catecholamine production, and tumor site

Enhanced excretion	Site of Tumor (s)		
	Adrenal	Extra-adreal	Adrenal + extra-adrenal
Norepinephrine	61%	31%	8%
Epinephrine	100%	—	—
Norepinephrine + Epinephrine	95%	—	5%

Finally, the quantitative pattern of single catecholamines gives very useful indications about the location of the tumor (Table 4). Indeed, epinephrine- or epinephrine- and norepinephrine-producing tumors are always located at intra-adrenal sites, while exclusively norepinephrine-excreting tumors may also be found at extra-adrenal sites.

For the more accurate localization of a biochemically diagnosed pheochromo-cytoma, more precise methods are needed. The conventional radiologic methods (i.e., urography, tomography, angiography) do not always allow a precise localization, and therefore, especially in adults, computed tomography is preferred. Even echosonography yields good results if performed by an experienced technician (Otto 1983). Unfortunately, the latter two methods do not detect a small tumor of less than 1 cm in diameter or multifocal processes. Scintigraphy, using radiolabeled metaiodobenzylguanidine (MIBG), should then be used since this chemical accumulates mainly in the sympatho-adrenomedullary tissue (Beierwaltes 1985; Chatal and Charbonnel 1985; Fisher et al. 1985). Very few data are presently available on nuclear spin resonance tomography (Fink et al. 1985; Schmedtje et al. 1987), thus preventing assessment of the utility of this method.

Pheochromoblastoma

Pheochromoblastomas are malignant tumors which infiltrate the surrounding tissues and may develop metastases. Their frequency (Fig. 4) is about ten times less than that of pheochromocytomas. Similar to the latter, they develop from intra- or extra-adrenal chromaffin cells, but they are less frequently located in the adrenal medulla (Table 5). They also occur at any age, and they seem to be more frequent in women than in men (Niklaus 1986; Robinson 1980).

The symptoms are similar to those in pheochromocytoma. At later stages, however, additional signs, such as anemia, hepatomegaly, and pain due to bone metastases and/or cachexia, may be observed which are due to the neoplastic process. The presence of a pheochromoblastoma is diagnosed in the same way as a pheochromocytoma, namely by means of chemical quantitation of catecholamines. In this regard, the fact that in addition to norepinephrine and/or epinephrine and their metabolites, dopa, dopamine, methoxytyramine, and/or homovanillic

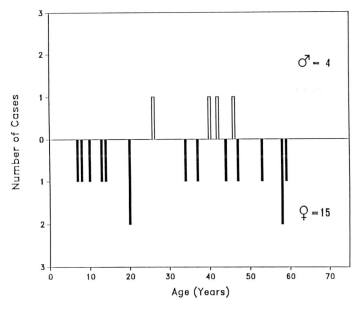

Fig. 4. Age of diagnosis and sex of 19 patients with pheochromoblastoma

Table 5. Clinical differences between benign and malignant chromaffin tumors

	Pheochromocytoma	Pheochromoblastoma
Incidence	90%	10%
Adrenal origin	80%	50%
Male: female ratio	~1:1	~1:5
Diagnostic criteria	NE/E↑	NE/E + DA↑

NE/E ↑, elevated nor- and/or epinephrine levels; DA↑, elevated DOPA, dopamine, and/or corresponding breakdown product levels.

In contrast to the case with pheochromocytoma, scintigraphy with radiolabeled MIBG is the preferred method to localize the tumor, estimate its spread, and detect metastases (Shapiro et al. 1985; Shulkin et al. 1987).

The definite surgical removal of all tumor foci is the only way to cure a patient. This succeeds if there are no or only local metastases to the lymph nodes; this occurs in about one out of three patients. For the other patients, radiotherapy and the use of receptor blockers or inhibitors of catecholamine synthesis are able to moderate the symptoms. Unfortunately, cytostatics are of almost no help. Whether the therapeutic use of radiolabeled MIBG or similar substances works merely as a palliative, or whether it leads to recovery is not yet known (Beutter et al. 1987; Bouvier et al. 1987; Grunwald et al. 1988; McDougall 1984). Generally the disease progresses slowly, and survival time is less than 5 years.

References

Beierwaltes WH (1985) A new method of identifying pheochromocytoma and proving that a "mass" is a "Pheo". J Urol 134: 105

Beutter D, Chatal JF, Brunet G, Charbonnel B (1987) Treatment of malignant pheochromocytoma with I-131 metaiodobenzylguanidine. Ann Endocrinol 48: 53–57

Bouvier JF, Maiassi N, Fleury MC, Mornex R, Lahneche BE (1987) Diagnosis and treatment of metastatic pheochromocytomas by I-131 MIBG. Tumour Biol 8: 362–363

Bravo EL, Tarazi RC, Gifford RW, Steward BH (1979) Circulating and urinary catecholamines in pheochromocytoma. N Engl. J. Med. 301: 682–686

Chatal JF, Charbonnel B (1985) Comparison of jodobenzylguanidine imaging with computed tomography in locating pheochromocytoma. J. Clin. Endocrinol Metab 61: 769–772

Cordes U (1985) Nebennierenmark. In: Kümmerle F, Lenner V (eds) Erkrankungen der Nebennieren. Thieme, Stuttgart, pp 96–120

Coupland RE (1965) The natural history of the chromaffin cell. Longmans, Green, London

Coupland RE (1981) Catecholamine secreting tissues. In: Fotherby K, Pal SB (eds) Hormones in normal and abnormal human tissues, De Gruyter, Berlin, pp 589–633

Fink IJ, Reining JW, Dwyer AJ, Doppman JL, Marston-Linehan W, Keiser HR (1985) MR – imaging of pheochromocytomas. J. Comput Assist Tomogr. 9: 454–458

Fischer M, Galanski M, Winterberg B, Vetter H (1985) Localization procedures in pheochromocytoma and neuroblastoma. Cardiology 72 (Suppl 1): 143–146

Fries JG, Chambertin JA (1968) Extra-adrenal pheochromocytoma: literature review and report of a cervical pheochromocytoma. Surgery 63: 268–279

Gauer J.-M, Käser H, Zingg EJ (1988) Klinik, Diagnose und Therapie des Phäochromozytoms. Aktuel Urol 19: 7–12

Gifford RW, Bravo EL, Manger WM (1985) Diagnosis and management of pheochromocytoma. Cardiology 72 (Suppl 1): 126–130

Grunwald F, Ruhlmann J, Kozak B, Overlack A, Christ F, Hotze A, Biersack H (1988) I–131 labeled metaiodobenzylguanidine in the diagnosis and treatment of distant metastases of a pheochromocytoma. Dtsch Med Wochenschr 113: 297–299

Käser H, (1985) Pathophysiologie und Klinik des Phaeochromocytoms und des Phaeochromoblastoms. In: Hauri D, Schmucki O (eds) Erkrankungen der Nebenschilddrüsen und Nebennieren. Fischer, Stuttgart, pp 195–207

Käser, H. (1987) Nebennierenmark-Funktion und -Störungen, In: Ziegler R (ed) Hormon- und Stoffwechselerkrankungen in der Praxis. Edition Medizin, Weinheim- Deerfield-Beach, Basel, pp 345–366

Käser H, Wagner HP (1982) Chromaffin tumors in childhood: experiences with 29 cases. In: Pediatric Oncology. Excerpta Medica, Amsterdam

Labhart A (1971) Das Nebennierenmark. In: Klinik der inneren Sekretion, Springer, Berlin Heidelberg New York

Langmann J (1970) Medizinische Embryologie. Thieme, Stuttgart

Manger WM, Gifford RW (1977) Pheochromocytoma. Springer, Berlin Heidelberg New York

McDougall IR (1984) Malignant pheochromocytoma treated by I–131 MIBG. J. Nucl. Med. 25: 249

Niklaus T (1986) Chromaffine Tumoren im Kindesalter. Inauguraldissertation, University of Berne, Switzerland

Otto R (1983) Die Sonographie der Nieren, der ableitenden Harnwege und der Nebennieren. Schweiz. Rundsch Med Prax 72: 227–232

Plouin PF, Duclos JM, Menard J, Comoy E, Bohuon C, Alexandre JM (1981) Biochemical tests for diagnosis of pheochromocytoma: urinary versus plasma determinations. Br Med J 282: 853–854

Robinson R (1980) Tumours that secrete catecholamines. Wiley, Chichester

Schmedtje JF, Sax S, Pool JL, Goldfarb RA, Nelson EB (1987) Localization of ectopic pheochromocytomas by magnetic-resonance imaging. J Med. 83: 770–772

Shapiro B, Copp JE, Sisson JC, Eyre PL, Beierwaltes WH (1985) 131–I metaiodobenzylguanidine for the locating of suspected pheochromocytoma. Experience in 400 cases. J Nucl Med 26: 576–585

Shulkin BL, Shen SW, Sisson JC, Shapiro B (1987) Iodine–131 MIBG scintigraphy of the extremities in metastatic pheochromocytoma and neuroblastoma. J Nucl Med 28: 315–318

Stenström G, Svärdsudd K (1986) Pheochromocytoma in Sweden 1981–1985. Acta Med Scand 220: 225–232

Sutton MG St J, Sheps SG, Lie JT (1981) Prevalence of clinically unsuspected pheochromocytoma. Review of a 50-year autopsy series. Mayo Clin Proc 56: 354–360

Tippett PA, West RS, McEwan AJ, Middleton JE, Ackery DM (1987) A comparison of dopamine and homovanillic acid excretion, as prognostic indicators in malignant phaeochromocytoma. Clin. Chim. Acta 166: 123–133

Ziegler W (1985) Diagnostik des Phäochromocytoms. In: Hauri D, Schmucki O (eds) Erkrankungen der Nebenschilddrüsen und Nebennieren. Fischer, Stuttgart, pp 208–216

Adrenocortical Tumors: Clinical and Diagnostic Findings

J. Müller

Medizinische Klinik, Universitätsspital, 8091 Zürich, Switzerland

Clinical Classification

From the clinical point of view (Table 1), hormone-secreting adrenocortical tumors are of particular interest because autonomous excessive secretion of steroid hormones causes characteristic clinical syndromes. Thus, excessive production of aldosterone leads to the syndrome of hypermineralocorticoidism and excessive cortisol secretion to Cushing's syndrome, whereas the inappropriate secretion of androgens and estrogens by adrenocortical tumors may cause virilization of female patients (Gabrilove et al. 1981), feminization of male patients (Gabrilove et al. 1965), and precocious puberty in children. If present, inappropriate hormone secretion dominates the clinical picture, leads to elaborate differential diagnostic procedures, and gives an unequivocal indication for the localization and removal of adrenocortical tumors, while the question of malignancy often seems to be of secondary interest. However, approximately half of hormone-producing adrenocortical tumors are malignant, with a great tendency for metastatic spread and often showing a poor response to radiotherapy and chemotherapy.

Metastases may secrete the same hormones as the primary tumors and lead to recurrence of an apparently cured clinical syndrome. In these instances, steroid hormones become tumor markers and can be used for monitoring tumor growth and effectiveness of therapy. Even if active hormones are secreted by an adrenocortical tumor, they do not always lead to endocrine manifestations. Androgen-producing tumors are not clinically apparent in male patients, whereas an estrogen-producing adrenocortical carcinoma may not lead to an endocrine manifestation in a mature woman. Most aldosterone-producing adenomas also produce considerable amounts of cortisol under in vitro conditions but do not generally cause Cushings's syndrome in vivo. Apparently silent adrenocortical carcinomas often produce considerable amounts of inactive precursor steroids, which lead to an increased urinary excretion rate of 17–ketosteroids. Other adrenocortical tumors are completely inactive.

Adrenocortical adenomas are frequently (in approximately 10% of cases) found at autopsy of patients who have never shown any manifestation of steroid

Table 1. Clinical classification of adrenocortical tumors

Excessive hormone production
    Aldosterone-producing adenomas and carcinomas
    Cortisol-producing adenomas and carcinomas
    Androgen-producing adenomas and carcinomas
    Estrogen-producing adenomas and carcinomas
    Mixed-activity steroid-producing adenomas and carcinomas

No excessive hormone production
    Inactive steroid-producing adenomas and carcinomas
    Non – steroid – producing adenomas and carcinomas
    Adrenal metastases
        No endocrine manifestations
        Addison's disease

---

hormone excess (Hedeland et al. 1968). With increasing frequency, nonfunctioning adenomas or carcinomas of the adrenal cortex are incidentally discovered by computed tomography during abdominal scanning for unrelated clinical problems (Belldegrun et al. 1986). In patients without endocrinological abnormality, an adrenal mass of less than 3.5 cm in diameter can be left in situ and controlled by serial computed tomography scans, whereas larger tumors should be removed for pathohistological classification or at least be checked for malignancy by percutaneous fine-needle biopsy. In patients with established extra-adrenal malignant tumors, adrenal masses should always be suspected of metastases. Only in rare instances, bilateral adrenal metastases lead to Addison's disease.

Primary Aldosteronism

Primary aldosteronism (Table 2), i.e., excessive and largely autonomous secretion of aldosterone, is a rare cause of arterial hypertension (less than 0.5% of cases) and is usually characterized by the combination of elevated blood pressure and chronic potassium depletion (Bravo et al. 1983; Vaughan et al. 1981; Weinberger et al. 1979). In approximately two-thirds of all cases, the disorder is due to an aldosterone-producing, generally benign adrenocortical tumor (adenomas 95%, carcinomas 5%). The majority of these cases can be completely cured by unilateral adrenalectomy. In cases without an adrenal tumor, the condition is associated with bilateral diffuse or nodular hyperplasia of the adrenal cortex of unknown etiology. In this so-called idiopathic hyperaldosteronism, blood pressure does not become normalized upon unilateral or bilateral adrenalectomy and must be lowered by a combination of spironolactone and other antihypertensive medication. In a rare, often familial form of primary aldosteronism, i.e., glucocorticoid-suppressible hyperaldosteronism, aldosterone secretion becomes normal under long-term therapy with a glucocorticoid.

Table 2. Primary aldosteronism

Etiology
Aldosterone-producing adenomas (63%)
Aldosterone-producing carcinomas (3%)
Idiopathic hyperaldosteronism (bilateral adrenocortical hyperplasia; 33%)
Glucocorticoid-suppressible hyperaldosteronism (1%)

Main clinical manifestations
Arterial hypertension
Hypokalemia, hyperkaluria, metabolic alkalosis

Differential diagnosis
Essential hypertension treated with diuretics
Malignant hypertension
Renovascular hypertension
Licorice abuse
Ectopic ACTH secretion

Diagnosis
Inappropriately elevated plasma and urinary aldosterone
Suppressed plasma renin activity

Therapy
Aldosterone-producing tumors: unilateral adrenalectomy
Idiopathic hyperaldosteronism: spironolactone combined with other antihypertensive
  medication
Glucocorticoid-suppressible hyperaldosteronism: dexamethasone

---

Primary aldosteronism is suspected when hypokalemia is found in a hypertensive patient. The definite diagnosis is based on the combined finding of inappropriately high plasma levels and/or urinary excretion rates of aldosterone and inappropriately suppressed plasma renin activity. Only if these criteria are met, is a radiological search for an adrenocortical tumor indicated. It must be kept in mind that hypokalemia in a hypertensive patient is most frequently due to diuretic therapy, and that aldosterone-secreting adrenocortical adenomas are rare. Thus, the combination of hypokalemic hypertension with an adrenal adenoma does not prove a causal relationship unless autonomous hypersecretion of aldosterone has been established. In proven primary aldosteronism, lateralization of aldosterone-secreting tumors is generally based on computed tomography and/or scintiscan of the adrenal glands with a radioiodinated cholesterol analogue. Only in rare instance is the catheterization of the adrenal veins indicated for measuring aldosterone in the effluent blood.

Table 3. Etiology of spontaneous Cushing's syndrome

Pituitary-dependent (65%)
  ACTH-producing pituitary adenoma
  Ectopic CRF secretion
  Dysregulation of ACTH secretion (?)

Adrenal (20%)
  Cortisol-producing adrenocortical adenoma (10%)
  Cortisol-producing adrenocortical carcinoma (9%)
  Bilateral nodular adrenocortical dysplasia (1%)

Ectopic ACTH secretion (15%)
  Bronchial carcinoma (7.5%)
  Thymic carcinoma (1.5%), pancreatic carcinoma (1.5%)
  Medullary thyroid carcinoma (0.75%), bronchial carcinoid (0.75%), pheochromocy-
    toma, neuroblastoma (0.75%)
  Other tumors (2.25%)

Cushing's Syndrome

In contrast to primary aldosteronism, Cushing's syndrome is due to an adrenocortical adenoma or carcinoma only in a minority of cases, i.e., in about 20% of adult patients with spontaneous forms of Cushing's syndrome (Table 3). However, in children a cortisol-secreting adrenocortical carcinoma is the most common etiology. According to the contemporary view, the pituitary-dependent form of Cushing's syndrome ('Cushing's disease') is generally caused by a semiautonomous ACTH-secreting pituitary adenoma and not by a hypothalamic disorder of corticotropin-releasing factor (CRF) secretion, as had been previously assumed. Several cases of ectopic CRF secretion by malignant tumors have been reported, but it is still uncertain whether a truly hypothalamic form of the disease exists. Removal of an ACTH-producing microadenoma by transsphenoidal microsurgery is generally followed by a period of secondary adrenocortical failure before a normal cortisol secretion pattern is reestablished after a few months (Fitzgerald et al. 1982). Similarly, the removal of a cortisol-producing adrenocortical tumor is followed by a period of secondary adrenocortical failure. This period may vary from a few days to several years (Müller et al. 1967). Among our patients with a cortisol-producing adrenocortical adenoma, four needed a life-long substitution therapy with cortisone upon unilateral adrenalectomy, although their remaining adrenals were fully responsive to high doses of exogenous ACTH.

    A stepwise approach is recommended for the diagnostic work-up of patients suspected of having Cushing's syndrome (Table 4; Müller 1986). The clinicallly important discrimination between Cushing's syndrome and patients with normal adrenocortical function can be reliably made in ambulatory practice with a simple overnight dexamethasone (1 mg) suppression test. A pathological outcome of this test should be confirmed by a classical 2-day dexamethasone (2 mg per day)

Table 4. Stepwise diagnosis of Cushing's syndrome

Clinical suspicion
  History
  Appearance
  Physical examination

Cushing's syndrome: yes or no?
  Single-dose (1 mg) overnight dexamethasone suppression test
  Two-day 2 mg per day dexamethasone suppression test
  Urinary free cortisol

Established diagnosis of Cushing's syndrome: which form?
  Two-day 8 mg per day dexamethasone suppression test
  Plasma ACTH
  Depending on outcome of above two:
    Computed tomography and/or magnetic resonance imaging of pituitary gland
    Computed tomography and/or scintiscan of adrenal glands
    Search for ectopic ACTH source

Table 5. Androgen excess in women

Manifestations
  Hirsutism
  Acne
  Oligomenorrhea, amenorrhea
  Clitoral hypertrophy
  Deepening of the voice
  Frontal baldness
  Muscular hypertrophy
  Increased libido

Differential diagnosis
  Idiopathic hirsutism
  Polycystic ovary syndrome
  Congenital adrenal hyperplasia (21-hydroxylase deficiency, 11-β-hydroxylase deficiency)
  Androgen-producing ovarian tumors (arrhenoblastoma, Leydig cell adenoma)
  Androgen-producing adrenocortical tumors (adenoma, carcinoma)
  Cushing's syndrome
  Prolactinoma
  Exogenous androgens (anabolics)

Table 6. Hirsutism with or without virilization: diagnostic work-up

---

In all cases
  Serum testosterone
  Urinary 17-ketosteroids (or serum androstenedione and dehydroepiandrosterone)
  Serum prolactin

Only if androgens (serum testosterone and/or urinary 17-ketosteroids) are elevated
  Repeat measurement(s) after 4 days of dexamethasone (2 mg per day in divided doses).
  Elevated androgens unequivocally suppressible by dexamethasone: idiopathic hirsutism,
    polycystic ovary syndrome, congenital adrenal hyperplasia

Only if androgens are elevated and not suppressible
  Search for ovarian or adrenocortical tumor (computed tomography of ovaries and
  adrenals, laparascopy)
Only if serum prolactin is elevated
  Computed tomography of pituitary gland

---

suppression test and by measuring the excretion rate of free urinary cortisol. Only if the diagnosis of Cushing's syndrome has been unequivocally established by these procedures, should a differentiation of the various forms of the syndrome be attempted by a high-dose dexamethasone (8 mg per day) suppression test and by measuring plasma ACTH (Findling and Tyrell 1986; Labhart 1986). Failure of suppression of plasma cortisol and urinary 17-hydroxycorticoids by high doses of dexamethasone and immeasurably low plasma ACTH concentrations characterize the adrenal forms of Cushing's syndrome and require a search for an adrenocortical tumor by radiological methods (sonography, computed tomography, scintiscan).

Virilization

Clinical manifestations of hyperandrogenism in women are listed in Table 5. The most common one among them is hirsutism, which is in most instances due to a constitutional disorder and associated with only a minor abnormality in testosterone production and metabolism not correctable by a surgical intervention (idiopathic hirsutism). In patients with idiopathic hirsutism, treatment with dexamethasone for a few days generally suppresses elevated plasma androgens into the normal range (Table 6). Similarly, elevated plasma androgens and urinary 17-ketosteroids are lowered by dexamethasone in patients with polycystic ovary syndrome or with congenital adrenal hyperplasia (21-hydroxylase or 11-hydroxylase deficiencies). Only elevated plasma androgens and/or urinary 17-ketosteroids not suppressible by dexamethasone justify a search for androgen-producing ovarian or adrenococrtical tumors by sonography, computed tomography, laparascopy and – in exceptional instances – catheterization of the ovarian and adrenal veins for localized plasma androgen determinations.

References

Belldegrun A, Hussain S, Seltzer SE, Loughlin KR, Gittes RF, Richie JP (1986) Incidentally discovered mass of the adrenal gland. Surg Gynecol Obstet 163: 203–208

Bravo EL, Tarazi RC, Dustan HP, Fouad FM, Textor SC, Gifford RW, Vidt DG (1983) The changing clinical spectrum of primary aldosteronism. Am J Med 74: 641–651

Findling JW, Tyrrell JB (1986) Occult ectopic secretion of corticotropin. Arch Intern Med 146: 929–933

Fitzgerald PA, Aron DC, Findling JW, Brooks RM, Wilson CB, Forsham PH, Tyrrell JB (1982) Cushing's disease: transient secondary adrenal insufficiency after selective removal of pituitary microadenomas; evidence for a pituitary origin. J Clin Endocrinol Metab 54: 413–422

Gabrilove JL, Sharma DC, Wotiz HH, Dorfman RI (1965) Feminizing adrenocortical tumors in the male. A review of 52 cases including a case report. Medicine 44: 37–79

Gabrilove JL, Seman AT, Sabet R, Mitty HA, Nicolis GL (1981) Virilizing adrenal adenoma with studies on the steroid content of the adrenal venous effluent and a review of the literature. Endocr Rev 2: 462–470

Hedeland H, Oestberg G, Hökfelt B (1968) On the prevalence of adrenocortical adenomas in an autopsy material in relation to hypertension and diabetes. Act Med Scand 184: 211–214

Labhart A (1986) Clinical endocrinology. Theory and practice, 2nd ed. Springer, Berlin Heidelberg New York London Paris Tokyo

Müller J, Froesch ER, Meyer UA, Labhart A (1967) Persistierende Störung der ACTH-Sekretion nach Operation eines Nebennierenrinden-Adenoms bei drei Fällen von Cushing-Syndrom. Schweiz Med Wochenschr 97: 861–865

Müller J (1986) Cushing-Syndrom 1985: neue Erkenntnisse und Möglichkeiten. Schweiz Med Wochenschr 116: 262–265

Vaughan NJA, Jowett TP, Slater JDH, Wiggins RC, Lightman SL, Ma JTC, Payne NN (1981) The diagnosis of primary hyperaldosteronism. Lancet 1: 120–125

Weinberger MH, Grim CE, Hollifield JW, Kem DC, Ganguly A, Kramer NJ, Yune HY, Wellman H, Donohue JP (1979) Primary aldosteronism. Diagnosis, localization, and treatment. Ann Intern Med 90: 386–395

Contributions of Nuclear Endocrinology to the Diagnosis of Adrenal Tumors*

B. Shapiro, L.M. Fig, M.D. Gross, and F. Khafagi

Division of Nuclear Medicine, University of Michigan Medical Center,
Ann Arbor, MI 48109, USA

Introduction

The scintigraphic evaluation of the adrenal cortex with [^{131}I] 6β-iodomethylnor-cholesterol (NP-59) and the sympathomedullary system with [^{131}I]- or [^{123}I]-metaiodobenzylguanidine (MIBG) provides a unique means of depicting the in vivo functional status of these tissues. This functional depiction is complementary to the high-resolution anatomical studies such as computed tomography (CT), ultrasound and magnetic resonance imaging (MRI; Shapiro et al. 1987; Thrall et al. 1978; McEwan et al. 1985). A fundamental principle is that localizing procedures should be performed only when clinical suspicion has led to the performance of appropriate biochemical testing, the results of which support the diagnosis of an endocrine hypersecretory state.

Radiopharmaceuticals

The clinically useful adrenocortical radiopharmaceuticals are radiolabeled analogs of cholesterol and include [^{131}I]- 6β-iodomethylnorcholesterol (NP-59). [^{75}Se]-6β- selenomethylnorcholesterol (Scintadren), and the older, less suitable [^{131}I]-19-iodocholesterol (Shapiro et al. 1987; Thrall et al. 1978; Shapiro et al. 1981). Like native cholesterol, these radiopharmaceuticals are transported through the circulation bound to low-density lipoproteins (LDL) which in turn bind to specific receptors on cells from which the cholesterol and NP-59 are internalized. The cholesterol is then esterified and forms a pool of substrate for all adrenal steroid synthesis (a minor fraction of cholesterol is synthesized in situ). NP-59 is esterified but not further metabolized into steroid hormone analogs (Shapiro et al. 1987; Thrall et al. 1978). Substrate LDL cholesterol and NP-59 uptake are influenced by

* Supported by grants NCI (CA-09015), NIAMDD (R01-AM 21477RAD), GCRC (HEW3M01-RR-0042-21CLR), NIH(R01-CA-43300), the Veterans Administration Research Service, and the Nuclear Medicine Research Fund.

adrenocortical secretogogues (e.g., ACTH and angiotensin II increase while dex-amethasone and op DDD reduce tracer uptake; Shapiro et al. 1987; Thrall et al. 1978). Biliary excretion of NP-59 and its metabolic products often results in significant gut activity which may interfere with adrenal visualization (Lynn et al. 1986; Shapiro et al. 1983). The use of laxatives eliminates this and improves the quality of studies (Lynn et al. 1986; Shapiro et al 1983).

MIBG is an analog of the endogenous neurotransmitter and hormone norepin-ephrine and shares its energy- and sodium-dependent specific uptake mechanism (type 1 uptake; Shapiro et al. 1984b). (A fraction also enters cells by a nonspecific diffusional mechanism; Shapiro et al. 1984b). Once MIBG enters the cell, it is concentrated into the intracellular hormone storage vesicles by an energy-depend-ent specific process distinct from the cell membrane type 1 uptake mechanism (Shapiro et al. 1984b; Sisson et al. 1987b). Thus, drugs which inhibit type 1 uptake (cocaine and tricyclic antidepressants), interfere with vesicular storage (reserpine), or displace intracellular amines (amphetamines and phenylpropanolamine) are all contraindicated if MIBG scintigraphy is to succeed (Shapiro et al. 1984b; Sisson et al. 1987b). Ordinary β-adrenergic blockers, minor tranquillizers, diuretics, and ACE inhibitors do not influence MIBG biodistribution (Shapiro et al. 1984b). The majority of MIBG is excreted by the kidneys in unchanged form, although minor degrees of deiodination and other metabolism occur (Mangner et al. 1986).

The usual doses of NP-59 is 1 mCi and that of [^{131}I]-MIBG 0.5–1.0 mCi; the radiation dosimetry (Lynn et al. 1984; Carey et al. 1979; Swanson et al. 1981) is presented in Tables 1 and 2. The favorable gamma ray energy, half-life of 13 h, and mode of decay by electron capture mean that [^{123}I] is a very suitable label for MIBG. A dose of 10 mCi may be administered for a radiation dose no greater than that from 0.5 mCi [^{131}I]-MIBG (Lynn et al. 1984).

In both NP-59 and MIBG scintigraphy the thyroid gland radiation dosimetry may be minimized by the administration of iodides (e.g., SSKI 1 drop t.i.d. for 1 or 2 days before tracer administration and for 1 week thereafter; Lynn et al. 1984; Carey et al. 1979; Swanson et al. 1981). Alternative thyroid-blocking regimens have also been used (e.g., thyroxine and perchlorate). When NP-59 scintigraphy is

Table 1. Radiation dosimetry of [^{131}I] - 6β-iodomethyl-19-norcholesterol (NP-59). (From Carey et al. 1979)

Organ	Rad/mCi
Total Body	1.2
Adrenal	26.0[a]
Ovary	8.0[a]
Testes	2.3[a]
Liver	2.4

[a] A 50% decrease is seen on dexamethasone suppression.

Table 2. Estimated radiation-absorbed doses from $[^{131}I]$- and $[^{123}I]$ MIBG, estimated human dosimetry. (From Swanson et al. 1981)

Organs	Maximal uptake "pure" (% kg dose/g)	Time of maximal uptake (h)	rad/mCi		
			$[^{131}I]$MIBG	$[^{123}I]$MIBG	Contaminated $[^{123}I]$MIBG
Thyroid	3.40	24.0	35	2.20	2.55
Adrenal medulla	13.60	48.0	100	0.80	2.76
Heart wall	0.50	0.5	0.7	0.03	0.04
Liver	0.36	0.5	0.4	0.05	0.05
Spleen	0.30	0.5	1.6	0.14	0.15
Ovaries	0.14	2.0	1.0	0.06	0.07
Total body			0.1	0.02	0.02

performed in the face of dexamethasone administration, the absorbed radiation dose is halved (Lynn et al. 1984; Carey et al. 1979).

The Scintigraphy of Adrenocortical Disorders

The three main hypersecretory disorders of the adrenal cortex arise from the three functional zones of this organ: and are primary aldosteronism, Cushing's syndrome and adrenal hyperandrogenism (Nelson 1980).

Primary Aldosteronism

Aldosterone is the principal mineralocorticoid and is secreted from the outermost zone, the zona glomerulosa (Nelson 1980). Its secretion is modulated by the renin-angiotensin and atrial-naturetic factor systems. Autonomous aldosterone secretion is characterized by renal sodium retention and potassium and hydrogen ion wasting which leads to hypertension, hypokalemia, and alkalosis with elevated aldosterone and suppressed plasma renin activity levels (Weinberger et al. 1979). This syndrome may result from a tumor (almost always an adrenocortical adenoma) or bilateral hyperplasia. About 75% of cases are due to adenoma and 25% to hyperplasia. Because adenomas are best treated by surgical extirpation and hyperplasia by aldosterone antagonists, it is important to identify the causative pathology prior to therapy (Weinberger et al. 1979; Gross et al. 1984a). Adrenocortical carcinoma causing primary aldosteronism is very rare (Weinberger et al. 1979; Gross et al. 1984a).

NP-59 scintigraphy has proven efficacious in the location of abnormal tissue in primary aldosteronism (Gross et al. 1984a). Because the adenomas are often small, typically 1.6–1.8 cm, the sensitivity of NP-59 scintigraphy can often be enhanced by dexamethasone suppression (Conn et al. 1976). Dexamethasone by suppressing ACTH reduces NP-59 uptake into the glucocorticoid synthesizing layer, the zona fasciculata, and thus permits the detection of small (dexamethasone-nonsuppressible) adenomas because the background uptake in the remainder of the adrenal is reduced (Conn et al. 1976). Dexamethasone (1 mg q.i.d.) is administered for 7 days prior to NP-59 administration and continued through the imaging interval. Images are obtained at 3, 4, 5, and if necessary 7 days following injection (Gross et al. 1984a; Conn et al. 1976). In the face of dexamethasone suppression the normal adrenal cortex is not visualized before the 5th day, while adenomas are depicted by early (prior to the 5th day) unilateral imaging, and bilateral hyperplasia as bilateral early imaging (Gross et al. 1984a; Conn et al. 1976). Bilateral adrenal imaging on or after the 5th day in a patient with biochemically confirmed primary aldosteronism is nondiagnostic and is fortunately rare (Gross et al. 1984a; Conn et al. 1976).

In addition to observing these characteristic patterns of imaging the adrenals, NP-59 uptake may be quantified using a semi – operator – independent computer algorithm and measurements of adrenal depth (for attenuation) on a lateral image (Koral and Sarkar 1977). Although such quantification may only add slight, if any, improvement in diagnostic accuracy (Gross et al. 1985a), these data have been used to show that NP-59 uptake in primary aldosteronism (due to both adenomas and bilateral hyperplasia), is proportional to the degree of aldosterone hypersecretion (Gross et al. 1983).

When the efficacy of NP-59 scintigraphy for the characterization and localization of the causative lesion in primary aldosteronism is compared to other available modalities, the following conclusions may be drawn (Shapiro et al. 1987; Gross et al. 1984a):

1. Intravenous urography (with and without nephrotomography), retroperitoneal air insufflation, and arteriography are obsolete.
2. Venography with venous sampling is invasive, technically demanding, and has a significant failure rate.
3. Given the small size of many of the lesions, ultrasound is insensitive.
4. CT scanning is efficacious but requires meticulous attention to detail, and thin sections and may fail in lesions smaller than 1.0 cm. Furthermore, the diagnosis of bilateral adrenal hyperplasia is often made by exclusion, in that the morphological abnormalities are not delineated by CT (Gross et al. 1984a). A recent review of many series of CT scans yielded an average sensitivity of 68% and average specificity of 66% although experienced radiologists with modern equipment may achieve sensitivity of 85% and specificity of 94% (Gross et al. 1984a).
5. MRI, while having a potential for tissue characterization and not subjecting the patient to ionizing radiation, has not been shown to be superior to CT (Shapiro et al. 1987).
6. NP-59 scintigraphy when performed with dexamethasone suppression is equal or superior to CT and has the advantage of frequently permitting the positive diagnosis of bilateral hyperplasia to be made (Gross et al. 1984a). A recent

Table 3. Localization in primary aldosteronism: results of dexamethasone scintigraphy. (From Gross et al. 1984a)

Reference	Total scans	Adenoma	Hyperplasia	Localization[a]	Specificity[b]
Dige-Petersen et al. 1975	4	3	1	3 (100%)	1/1 (100%)
Conn et al. 1976	37	25	12	21 (84%)	11/12 (92%)
Troncone 1980	8	7	—	7 (87%)	—
Ryo et al. 1978	7	5	2	5 (100%)	2/2 (100%)
Freitas et al. 1979	20	10	10	9 (90%)	9/10 (90%)
Weinberger et al. 1979	18	13	5	6 (47%)	2/7 (28%)
Miles et al. 1979	17	9	8	9 (100%)	8/8 (100%)
Herf et al. 1979	11	8	3	8 (100%)	3/3 (100%)
Leger et al. 1981	42	22	20	17 (77%)	19/19 (100%)
Hoefnagel et al. 1981	10	9	—	8 (89%)	—
Guerin et al. 1983	44	18	26	15 (83%)	24/26 (92%)
Gross et al. 1984a	87	50	37	48 (96%)	35/37 (94%)
Total	305	179	126	88%	90%

[a] Total number of adrenal cortical adenomas localized/total number of adrenal cortical adenomas.

[b] Total number of bilateral adrenal hyperplasia patterns/total number of bilateral adrenal hyperplasia + false positive results.

review of many series yielded an average sensitivity of 87% and average specificity of 89% (Gross et al. 1984a; see Table 3). This is compared to a sensitivity of 68% and specificity of 63% if studies are performed without dexamethasone suppression (Gross et al. 1984a).

Thus, we recommend dexamethasone NP-59 scintigraphy as the primary imaging modality for primary aldosteronism, with CT being used in complementary fashion to solve the problem of equivocal scintigraphy or to provide confirmation. Where NP-59 is not readily available, we advocate the reverse sequence of studies (Shapiro et al. 1987; Gross et al. 1984a).

Cushings's Syndrome

Cortisol, the glucocorticoid steroid hormone in man, is secreted principally from the zona fasiculata (Nelson 1980). The modulation of cortisol secretion is under the control of pituitary ACTH which is itself the cleavage product of a larger parent peptide, proopiomelanocortin, and is itself controlled by hypothalamic corticotrophin-releasing factor (CRF). The CRF-ACTH axis serves as a common pathway for integrating a large number of factors influencing cortisol secretion. The most important of these is a negative feedback loop in which cortisol inhibits ACTH and CRF secretion. Other factors include a normal diurnal rhythm and responses to psychic stress, hypotension, hypoglycemia, pyrexia, and pain (Shapiro et al. 1987; Thrall et al. 1978; Scott et al. 1984; Chrousos 1985).

An excessive secretion of cortisol results in Cushing's syndrome, which results in a characteristic constellation of effects, including glucose intolerance, obesity and fat redistribution, negative nitrogen balance (e.g., muscle wasting, skin atrophy, striae, and osteoporosis), and psychological effects (Scott et al. 1984; Chrousos 1985).

This excessive secretion may arise from: (a) primary adrenal lesions (e.g., adenomas), (b) orthotopic ACTH hypersecretion (Cushing's disease), (c) ectopic ACTH secretion, or (d) very rarely, ectopic CRF secretion (Scott et al. 1984; Chrousos 1985). In the cases of b, c, and d there is a symmetrical bilateral stimulation of both adrenal cortexes which leads to bilateral hyperplasia, the severity of which is proportional to the strength of the stimulus (Shapiro et al. 1987; Thrall et al. 1978; Miles et al. 1979). The symmetrical bilateral hyperplasia is depicted as symmetrical increased NP-59 uptake (Shapiro et al. 1987; Thrall et al. 1978; Miles et al. 1979). These studies are typically performed without dexamethasone suppression, and images are obtained 5 or 7 days following tracer injection (Shapiro et al. 1987; Thrall et al. 1978; Miles et al. 1979). The adrenal NP-59 uptake may be quantified, and the level of uptake is proportional to the degree of cortisol hypersecretion (as evaluated by urinary free cortisol excretion rate; Gross et al. 1981). While the highest uptakes are encountered in the ectopic ACTH syndrome, there is considerable overlap between types (Gross et al. 1981). Thus, for those forms of Cushing's syndrome with elevated ACTH levels, localization efforts are best directed towards the sites of the trophic hormone production (e.g., CT of pituitary, lung, and other potential sites of ectopic ACTH secretion; Shapiro et al 1987; Thrall et al. 1978). The exception may be the now decreasingly important group of patients who have been subjected to previous adrenalectomy, and in whom postoperative remnants of adrenal tissue are sought (Shapiro et al. 1987; Thrall et al. 1978; Miles et al. 1979).

The main utility of NP-59 scintigraphy in Cushing's syndrome is in primary adrenal lesions in which ACTH is suppressed (ACTH-independent Cushing's syndrome). The commonest cause is benign, unilateral adenoma which gives rise to a highly characteristic pattern of NP-59 uptake with intense uptake in the lesion and no uptake on the contralateral side (due to the suppression of ACTH stimulation; Shapiro et al. 1987; Thrall et al. 1978; Miles et al. 1979). Because most of these adenomas are relatively large (2–5 cm), they are also well-depicted by CT scanning. Both NP-59 scintigraphy and CT have close to 100% sensitivity in this setting (see Table 4).

Less frequently, the causative lesion is a carcinoma. These are usually large (5–10 cm or larger), are readily located by CT, and on NP-59 scintigraphy show a pattern of no visible adrenal uptake because normal adrenocortical tissue is suppressed, and the per gram uptake of NP-59 is so low that the lesion itself is not visualized. Occasionally, well-differentiated carcinomas are visualized like adenomas, and minimal uptake has been reported in some metastases, although this is exceptional. The least common but most problematic type of Cushing's syndrome is ACTH-independent bilateral cortical nodular hyperplasia (AIBCNH)

Table 4. Localization in ACTH-independent Cushing's syndrome: results of scintigraphy

Reference	Agent	Adenoma	Carcinoma[a]	CNH
Ryo et al. 1978	19-IC/NP-59	7/7		
Sarkar et al. 1977	NP-59	3/3		
Dunnick et al. 1979	NP-59	3/3		
Miles et al. 1979	NP-59	2/2		1/1
Leger et al. 1981	75-Se	7/7	3/3	
Shapiro et al. 1982b	75-Se			1/1
Baba et al. 1982	19-IC/NP-59	5/5		4/4
Guerin et al. 1983	19-IC/NP-59	6/6	5/5	
Joffe and Brown 1983	75-Se			2/2
Watson et al. 1985	75-Se	6/6		
Sudell et al. 1985	75-Se		3/3	2/2
Sarkar et al. 1987	NP-59	7/7		4/4
Total		46/46[b]	11/11[b]	14/14[b]

19-IC, 19-iodocholestol; 75-Se,[^{75}Se] selenomethylnorcholesterol; CNH, cortical nodular hyperplasia.
[a] Characteristic pattern of bilateral nonvisualization in a patient with an adrenal mass.
[b] Correctly localized/total studied.

which contributes about 10% of cases (Shapiro et al. 1987; Thrall et al. 1978; Miles et al. 1979; Joffe and Brown 1983). The NP-59 scintigraphic pattern is one of bilateral adrenal tracer uptake which is often assymmetrical, and which clearly depicts the bilateral nature of the disease process (Shapiro et al. 1987; Thrall et al. 1978; Miles et al. 1979; Fig et al. 1987). CT scanning which relies on morphology alone frequently (up to 40% of cases) incorrectly depicts only the larger nodule on one side as "an adenoma" rather than the bilateral nature of the process (Fig et al. 1987). This can lead, incorrectly, to unilateral rather than bilateral, curative, adrenalectomy.

In our experience with ACTH-independent Cushing's syndrome we have found that NP-59 correctly yields the characteristic patterns described above in all 100% of 24 patients (6 AIBCNH). CT was correct in all cases of adenoma and carcinoma but in only one of four AIBCNH cases so studied (Fig et al. 1987).

MRI at the present time, does not appear to offer an obvious advantage over CT or NP-59, except for the lack of ionizing radiation (Shapiro et al. 1987).

Adrenal Hyperandrogenism

The innermost layer of the adrenal cortex, the zona reticularis, is the main site of adrenal androgen secretion (Nelson 1980). These hormones include androstenedione and dehydroepiandrosterone (DHEA) which are biologically weak androgens secreted in relatively large quantities and responsible for secondary sexual hair growth in women. The secretion of these androgens is partly modulated by ACTH

and possibly by leutinizing hormone. Adrenal hyperandrogenism leads to virilization and hirsuitism in women (Givens 1976). This is occasionally due to unilateral
autonomous adrenal adenomas but more frequently to bilateral adrenal hyperplasia (Givens 1976). The latter may be due to classical or late-onset adrenal
hyperplasia due to various defects in adrenal hormone synthetic pathways (e.g.,
21-hydroxylase deficiency), or it may be associated in some patients with ovarian
androgen hypersecretion as part of the polycystic ovarian syndrome.

Studies are performed with dexamethasone suppression, and the patterns of
imaging are exactly analogous to those encountered in primary aldosteronism. As
is the case with mineralocorticoid and glucocorticoid hypersecretion, the adrenal
uptake of NP-59 has been shown to be proportional to an index of adrenal
androgen secretion (17-OH steroid excretion; Gross et al. 1984b).

A number of cases of ovarian androgen secreting tumors and ovarian hyper-
thecosis have been depicted by NP-59 scintigraphy of the pelvis (Gross et al.
1985b).

If this is attempted, potential interference by radioactivity in the feces must be
considered, and adequate bowel preparation with laxatives and enemas is required
(Gross et al. 1985b).

The Problem of the Incidentally Discovered Adrenal Mass Lesion

The wide application of high-resolution anatomical imaging with CT, and to a
lesser extent MRI and ultrasound, has given rise to what is perhaps the most
vexing problem in the study of the adrenal gland. This is the incidental discovery of
an adrenal mass lesion (incidentaloma) in a patient with no clinical features of a
hypersecretory adrenocortical or adrenomedullary syndrome (Copeland 1983).
The commonest indications for the original CT scan are abdominal pain or the
diagnosis and staging of tumors. In the latter case the question of possible
metastasis is critical in that, if present, the disease is systemic and incurable
(Copeland 1983).

Both metastases to and primary carcinoma of the adrenal as well as adrenal
hypersecretory syndromes are relatively rare, but incidentalomas are surprisingly
common and observed in 1%–5% of patients. The vast majority of lesions are
benign "nonfunctional" adrenocortical adenomas. Neither the CT or MRI characteristics of such lesions are sufficiently specific to distinguish their nature (Copeland 1983). Thus, following screening biochemical studies to diagnose any sub-
clinical endocrine hypersecretory states, two approaches have been taken: (a)
excision of all lesions greater than 5 cm (because of the risk of cancer) and in
lesions of less than 5 cm serial CT scans with excision of lesions that show growth;
and (b) percutaneous needle biopsy that may permit the diagnosis of metastasis
but cannot readily distinguish normal from neoplastic adrenal cortex (Berkman et
al. 1984). Furthermore the latter procedure is invasive and carries a low but
significant morbidity.

We have thus sought to characterize adrenal incidentalomas by means of NP-
59 scintigraphy (Gross et al. 1987). Studies of unilateral lesions using baseline,

unsuppressed NP-59 scintigraphy now number over 100 cases and have revealed three imaging patterns (Gross et al. 1987):

1. "Concordant lesions" in which there was increased NP-59 uptake on the side of the CT abnormality. Every instance in which the mass was 2 cm or larger was due to "nonfunctioning" adrenocortical adenomas which concentrate NP-59 but do not hypersecrete any hormone.
2. "Discordant lesions" in which there was decreased, absent, or distorted NP-59 uptake on the side of the CT abnormality have, in many instances in which the lesion is 2 cm or larger, been associated with destructive lesions, including adrenocortical cancers, lymphomas, metastasis, and hemorrhages.
3. "Nondiagnostic studies" in which NP-59 uptake was within the normal range of assymmetry. If the mass is 2 cm in diameter or greater such a pattern strongly suggested that the lesion was a pseudoadrenal mass (e.g., a renal, pancreatic, or para-adrenal lesion). In lesions less than 2 cm in diameter the somewhat limited resolution of NP-59 scintigraphy may lead to this pattern in the face of both destructive lesions and nonfunctioning adrenocortical adenomas.

Thus, although results are preliminary, we believe NP-59 scintigraphy has an important role to play in the management of so-called "incidentalomas" (Gross et al. 1987).

The Scintigraphy of Sympathomedullary and Other Neuroendocrine Tumors

Diagnostic [^{131}I]MIBG scintigraphy is performed following the intravenous injection of 0.5 mCi [^{131}I]MIBG per 1.73 m^2 body surface area to a maximum of 0.5 mCi (Shapiro et al. 1982a; McEwan et al 1985). More recently 1.0 mCi per 1.73 m^2 body surface area to a maximum of 1.0 mCi has been used in patients with known or suspected metastatic disease or obesity.

Images are usually obtained for 100 000 counts or 20 min imaging time 1, 2, and 3 days after injection. Multiple overlapping views are obtained to include the head, neck, chest, abdomen, and pelvis including the proximal femurs (Shapiro et al. 1982a, 1987, McEwan et al. 1985)

Anatomic location of abnormal foci of MIBG uptake is provided by liberal use of radioactive markers on shoulders, costal margins, and iliac crests (Shapiro et al. 1982a, 1987, McEwan et al. 1985). Simultaneous images of the kidney and bladder (^{99m}Tc-labeled DTPA), skeleton (^{99m}Tc-labeled methylenediphosphonate), blood pool (^{99m}Tc-labeled red blood cells), liver and spleen (^{99m}Tc-labeled sulfur colloid), and myocardium (^{201}Tl) may also be helpful (Shapiro et al. 1984c). The images are presented in analog form on film or digitized (with or without moderate background subtraction), and the simultaneously acquired images of other systems may be superimposed on or subtracted from the MIBG image (McEwan et al. 1985; Shapiro et al. 1982a, 1984c, 1987).

Normal MIBG distribution in man includes uptake by a number of sympathetically innervated structures including the salivary glands, nasopharynx, heart, and spleen, as well as uptake in the liver and excretion through the urinary tract (Nakajo et al. 1983a). Cardiac MIBG uptake is reduced in the presence of the hypercatecholaminemia of pheochromocytoma (Nakajo et al. 1983b). Due to their small size and the unfavorable imaging characteristics of ^{131}-I the normal adrenal medullae are visualized in only a minority of subjects (fewer than 20%), and this tends to be faint and seen only on the 2nd and 3rd postinjection days (Nakajo et al. 1983a); faint imaging at 24 h was not initially observed (Nakajo et al. 1983a) but is now recognized to occur very occasionally. The lung bases and colon are occasionally visualized, and recent studies have shown the colonic activities to result from fecal radioactivity (Nakajo et al. 1983a).

Any focal accumulation of tracer other than those described must be considered to be abnormal (Shapiro et al. 1982a 1987, McEwan et al. 1985; Nakajo et al. 1983a). Some abnormal tumorous uptake of MIBG becomes evident only at 2 or 3 days.

Diagnostic studies with [^{123}I]MIBG utilize 3–10 mCi and imaging at 2–4 h, 17–20 h, and in some cases 40–48 h postinjection (McEwan et al. 1985; Lynn et al. 1984, 1985). Multiple overlapping views of 10–15 min each are acquired (Lynn et al. 1984, 1985). Single photon-emission computed tomography (SPECT) may also be performed, typically using a rotating gamma camera, 64 projections over 360° at 15–20 s per projection (Lynn et al. 1985). Images are then reconstructed as transaxial, sagittal, and coronal sections. In addition, examination of the rotating cine image may be helpful (Lynn et al. 1984, 1985).

When compared to [^{131}I]MIBG we have found [^{123}I]MIBG to provide a far more useful photon flux resulting in a clearer depiction of normal structures, including the normal adrenal medullae in most subjects. Lesion detection is. enhanced, and SPECT may offer some further advantages over planar imaging (Lynn et al. 1984, 1985).

In the 8 years since MIBG scintigraphy was introduced for the location of pheochromocytomas, its role has been established for: (a) sporadic intra-adrenal (Shapiro et al. 1985; McEwan et al. 1985; Shapiro 1987, 1988), (b) sporadic extra-adrenal (cervical, thoracic, abdominal, and pelvic; Shapiro et al. 1984c, 1985, 1987; McEwan et al. 1985; Shapiro 1987, 1988), and (c) familial pheochromocytomas including those associated with multiple endocrine neoplasia (MEN) types 2a and 2b (Valk et al. 1981; Sisson et al. 1984a), neurofibromatosis (Kalff et al. 1982); von Hippel-Lindau disease (Shapiro et al. 1985; Shapiro 1987, 1988), and simple familial pheochromocytoma (Shapiro 1987, 1988; Kalff et al. 1982). In adrenal medullary hyperplasia, which precedes frank pheochromocytoma in the MEN 2 syndromes, increased adrenal medullary uptake of [^{131}I]MIBG was frequently observed, although in some individuals this may overlap with the uptake which was occasionally seen in normal subjects (Nakajo et al. 1983a; Valk et al. 1981). And finally (d) its role has been established in the location of benign lesions and metastatic deposits (including lymph node, liver, lung, and the most frequent site, bone; Shapiro et al. 1984a). The pathophysiology of pheochromocytoma is primarily related to the hypersecretion of the hormones norepinephrine and epinephrine which lead to hypertension (sustained or paroxysmal), tachycardia, headache, sweating, chest pain, and anxiety (Manger and Gifford 1982). The ability to accurately depict the location and extent of pheochromocytoma is essential because surgical extirpation is the only curative therapy (Manger and Gifford 1982; Bravo and Gifford 1984). MIBG scintigraphy provides a safe noninvasive procedure to screen the entire body for pheochromocytoma deposits which can arise from chromaffin tissue anywhere from the base of the skull to the pelvic floor (Shapiro et al. 1982a, 1985 1987; McEwan et al. 1985). The largest component of the system (and commonest site of pheochromocytoma) is the adrenal medulla (Shapiro et al. 1985; Shapiro 1987, 1988; Manger and Gifford 1982). MIBG scintigraphy is especially useful for extra-adrenal and metastatic disease, for which CT is less successful (Shapiro et al. 1984a, 1987; McEwan et al. 1985; Shulkin et al. 1986a). Adrenal lesions are readily disclosed by both CT and MIBG (Shapiro et al. 1985, 1987; McEwan et al. 1985). MRI is of interest in that

Table 5. University of Michigan experience: results of [^{131}-I-]MIBG scintigraphy for suspected pheochromocytoma by cases (1980–1988). (From Shapiro 1987, 1988)

	Total	True Positive	True Negative	False Positive	False Negative
Sporadic intra-adrenal pheochromo-cytoma	47	44	0	0	3
Sporadic extra-adrenal abdominal pheochromocytoma	15	13	0	0	2
Sporadic extra-adrenal thoracic pheochromocytoma	11 (1 malig)	11	0	0	0
Sporadic extra-adrenal cervical pheochromocytoma	3	2	0	0	1
Sporadic malignant pheochromo-cytoma	71	64	0	0	7
Familial syndromes MEN 2a and 2b	39 (2 malig)	23	15	0	1
Neurofibromatosis	17 (1 malig)	9	8	0	0
von Hippel-Lindau Disease	4 (1 malig)	3	0	0	1
Simple Familial	10 (5 malig)	5	4	0	1
Unknown site	6	0	0	0	6
"False positive"[a]	4	0	0	4	0
Pheochromocytoma excluded[b]	700	0	700	0	0
Total	927	174	727	4	22

[a] Suspected pheochromocytoma with positive scan were subsequently shown to have been due to one case each of: retroperitoneal secretory granule containing atypical schwannoma, metastatic choriacarcinoma, and probable dilated renal pelvis.
[b] Non diagnostically elevated catecholamines but negative radiology and follow-up or negative scan and entirely normal biochemistry.

Table 6. Comparison of results of [^{131}-I-]MIBG scintigraphy for suspected pheochromocytoma. (From Shapiro 1987, 1988)

Study/Reference	Number	TP	FP	TN	FN	Sens	Spec	−PDA	+PDA	Prevalence
Michigan: most recent summary of data by cases	927	174	4	727	22	88	99	97	98	20
Michigan: most recent summary of data by studies	1109	312	4	768	25	93	99	97	99	30
Michigan: previously published experience (Shapiro 1987)	600	152	3	424	21	88	99	95	98	29
Michigan: previously published experience (Shapiro et al. 1987)	475	124	3	329	19	87	99	95	97	30
Combined German series (Anonymous 1983)	191	56	1	126	8	88	99	94	98	34
Combined French series[a] (Chatal and Charbonnel 1985)	99	42	2	51	4	91	96	95	92	46
Southampton, UK (Ackery et al. 1984)	46	21	1	21	3	88	95	88	95	52
Mayo Clinic, USA (Swensen et al 1985)	42	15	1	22	4	79	96	85	94	45
Tours, France (Baulieu et al. 1984)	27	8	1	17	1	89	94	94	89	33

TP, True positive; FP, false positive; TN, true negative; FN, false negative; Sens, sensitivity; Spec, specificity; −PDA, negative predictive accuracy; +PDA, positive predictive accuracy.
[a] Equivocal negative added to true negative and equivocal positive added to true positive.

most pheochromocytomas have high signal intensity on T_2-weighted imaging (Shapiro et al. 1987).

The overall experience at the University of Michigan is presented in Table 5, and this is compared to the results of other institutions in Table 6.

Table 7. University of Michigan experience: results of [^{123}-I-]MIBG scintigraphy. (From Shapiro 1987)

	Total	True[b] positive	True negative	False positive	False negative
Primary pheochromocytoma	5	5[c] (Bilateral adrenal, 2 left atrial, 2 pararenal)	0	0	0
Locally recurrent pheochromocytoma	2	2 (abdominal, left atrial)	0	0	0
Malignant pheochromocytoma	11	11	0	0	0
Pheochromocytoma excluded	5	0	5[d] (3 following successful tumor resection, 2 essential hypertension)	0	0
Normal volunteers	12[a]				
Pharmacological intervention	7[e]				
Autonomic neuropathy	5[f]				

[a] Data previously presented in Shapiro (1987).

[b] In every instance without exception all the lesions depicted by [^{131}I]MIBG were more clearly depicted by [^{123}I]MIBG. In nine cases single photon-emission computed tomography revealed diagnostic information not appreciated from planar views.

[c] In two cases [^{123}I]MIBG depicted lesions not revealed by [^{131}I]MIBG scintigraphy. One pararenal and one left atrial lesion were clearly depicted.

[d] The normal adrenal medullae were scintigraphically depicted in 11 of 16 patients still having adrenal glands. In five of the remaining patients multiple intra-abdominal tumor deposits taking up [^{123}I]MIBG could not be differentiated from the normal adrenal medullae.

[e] In normal volunteers the adrenal medullae and sympathetic innervation of the heart were clearly depicted. Tricyclic antidepressants (four subjects) and the sympathomimetic drug phenylpropranolamine (three subjects) strikingly reduced cardiac [^{123}I]MIBG uptake.

[f] Cardiac [^{123}I]MIBG uptake was markedly reduced in cases of autonomic neuropathy (including diabetic autonomic neuropathy, Shy-Drager Syndrome, and idiopathic autonomic neuropathy).

Table 8. Comparison of results of [131I]MIBG scintigraphy for suspected neuroblastoma. (From Shapiro 1987, 1988)

Study/Reference	Number	TP	FP	TN	FN	Sens	Spec	−PDA	+PDA	Prevalence
Michigan: most recent summary of data by cases (Shapiro 1988)	63	45	2	9	7	87	82	56	83	83
Michigan: most recent summary of data by studies (Shapiro 1988)	96	68	4	14	10	87	78	58	94	81
Michigan: previously published experience (Shapiro 1987)	45	32	0	5	8	80	100	39	100	89
Michigan: previously published experience (Geatti et al. 1985)	10	9	0	0	1	90	—	—	100	100
Amsterdam, Holland (Hoefnagel et al. 1987)	26	21	0	4	1	95	100	80	100	85
Villejuif, France (Lumbroso et al. 1985)[a]	24	14	0	4	6	70	100	40	100	83
Philadelphia, USA (Hattner et al. 1984)[b]	19	8	2	3	6[c]	57	60	60	80	74
Copenhagen, Denmark (Munkner 1985)	16	12	0	0	4	75	—	—	100	100
Tübingen, FRG (Feine et al. 1984)	5	4	0	1	0	100	100	100	100	80

TP True positive; FP false positive; TN true negative; FN false negative; Sens sensitivity; Spec specificity; −PDA negative predictive accuracy; +PDA positive predictive accuracy.

[a]Majority of studies performed with 123-I-MIBG.

[b]19 listed sites of disease in 13 patients.

[c]In four cases tumor was present but had matured to ganglioneuroma or ganglioneuroblastoma.

The results with [^{123}I]MIBG are far more limited but are presented in Table 7. When available on a regular basis [^{123}I]MIBG must be considered superior to [^{131}I]MIBG but the cost and logistical problems in its supply limit its use (Lynn et al. 1984, 1985).

Detailed anatomical relationships of abnormal foci of MIBG uptake can be derived from MIBG-directed CT, MRI, and occasionally arteriography (Shapiro et al. 1984a, c, 1987; McEwan et al. 1985; Glowniak et al. 1985; Francis et al. 1983).

Following the initial success with the depiction of pheochromocytomas attention was directed towards neuroblastomas, which are highly lethal, and important childhood tumors derived from the sympathomedullary system (Jaffe 1976). The efficacy of [^{131}I]MIBG in neuroblastoma is similar to that in pheochromocytoma (Geatti et al. 1985; Treuner et al. 1984; Lumbroso et al. 1985; Shulkin and Shapiro 1988). The University of Michigan experience is depicted and compared to that of other investigators (Shapiro 1987, 1988; Shulkin and Shapiro 1988) in Table 8. Because of the predilection of neuroblastoma to spread to bone and bone marrow it is important to include the limbs in the scintigraphic field (Shulkin et al. 1987). In the majority of cases MIBG scintigraphy depicts the extent of disease as accurately as a combination of all other imaging modalities (CT, ultrasound, and bone scan; Geatti et al. 1985; Treuner et al. 1984; Lumbroso et al. 1985; Shulkin

Table 9. University of Michigan experience: results of [^{131}I]MIBG scintigraphy in neuroendocrine tumors other than pheochromocytomas and neuroblastoma (1980–1988). (From Shapiro 1987, 1988)

Tumor type	Total number studied	[^{131}I]MIBG positive	% [^{131}I]MIBG positive
Carcinoids	10	4	40
Nonsecretory paraganglioma	3	3	100
Chemodectoma (carotid body tumor)	5	2	40
Sporadic MCT[b]	7	1	14
Multiple endocrine neoplasia types 2a and 2b associated MCT[a]			
Cases with elevated calcitonin	12	1	8
Cases with normal calcitonin	8	0	0
Cases with unavailable calcitonin	6	0	0
Oat cell carcinoma of lung	4	0	0
Metastatic choriocarcinoma	1	1	100
Atypical schwannoma[a]	1	1	100
Merkel cell skin cancer	1	1	100
Islet cell tumor of pancreas	4	1[b]	25
Undifferentiated neuroendocrine tumors	2	0	0
Total	64	15	23

MCT, Medullary carcinoma of the thyroid.
[a] Tumor contained neurosecretory granules.
[b] Case of insulinoma studied in collaboration with Dr. O. Geatti, Udine, Italy.

and Shapiro 1988; Shulkin et al. 1987). In a small but important group of patients MIBG scintigraphy depicts lesions not detected by any other technique. As with pheochromocytoma, there may be a heterogeneity of MIBG uptake, with a minority of lesions showing no MIBG uptake (Geatti et al. 1985; Treuner et al. 1984; Lumbroso et al. 1985; Shulkin and Shapiro 1988; Shulkin et al. 1987). Extensive chemotherapy seems to reduce MIBG uptake in some cases, but this is far from a uniform finding (Geatti et al. 1985). As with pheochromocytoma, [^{123}I]MIBG may be the optimal tracer for neuroblastoma (Lumbroso et al. 1985).

Both neuroblastoma and pheochromocytoma are members of a larger family of neuroendocrine tumors derived from the neural crest or closely related embryonic tissues which share the property of amine precursor uptake and decarboxylation and are thus called APUDomas (Von Moll et al. 1987; Hoefnagel et al. 1987). In addition to synthesizing various hormonal peptides, many of these lesions have type 1 amine uptake mechanisms and cytoplasmic hormone storage vesicles which are both required for successful MIBG scintigraphy (Sission et al. 1987b; Von Moll et al. 1987; Hoefnagel et al. 1987). Thus far a number of these tumor types have been studied by [^{131}I]MIBG scintigraphy (Sisson et al. 1987b; Von Moll et al. 1987; Hoefnagel et al. 1987). This includes successful imaging of most nonfunctional paragangliomas, many carcinoids, a minority of medullary carcinomas of the thyroid, and islet cell tumors (Von Moll et al. 1987; Hoefnagel et al. 1987; Endo et al. 1984; Fischer et al. 1984). The experience at the University of Michigan is depicted in Table 9.

Therapeutic Administration of Radioiodinated Metaiodobenzylguanidine

Having observed intense and prolonged tracer uptake of [^{131}I]MIBG in certain cases of malignant pheochromocytoma, we were encouraged to administer large therapeutic doses of [^{131}I]MIBG for the treatment of selected malignant metastatic or inoperable pheochromocytomas (Sisson et al; 1983, 1987b).

Patients were selected on the basis of the following criteria: Pheochromocytoma untreatable by other therapeutic modalities, a prognosis such that even without therapy the patient was expected to survive at least 1 year, ability and willingness to return frequently, and, most importantly, intense and prolonged [^{131}I]MIBG uptake by all known tumor deposits such that whenever possible a calculated radiation dose of at least 20 rad/mCi to the tumor and no more than 0.5 rad/mCi to the blood or whole body was obtained (Shapiro 1987; Sisson et al. 1983, 1984b). Dosimetric studies made use of a conjugate view technique which was enhanced by the addition of external standard sources (mock tumors) to the field of view encompassing the tumor (Shulkin et al. 1988). Serial studies were performed over 5–8 days. Tumor volume was obtained from CT, MRI, or ultrasound. Accurate determination of tumor volume was often difficult especially as metastases were often present in bone where this was problematic (Sisson et al. 1983, 1984b; Shulkin et al. 1988). Tumor dosimetry was then calculated using standard medical internal radiation dose (MIRD) formalism (Sisson et al. 1983,

1984b; Shulkin et al. 1988). In addition, blood dosimetry was calculated from serial blood samples over several days and whole body dosimetry from serial measurements using a scintillation probe or uncollimated gamma camera over a period of 5–8 days following the tracer dose (Sisson et al. 1983, 1984b, 1987a). The therapeutic doses of [^{131}I]MIBG were individually synthesized and administered within 24 h. They had specific activities of 41–53 mCi/mg (Sisson et al. 1983, 1987b). Administration was by infusion over 90 min. Patients were subjected to continuous BP, EKG, pulse rate, and frequent temperature monitoring during the infusion and for 24 h thereafter. Initially, doses of 90–100 mCi were used, and subsequently this was increased to 200–262 mCi (Shapiro 1987; Sisson et al. 1983, 1984b). Thyroidal uptake of free ^{131}-I was blocked by iodides which were administered for 4 weeks following the therapy dose. Doses have been administered at 2–12 months intervals (typically 6–12 months) to a total of 2–6 doses. Cumulative doses in a number of subjects have exceeded 800 mCi.

Because of the potential of radiation-induced injury, baseline and serial studies of hepatic, renal, thyroid, adrenocortical, and autonomic nervous system function have been performed (Shapiro 1987; Sisson et al. 1983, 1984b, 1987b). To date no abnormalities have been encountered except hypothyroidism in three cases. Serial observations of hematological parameters have shown mild transient leukopenia and thrombocytopenia in adults treated with [^{131}I]MIBG (Sisson et al. 1983, 1984b, 1987a).

Tumor response to therapy has been evaluated by serial tumor volume measurements using CT or MRI, tumor extent by serial [^{131}I]MIBG scintigraphy, and hormonal secretion by multiple plasma catecholamine concentrations and urinary catecholamine and catecholamine metabolite excretion rates. A partial response was defined as a 50% reduction in tumor volume and/or hormonal rates. Additional evaluation factors were: functional status, dose of α-blockers required, adequacy of BP control, and doses of narcotic analgesics in the case of painful metastases (Shapiro 1987; Sisson et al. 1983, 1984b).

Thus far a total of 28 patients with malignant or unresectable pheochromocytoma have been treated using the protocol described above (Shapiro 1987). Preliminary evaluation of these cases has revealed stable disease in ten cases, deterioration in ten, and partial responses in eight. The partial response would appear to be related to the therapy because spontaneous regressions do not occur. The current status of the patients with partial responses is that in five cases recurrences occurred after periods of 1–3 years. In two cases these responded to further [^{131}I]MIBG therapy but failed to do so in three which eventually succumbed to the disease. All the patients with stable disease are still alive, and five of the ten who deteriorated despite MIBG therapy have died (Shapiro 1987). A possible factor in the low response rates may be the high intrinsic radioresistance and slow growth rate of pheochromocytomas (Shapiro 1987; Sisson et al. 1983, 1984b; Sisson 1986).

Therapeutic use of [^{131}I]MIBG has been extended to neuroblastoma, an intrinsically more radiosensitive lesion than pheochromocytoma (Jaffe 1976). The protocol followed was basically the same as that for pheochromocytoma but differed in the following respects. Patients had stage 4 disease which had failed to respond to surgery, radiotherapy, and chemotherapy (the latter frequently including both standard and experimental protocols; Shapiro 1987; Shulkin and Shapiro 1988; Shulkin et al. 1988; Sisson et al. 1987a). The prognostic projections for the patients with this highly lethal tumor were far shorter than for those with malignant pheochromocytoma. The doses delivered varied from 60 to 200 mCi, and the doses were administered at 3 to 12-months intervals. Up to five doses were administered in some cases (Shapiro 1987; Sisson et al. 1987a). Because of the small body mass of the patients the whole body absorbed radiation doses were greater than with adults, and significant leukopenia and even more marked

Table 10. Comparison of results of [^{131}I]MIBG therapy of neuroblastoma[a]

Reference	n	Objective complete response[b]	Objective partial response[b,f]	Minor or subjective response	No response (stable or progressive disease or unevaluable)
1. Shapiro 1987; Ann Arbor, USA	14	0	3	5	6
2. Belerwaltes 1987; Ann Arbor, USA	11	0	3	—	8
3. Voute et al. 1987; Amsterdam Holland	18	2	10	—	6[c]
4. Hoefnagel et al 1987; Amsterdam, Holland	16	2[d]	8	—	6[c]
5. Fischer et al 1987; Münster/Kassel FRG	3	1[d]	1	—	1
6. Treuner et al 1987; Tübingen FRG	10	0	4	—	6
7. Feine et al 1987; Tübingen FRG	8	0	1	3	4
8. Hartman et al 1987; Villejuif, France	9	0	2[g]	—	7
9. Bestagno et al 1987; Italian MIBG Study group	8	1[e]	2	2	3
10. Sanguineti 1987; Genoa, Italy	6	1	0	—	5
11. Troncone et al. 1987; Rome, Italy	7	1	3	—	3
Summation nonoverlapping cases in 1, 3, 5, 6, 8, 9, 10, 11	75	6	25	7	37

[a] There is considerable variation in the definition and documentation of what constitutes complete, partial, minor response, stable, or progessive disease.
[b] Majority of cases show subsequent relapse and progression.
[c] One case lost to follow-up.
[d] Subsequent relapse.
[e] MIBG therapy led to partial response which made curative surgery possible.
[f] Variously defined as >50% or >20% reduction in tumor.
[g] Tumor reduction by >25% but <50%.

thrombocytopenia occurred (Shapiro 1987; Sisson et al. 1987a). The nadir occurs between 4 and 8 weeks after therapy and is followed by a slow recovery (Sisson et al. 1987a). At the nadir, values can be in the potentially dangerous range, especially in patients in whom the pretherapy levels were subnormal due to chemotherapy and/or marrow infiltration (Shapiro 1987; Sisson et al 1987a). Radiation protection in young, incontinent patients may be more difficult, and catheterization may be required. The parents may have to participate in the care of these very ill patients, but the radiation exposures to the parents have been surprisingly small (Shulkin and Shapiro 1988).

We have found that [^{131}I]MIBG therapy is without benefit to moribund patients with large tumor burdens, but some patients with more limited stage 4 disease may benefit although this may be only temporary (Shapiro 1987; Shulkin and Shapiro 1988). Some workers have reported occasional complete remissions (Hoefnagel et al. 1985).

The results of our experience at the University of Michigan are presented in Table 10, where they are compared to those of other workers.

The physical properties of ^{125}I are such that it may be superior to ^{131}I as a label for therapeutic MIBG used to treat diffuse infiltrative neuroblastoma of the bone marrow, and its use is being planned for the near future (Shulkin and Shapiro 1988; Shapiro and Gross 1987).

In addition to pheochromocytomas and neuroblastomas, other APUDomas which manifest good MIBG uptake and retention may be treatable by [^{131}I]MIBG. A small number of carcinoids and medullary carcinomas of the thyroid have been treated with [^{131}I]MIBG although it is too early to define its role in these lesions (Von Moll et al. 1987; Hoefnagel et al. 1986, 1987).

The optimal case selection criteria, dose and dose frequency, and the determination of dosimetry remain to be developed in the optimum therapeutic use of radioiodobenzylguanidine, but preliminary data have been sufficiently encouraging to proceed to further studies (Shulkin and Shapiro 1988; Shapiro and Gross 1987).

Potential Future Developments

Many areas remain to be investigated and a few of these are listed below:

1. Adrenal cortical imaging
   (a) Confirmation of the role of NP-59 scintigraphy in unilateral "incidentalomas."
   (b) Studies of the natural history of "nonfunctioning adrenocortical adenomas." Do some evolve into endocrine hypersecretory lesions?
   (c) Is NP-59 uptake by "nonfunctioning adrenocortical adenomas" suppressible by dexamethasone or stimulable by ACTH, and do such responses have diagnostic significance?
   (d) Has NP-59 scintigraphy a role in the characterization of bilateral "incidentalomas?"

(e) Can adrenocortical tracers be developed which permit imaging within 24–48 h rather than the current 5–7 days (e.g., labels for LDL)?
2. Sympathomedullary imaging
   (a) Evaluation of more efficacious analogs of MIBG ([^{123}I]aminoiodo-benzylguanidine, which has been shown to be slightly inferior to [^{123}I]MIBG; Shulkin et al. 1986b).
   (b) Expansion of the experience with [^{123}I]MIBG and the role of SPECT.
   (c) Serial MIBG studies to examine the evolution of medullary hyperplasia in MEN 2a and 2b.
   (d) Expansion of the breadth and number of APUDomas studied by MIBG scintigraphy to determine the efficacy in each type of lesion.
   (e) Pharmacological interventions to enhance uptake or retention of MIBG in tumors (e.g., calcium channel blockers have been shown to prolong retention although they reduce initial uptake).
   (f) Refinement of dosimetric studies in the therapeutic use of MIBG.
   (g) Improved selection criteria, dosage schedules, and response criteria for lesions treated with MIBG (e.g., neuroblastoma, pheochromocytomas, and other APUDomas).
   (h) The use of [^{125}I]MIBG for the treatment of microscopic metastases (e.g., neuroblastoma deposits in bone marrow).
   (i) Development of relevant animal models for the study of MIBG therapy.
   (j) Expansion of studies of autonomic nervous system function in vivo, using [^{123}I]MIBG (e.g., autonomic neuropathy, cardiac arrhythmias, and cardiac failure).

Acknowledgements. The authors thank; Dr. T. Mangner and H. Anderson-Davis for the synthesis of [^{131}I]- NP-59 and, [^{123}I]- and [^{131}I]MIBG; Phoenix Memorial Laboratories for the use of their radiochemical facilities; J. Smith and the staff of the Laboratory Service, The Veterans Administration Medical Center, Ann Arbor; Ms. S. Mallette, the nurses of the Clinical Research Centre, and the nuclear medicine technologists for patient management and imaging, as well as Ms. T. Flaggs for her expert assistance in the preparation of the manuscript.

References

Ackery DM, Tippet P, Condon B (1984) New approach to the localization of pheochromo-cytoma: imaging with 131 I-MIBG. Br Med J 288: 1587–1591
Anonymous (1983) Clinical value of adrenomedullary scintigraphy with B1 I-MIBG. Nucl Compact 14: 318
Baba H (1982) CT of the normal adrenal glands and image diagnosis of the adrenal diseases. Nippon Iga Ku Hoshasen Gakkai Zasshi 42: 938–960
Balieu JL, Guilloteau C, Chambon C (1984) Meta-iodobenzyl 23 guanidine (MIBG) scintigraphy: a one year experience (abstract). J Nucl Med 25: 111
Beierwaltes WH (1987) Update on basic research and clinical experience with meta-iodobenzylguanidine. Med Pediatr Oncol 15: 163–169

Berkman WA, Bernardino ME, Sewell CW, Price RB, Sones PJ (1984) The computed tomography-guided adrenal biopsy. An alternative to surgery in adrenal mass diagnosis. Cancer 53: 2098–2103

Bestagno M. Guerra P, Puricelli G, Colombo L, Calculli I (1987) Treatment of neuroblastoma with 131-I-metaiodobenzylguanidine: the experience of an Italian study group. Med Pediatr Oncol 15: 203–204

Bravo EL, Gifford RW (1984) Pheochromocytoma: diagnosis; localization and management. N Engl J Med 311: 1298–1303

Carey JE, Thrall JH, Freitas JE, Beierwaltes WH (1979) Absorbed dose to the human adrenal from iodomethylnorcholesterol (I-131) "NP-59". J Nucl Med 20: 60–61

Chatal JF, Charbonnel B (1985) Comparison of iodobenzylguanidine imaging with computed tomography in locating pheochromocytoma. J Clin Endocrinol Metab 61: 769–772

Chrousos G (1985) Differential diagnosis of Cushing's syndrome. Ann Intern Med 102: 346–347

Conn JW, Cohen EL, Harwig KR (1976) The dexamethasone-modified adrenal scintiscan in hyporeninemic aldosteronism (tumor vs hyperplasia). A comparison with adrenal venography and adrenal venous aldosterone. J Lab Clin Med 88: 841–855

Copeland PM (1983) The incidentally discovered adrenal mass. Ann Intern Med 98: 940–945

Dige-Petersen H, Munkner T, Fogh J, Blichert-Toft M, Lund JO (1975) [131]I-19 iodocholesterol scintigraphy of the adrenal cortex. Acta Endocrinol 80: 81–94

Dunnick NR, Schaner EG, Doppman JL, Strott CA, Gill JR, Javadpour N (1979) Computed tomography in adrenal tumors. AJR 132: 43–46

Endo K, Shiomi K, Kasagi K, Konishi J, Torizuka K, Nakao K, Tanimura H (1984) Imaging of medullary carcinoma of the thyroid with 131-I-MIBG. Lancet ii: 233

Feine U, Treuner J, Niethammer (1984) Erste Untersuchungen zur scintigraphischen Darstellung von Neuroblastomen mit 131-I-Metabenzylguanidin. Nucl Compact 15: 23–26

Feine U, Muller-Schauenburg W, Treuner J, Klingebiel T (1987) Metaiodobenzylguanidine (MIBG) labeled with 123-I/131-I in neuroblastoma diagnosis and follow-up treatment with a review of the diagnostic results of the International workshop of pediatric oncology held in Rome, September 1986. Med Pediatr Oncol 15: 181–187

Fig LM, Gross MD, Shapiro B, Ehrmann D, Freitas JE, Schteingart DE, Glazer G (1987) Scintigraphic localization of the abnormal adrenals in ACTH independent Cushing's syndrome. J Nucl Med 28: 640 (Abstract 348)

Fischer M, Kamanabroo D, Sonderkamp H, Proske T (1984) Scintigraphic imaging of carcinoid tumors with 131-I-metaiodobenzylguanidine. Lancet ii: 165

Fischer M, Wehinger H, Kraus C, Ritter J, Schroter W (1987) Treatment of neuroblastoma with ^{131}I-metaiodobenzylguanidine: experience of the Munster/Kassel group. Med Pediatr Oncol 15: 196–198

Francis IR, Glazer GM, Shapiro B, Sisson JC, Gross BH (1983) Complementary roles of CT scanning and 131-I-MIBG scintigraphy in the diagnosis of pheochromocytoma. AJR 141: 719–725

Freitas JE, Grekin RJ, Thrall JH, Gross MD, Swanson DP, Beierwaltes (1979) Adrenal imaging with iodomethyl-norcholesterol (1–131) in primary aldosteronism. J Nucl Med 20: 7–12

Geatti O, Shapiro B, Sisson JC, Hutchinson RJ, Mallette S, Eyre P, Beierwaltes WH (1985) 131-I-metaiodobenzylguanidine (131-I-MIBG) scintigraphy for the location of neuroblastoma: preliminary experience in 10 cases. J Nucl Med 26: 736–742

Givens JR (1976) Hirsutism and hyperandrogenism. Adv Intern Med 1: 221–247

Glowniak JV, Shapiro B, Sisson JC, Thompson NW, Coran AG, Lloyd RV, Kelsch RC, Beierwaltes WH (1985) Familial extra-adrenal pheochromocytoma: a new syndrome. Arch Intern Med 145: 257–261

lguanidine (131-I-MIBG) scintigraphy for the location of neuroblastoma: preliminary experience in 10 cases. J Nucl Med 26: 736–742

Givens JR (1976) Hirsutism and hyperandrogenism. Adv intern Med 1: 221–247

Glowniak JV, Shapiro B, Sisson JC, Thompson NW, Coran AG, Lloyd RV, Kelsch RC, Beierwaltes WH (1985) Familial extra-adrenal pheochromocytoma: a new syndrome. Arch Int Med 145: 257–261

Gross MD, Valk T, Freitas JE, Swanson DP, Schteingart DE, Beierwaltes WH (1981) The relationship of adrenal iodomethylnorcholesterol uptake to indices of adrenal cortical function in Cushing's syndrome. J Clin Endocrinol Metab 52: 10621066

Gross MD, Shapiro B, Grekin RJ, Meyers L, Swanson DP, Beierwaltes WH (1983) The relationship of adrenal gland iodomethyl- norcholesterol uptake to zona glomerulosa function in primary aldosteronism. J Clin Endocrinol Metab 57: 477481

Gross MD, Shapiro B, Grekin RJ, Freitas JE, Glazer G, Beierwaltes WH, Thompson NW (1984a) Scintigraphic localization of adrenal lesions in primary aldosteronism. Am J Med 77: 839844

Gross MD, Shapiro B, Freitas JE, Ayers J, Swanson DP, Woodbury MC, Schteingart DE, Beierwaltes WH (1984b) The relationship of 131-I-6β-iodomethyl-19- norcholesterol (NP-59) uptake to indices of androgen secretion in women with hyperandrogenism. Clin Nucl Med 9: 264–270

Gross MD, Shapiro B, Freitas JE (1985a) The limited significance of asymmetrical adrenal visualization on dexamethasone suppression scintigraphy. J Nucl Med 26: 43–48

Gross MD, Wortsman J, Shapiro B, Meyers LC, Woodbury MC, Ayers JWT (1985b) Scintigraphic evidence of adrenal cortical dysfunction in the polycystic ovary syndrome. J Clin Endocrinol Metab 62: 197–20

Gross MD, Wilton GP, Shapiro B, Cho K, Samuels BI, Bouffard JA, Glazer G, Grekin RJ, Brady T (1987) Functional and scintigraphic evaluation of the silent adrenal mass. J Nucl Med 28: 1401–1407

Guerin CK, Wahner HW, Gorman CA, Carpenter PC, Sheedy PF (1983) Computed tomographic scanning versus radioisotope imaging in adrenocortical diagnosis. Am J Med 75: 653–657

Hartmann O, Lumbroso J, Lemerle J, Schlumberger M, Ricard M, Aubert B, Coonaert S, Merline L, Olive D, De Lumley L, Parmentier C (1987) Therapeutic use of 131-I-metaiodobenzylguanidine (MIBG) in neuroblastoma: a phase II study in nine patients. Med Pediatr Oncol 15: 205–211

Hattner RS, Huberty JP, Engelstad BL, Gooding CA, Ablin AR (1984) Localization of m-iodo (131 I) benzylguanidine. Am J Rontgenol 143: 373–374

Herf SM, Teates DC, Tegtmeyer CJ, Vaughan ED, Ayers CR, Carey RM (1979) Identification and differentiation of surgically correctable hypertension due to primary aldosteronism. Am J Med 67: 397–402

Hoefnagel WH, Claessens RA, Corstens FH, Drayer JI, Kazem I, Kloppenborg P (1981) Adrenal scintigraphy in primary aldosteronism: improved visualization after long-term pretreatment with dexamethasone. Nuklearmedizin 20: 76–81

Hoefnagel CA, Dekraker J, Marcuse HR, Voute P (1985) Detection and treatment of neural crest tumors using 1-131-meta-iodobenzylguanidine. Eur J Nucl Med 11: A17 (Abstract A73)

Hoefnagel CA, Den Hartog Jager FC, Van Gennip AM, Marcuse HR, Taal BG (1986) Diagnosis and treatment of a carcinoid tumor using iodine 131 metaiodobenzylguanidine. Clin Nucl Med 3: 150

Hoefnagel CA, Voute PA, Dekraker J, Marcuse HR (1987) Radionuclide diagnosis and therapy of neural crest tumors using iodine- 131 metaiodobenzylguanidine. J Nucl Med 28: 308–314

Jaffe N (1976) Neuroblastoma: review of the literature and an examination of factors contributing to its enigmatic character. Cancer Treat Rev 3: 61–82

Joffe SN, Brown C (1983) Nodular adrenal hyperplasia and Cushing's syndrome. Surgery 94: 919–925

Kalff V, Shapiro B, Lloyd R, Sisson JC, Holland K, Nakajo M, Beierwaltes WH (1982) The spectrum of pheochromocytoma in hypertensive patients with neurofibromatosis. Arch Intern Med 142: 2092–2098

Koral KF, Sarkar SD (1977) An operator-independent method for background subtraction in adrenal uptake measurements. J Nucl Med 18: 925–928

Leger FA, Requeda E, Reach G, Plovin PF, Savoie JC (1981) Scintigraphic corticosurrenal-inenne au ^{131}I-19-iodocholesterol. Nouv Presse Med 10: 395–399

Lumbroso J, Hartmann O, Lemerle J, Coornaert S, Desplanches G, Menard F, Gardet P, Schlumberger M, Parmentier C (1985) Scintigraphic detection of neuroblastoma using 131-I and 123-I labelled metaiodobenzylguanidine. Eur J Nucl Med 11: A16 (Abstract 71)

Lynn MD, Shapiro B, Sisson JC, Swanson DP, Mangner TJ, Wieland DM, Meyers LJ, Beierwaltes WH (1984) Portrayal of pheochromocytoma and normal human adrenal medulla by 123-I-metaiodobenzylguanidine (123-I-MIBG). J Nucl Med 25: 436–440

Lynn MD, Shapiro B, Sisson JC, Beierwaltes WH, Meyers LJ, Ackerman R, Mangner TJ (1985) Pheochromocytomas and normal adrenal medulla: improved visualization with 123-I-MIBG scintigraphy. Radiology 156: 789–792

Lynn MD, Gross MD, Shapiro B (1986) Enterohepatic circulation and distribution of 131-I-6β- iodomethyl- 19-norcholesterol (NP-59). Nucl Med Commun 7: 625–630

Mangner WM, Gifford RW (1982) Hypertension secondary to pheochromocytoma. Bull N Y Acad Med 58: 139–158

Mannger TJ, Tobes MC, Wieland DM, Sisson JC, Shapiro B, Beierwaltes WH (1986) Metabolism of meta-I-131-iodo-benzylguanidine in patients with metastatic pheochromocytoma: concise communication. J Nucl Med 27: 37–44

McEwan AJ, Shapiro B, Sisson JC, Beierwaltes WH, Ackery DM (1985) Radioiodobenzylguanidine for the scintigraphic location and therapy of adrenergic tumors. Semin Nucl Med 15: 132–153

Miles JM, Wahner HW, Carpenter PC, Salassa RM, Northcutt RC (1979) Adrenal scintiscanning with NP-59, a new radioiodinated cholesterol agent. Mayo Clin Proc 54: 321–327

Munker T (1985) 131 I-metaiodobenzylguanidine (131 I-MIBG) scintigraphy of neuroblastomas. Sem Nucl Med 15: 154–160

Nakajo M, Shapiro B, Copp JE, Kalff V, Gross MD, Sisson JC, Beierwaltes WH (1983a) The normal and abnormal distribution of the adreno-medullary imaging agent m-(I-131)iodobenzylguanidine (I-131-MIBG) in man: evaluation by scintigraphy. J Nucl Med 24: 672–682

Nakajo M, Shapiro B, Glowniak JV, Sisson JC, Beierwaltes WH (1983b) Inverse relationship between cardiac accumulation of metal- 131-I-iodobenzylguanidine (I-131-MIBG) and circulating catecholamines: observations in patients with suspected pheochromocytoma. J Nucl Med 24: 1127- 1134

Nelson DH (1980) The adrenal cortex: physiological function and disease. Saunders, Philadelphia

Ryo U, Johnston AS, Kim I, Pinsky S (1978) Adrenal scanning and uptake with [131]I-6β-iodomethyl-norcholesterol. Radiology 128: 157–161

Sanguineti M (1987) Considerations of 131-I-metaiodobenzylguanidine therapy of six children with neuroblastoma. Med Pediatr Oncol 15: 212–215

Sarkar S, Simmons B, Kazam E (1987) Iodocholesterol scintigraphy and computed tomography (CT) in Cushing's syndrome and primary aldosteronism (abstract) J Nucl Med 28: 640

Sarkar SD, Cohen EL, Beierwaltes WH, Ju RD, Casper R, Gold EN (1977) A new and superior adrenal imaging agent 131-I-6β-iodomethyl-19-norcholesterol (NP-59): evaluation in humans. J Clin Endocrinol Metab 45: 353–362

Scott HW, Abumrad NN, Orth DN (1984) Tumors of the adrenal cortex and Cushing's syndrome. Ann Surg 201: 586–596

Shapiro B (1987) MIBG in the diagnosis and therapy of neuroblastoma and pheochromocytoma. In: Cattaruzzi E, Englaro E, Geatt, O (eds) Proceedings of the international symposium on recent advances in nuclear medicine, Udine, Italy October 2–3.

Shapiro B (1988) MIBG in the management of neuroendocrine tumors. International congress and advances in management of malignancies. Ascoli Piceno, Italy, May 3–6. Conference abstracts: APRIM, Pisa, Italy, p 129

Shapiro B, Gross MD (1987) Radiochemistry, biochemistry, and kinetics of 131-I-metaiodobenzylguanidine (MIBG) and 123-I-MIBG: clinical implications of the use of 123-I-MIBG. Med Pediatr Oncol 15: 170–177

Shapiro B, Britton KE, Hawkins LA, Edwards CE (1981) Clinical experience with ^{75}Se-selenomethylnorcholesterol adrenal imaging. Clin Endocrinol 15: 19–27

Shapiro B, Sisson JC, Beierwaltes WH (1982a) Experience with the use of 131-I-metaiodobenzylguanidine for locating pheochromocytomas. In: Raynaud (ed.) Nuclear Medicine and Biology. Proceedings of the Third World Congress of Nuclear Medicine and Biology, Vol II. Pergamon, Paris, pp 1265–1268

Shapiro B, Grant DB, Britton KE (1982b) ^{75}Se-selenomethylcholesterol uptake in familial congenital Cushing's syndrome. J Nucl Med 23: 799–800

Shapiro B, Nakajo M, Gross MD, Freitas JE, Copp JE, Beierwaltes WH (1983) Value of bowel preparation in adrenocorticol scintigraphy with NP-59. J Nucl Med 24: 732–734

Shapiro B, Sisson JC, Lloyd R, Nakajo M, Satterlee W, Beierwaltes WH (1984a) Malignant pheochromocytoma: clinical, biochemical and scintigraphic characterization. Clin Endocrinol 20: 189–203

Shapiro B, Wieland DM, Brown LE, Nakajo M, Sisson JC, Beierwaltes WH (1984b) 131-I-meta-iodobenzylguanidine (MIBG) adrenal medullary scintigraphy: interventional studies. In: Spencer RP (ed) Interventional nuclear medicine. Grune and Stratton, New York. Chap 19, pp 451–481

Shapiro B, Sisson JC, Kalff V, Glowniak J, Satterlee W, Glazer G, Francis I, Bowers R, Thompson N, Orringer M (1984c) The location of middle mediastinal pheochromocytomas. J Thorac Cardiovasc Surg 87: 816–820

Shapiro B, Copp JE, Sisson JC, Eyre PL, Wallis J, Beierwaltes WH (1985) Iodine-131-metaiodobenzylguanidine for the locating of suspected pheochromocytoma: experience in 400 cases. J Nucl Med 26: 576–585

Shapiro B, Gross MD, Sandler MP, Falke THM, Shaff MI (1987) The adrenal scan revisited: a current status report on radiotracers and clinical utility, correlative imaging In: Freeman LM, Weissmann HS (eds) Nuclear medicine annual. Raven, New York, pp 193–232

Shulkin BL, Shapiro B (1988) Radio-iodinated Metaiodobenzylguanidine in the Management of Neuroblastoma. In: Pochedly C, Tebbe C (eds) Neuroblastoma: tumor biology and treatment. CRC, Boca Raton

Shulkin B, Shapiro B, Francis, I, Dorr R, Shen S-W, Sisson JC (1986a) Primary extraadrenal pheochromocytoma: a case of positive 123-I-MIBG scintigraphy with negative 131-MIBG scintigraphy. Clin Nucl Med 11: 851–854

Shulkin BL, Shapiro B, Tobes MC, Shen S-W, Wielland DM, Meyers LJ, Lee HT, Petry NA, Sisson JC, Beierwaltes WH (1986b) Iodine 123-4-amino-3-iodobenzylguanidine (123-I-AIBG), a new sympathoadrenal imaging agent: comparison with 123-I-metaiodobenzylguanidine (123-I-MIBG). J Nucl Med 27: 1138–1142

Shulkin B, Shen S-W, Sisson JC, Shapiro B, Hutchinson R, Beierwaltes WH (1987) Normal and abnormal 131-I-metaiodobenzyl-guanidine scintigraphy of the extremities. J Nucl Med 28: 315–318

Shulkin BL, Sisson JC, Koral KF, Shapiro B, Wang X, Johnson J (1988) Conjugate-view gamma camera method for estimating tumor uptake of iodine-131-metaiodobenzylguanidine. J Nucl Med 29: 542–548

Sisson JC (1986) Radionuclide therapy for Malignancy: Influences of physical characteristics of Radionuclides and Experience with Radiolabelled meta-iodobenzylguanidine. In: Ackery D, Batty V (eds) Nuclear Medicine in Oncology. Saunders, London, pp 1–21 (Clinics in oncology, Vol 5)

Sisson JC, Shapiro B, Beierwaltes WH, Nakajo M, Glowniak J, Mangner T, Swanson DP, Copp J, Satterlee W, Wieland DM (1983) Treatment of malignant pheochromocytoma with a new radiopharmaceutical. Trans Assoc Am Physicians 96: 209–217

Sisson JC, Shapiro B, Beierwaltes WH (1984a) Scintigraphy with I-131 MIBG as an aid to the treatment of pheochromocytomas in patients with the MEN-2 syndromes. Henry Ford Hosp Med J 32: 254–261

Sisson JC, Shapiro B, Beierwaltes WH, Glowniak JV, Nakajo M, Mangner TJ, Carey JE, Swanson DP, Copp JE, Satterlee WG, Wieland DM (1984b) Radiopharmaceutical treatment of malignant pheochromocytoma. J Nucl Med 25: 197–206

Sisson JC, Hutchinson R, Johnson J, Mallette S, Carey J, Shapiro B, Beierwaltes WH (1987a) Acute toxicity of therapeutic 131-I-MIBG relates more to whole body than to blood radiation dosimetry. J Nucl Med 23: 618 (Abstract 254)

Sisson JC, Shapiro B, Meyers L, Mallette S, Mangner TJ, Wieland DM, Glowniak JV, Sherman P, Beierwaltes WH (1987b) Metaiodobenzylguanidine to map scintigraphically the adrenergic nervous system in man. J Nucl Med 28: 1625–1636

Sudell CJ, Blake GM, Gossage AAR, Cullen DR, Munro DS (1985) Adrenal Scintigraphy with ^{75}Se-selenonorcholesterol: a review. Nucl Med Commun 6: 519–527

Swanson DP, Carey JE, Brown LE, Kline RC, Wieland DM, Thrall JH, Beierwaltes WH (1981) Human absorbed dose calculations for iodine 131 and iodine 123-labeled metaiodobenzylguanidine (MIBG): a potential myocardial and adrenal medulla imaging agent. Proceedings of the third international radiopharmaceutical dosimetry symposium. Oak Ridge, Tennessee. FDA 81–8166. Department of Health and Human Services, Bethesda, Maryland, pp 213–224

Swensen SJ, Brown ML, Sheps SG (1985) Use of 131-I-MIBG scintigraphy in the evaluation of suspected pheochromocytoma. Mayo Clin Proc 60: 299–304

Thrall JH, Freitas JE, Beierwaltes WH (1978) Adrenal scintigraphy. Semin Nucl Med 8: 23–41

Treuner J, Feine U, Neithammer D, Muller-Schaumburg W, Meinke J, Eibach E, Dopfer R, Klingebiel T, Grumbach S (1984) Scintigraphic imaging of neuroblastoma with 131-I-metaiodobenzylguanidine. Lancet i: 333–334

Treuner J, Klingebiel T, Bruchelt G, Feine U, Niethammer D (1987) Treatment of neuroblastomas with metaiodobenzylguanidine: Results and side effects. Med Pediatr Oncol 15: 199–202

Troncone L (1980) Radioiodocholesterol scintigraphy in adrenal gland tumors. Eur J Nucl Med 5: 345–356

Troncone L, Rufini V, Riccardi R, Lasorella A, Salvini N, Montemaggi P, Falcinelli R, Mastrangelo R (1987) Radiometabolic treatment of neuroblastoma with 131-I-MIBG: preliminary results (abstract). Med Pediatr Oncol 15: 225

Valk TW, Frager MS, Gross MD, Sisson JC, Wieland DM, Swanson DP, Mangner TH, Beierwaltes WH (1981) spectrum of pheochromocytoma in multiple endocrine neoplasia: a scintigraphic portrayal using 131-I-metaiodobenzylguanidine. Ann Intern Med 49: 762–767

Voute P, Hoefnagel C, deKraker J, Evans A, Hayes A, Green A (1987) Radionuclide therapy of neural crest tumors. Med Pediatr Oncol 15: 192–195

Von Moll L, McEwan AJ, Shapiro B, Sisson JC, Gross MD, Lloyd R, Beals E, Beierwaltes WH, Thompson NW (1987) 131-I-MIBG scintigraphy of neuroendocrine tumors other than pheochromocytoma and neuroblastoma. J Nucl Med 28: 979–988

Watson NE, Cowan RJ, Chitton HM (1985) The utility of adrenal scintigraphy in Cushing's syndrome and hyperaldosteronism. Clin Nucl Med 10: 539–542

Weinberger MH, Grim CE, Hollifield JW (1979) Primary aldosteronism: diagnosis, localization and treatment. Ann Intern Med 90: 386–395

Aspects of Surgical Therapy of Adrenal Tumors

E.J. Zingg

Abteilung für Urologie, Universität Bern, 3004 Bern, Switzerland

Introduction

Familiarity with the surgical therapy of adrenal tumors is desirable for any surgeon, regardless to what surgical discipline endocrine surgery is assigned. The basic preconditions for surgical treatment include not only mastery of technique but also knowledge regarding the biology of the individual tumor and experience in dealing with endocrine tumors. Collaboration with radiologists, endocrinologists, and anesthetists is crucial. The surgeon is the last or next to last link in the long chain from diagnosis to therapy.

Detailed understanding of topographical relations is indispensable. The right adrenal adheres ventrally to the right lobe of the liver. Medially, it is partially covered by the vena cava; there is thus danger of invasion of the vena cava, especially in malignant adrenal tumors (Hoffmann et al. 1983). The relations to the peritoneum vary with the dorsal extent of liver adhesion. The upper part of the left adrenal is in contact with the peritoneum, the lower part with the pancreas and splenic vessels. The adrenals are organs of the retroperitoneal cavity, but large, invasively growing malignant adrenal tumors may spread to only the retroperitoneum (kidney, renal hilus, vena cava and aorta, dorsal regions of second part of duodenum, tail of pancreas), but also to intraperitoneal organs, such as liver, spleen, mesentery, and small intestine.

Approach Routes

Three of the possible surgical approach routes to the adrenals are of greatest importance (Edis et al. 1984): (a) the transabdominal approach (from the front), (b) the thoracoabdominal or subcostal approach (from the side), and (c) the dorsal approach according to Young. The choice of approach depends, inter alia, on: (a) the nature, size, and pathological status of the tumor; (b) unilateral or bilateral occurrence; (c) confirmed adrenal or possibly extra-adrenal location; (d) the degree

Recent Results in Cancer Research. Vol. 118
© Springer-Verlag Berlin·Heidelberg 1990

of obesity, thorax form and lung function of the patient; and (e) the surgeon's experience and preference.

Transabdominal Approach. The transabdominal approach involves a longitudinal or, preferentially, transverse laparotomy with wide opening of the abdominal cavity. This approach route allows bilateral exploration of the adrenals and revision of the abdomen. In large tumors, it also allows en bloc resection of intra-abdominal organs or parts of organ. The disadvantages of this approach route consists of technical difficulties in obese patients (Cushing's syndrome) and in invasive tumors, above all on the right, where exposure to cranial is more difficult in the direction of the crus of the diaphragm. (Sigel et al. 1987).

Indications include bilateral pheochromocytoma, extra-adrenal and adrenal pheochromocytoma, and large, bilateral tumors of the adrenal cortex.

Dorsal Approach of Young. The dorsal approach introduced by Young, and modified by Mayor (1984), is unknown to many surgeons; however, it is an elegant, technically sophisticated method. The patient lies prone, and angular incisions are made on both sides. The 11th rib is resected (key position). The pleura is exposed, detached sharply from Zuckerkandl's fascia, and then pushed bluntly upwards, creating access to the retroperitoneal cavity. The upper pole of the kidney is exposed, and the adrenals are dissected out. The advantages of this approach route are: (a) simple approach in obese patients, (b) possibility of bilateral exploration, (c) slight postoperative morbidity and mortality, and (d) shorter hospitalization time. The evident disadvantage is that no extension of the approach is possible; this technique is hence contraindicated in large tumors, carcinomas, and pheochromocytoma.

Indications include (a) primary aldosterone-producing adenomas, (b) bilateral hyperplasia in Cushing's syndrome, and (c) small, nonfunctional adrenal tumors.

Thoracoabdominal or Subcostal Approach Route. After thoracotomy in the eighth or ninth intercostal cavity and lateral incision of the diaphragm, the retroperitoneal space, adrenal and kidney, vena cava, and aorta are widely exposed. After opening of the abdominal cavity, the operation can be easily extended. A similarly broad exposure of the retroperitoneal cavity is attained by the subcostal incision. The advantages of these routes are: (a) readily surveyed approach, (b) possibility of en bloc resection, (c) simple mobilization of right lobe of liver, and (d) extension of approach as desired. The disadvantages of the method consist of the opening of the thoracic cavity, with raised postoperative morbidity, and the longer hospitalization time.

We regard this method as indicated in all adrenal tumors with a diameter of over 6–8 cm. In our hospital, the thoracoabdominal approach route is the method of choice in large pheochromocytomas and in large adrenocortical tumors of the right and left side, but especially in malignant tumors of the adrenals with suspicion of invasion. This facilitates regional lymphadenectomy and also en bloc resection if necessary.

Quite generally, the surgical technique has changed in recent years. Whereas the dissection and surgical treatment of vessels was formerly tedious and time consuming, these are treated today (depending on the caliber of the vessel) with bipolar coagulation or metal clips. Ligatures are applied only in larger vessels. The duration of operation has thus been appreciably reduced, and the loss of blood is minimal in benign tumors.

Surgical Treatment of Pheochromocytoma

Preparation of the Patient. Surgical removal is the only curative treatment for pheochromocytoma. Even today, this is still a high-risk operation. Hull (1986) notes "Pheochromocytoma remains one of the great challenges to anesthetists (and surgeons) in both the operating theater and the intensive-care unit." It is advantageous to carry out the operations in the appropriate centers (Sever et al. 1980). As shown by Atuk (1983), surgical stress can bring about a significant increase of catecholamine secretion not only in the patient but also in members of the surgical team. Today, preparation of the patient for operation by medication (Harris and Dela Roca 1984) is indispensable; this also applies to patients who are asymptomatic. Preoperative and perioperative risks may be minimized by blockade of adrenoreceptors. The blockade of α-receptors is performed with phenoxybenzamine (Dibenylin). The drug is given orally, has a relatively long half-life, and can be divided over two or three doses per day. As a rule, 30–80 mg distributed over 24 h is sufficient (Goldfien 1981). Duration of treatment is 1–2 weeks. Under this therapy, there is a normalization of hypovolemia and an improvement of clinical symptoms. Signs of sufficient α-blockade include blood pressure not over 165/90 mmHg and orthostatic hypotension not under 80/45 mmHg; in the ECG, there is no alteration in the ST segment and the T wave. Certain authors (Manger and Gifford 1977) dispute the appropriateness of complete α-blockade because additional tumors cannot be diagnosed perioperatively by palpation and because of the consequent rise in blood pressure. In complete blockade, dangerous blood pressure crises are rare intraoperatively, whereas a fall in blood pressure may occur after removal of the tumor. We do not have any experience in our hospital with prazosin (Minipress). In existing supraventricular tachycardia and arrhythmia, or supraventricular tachycardia or arrhythmia occurring under α-blockade, an additional β-blockade is indicated preoperatively. Propranolol (Inderal) may be used. Contraindications are manifest heart failure and asthma. An initial dose 30–40 mg per day is distributed over three to four doses. Duration of therapy is 3–7 days. β-Blockade must never be carried out before α-blockade because of the danger of hypertensive crises.

Surgical Technique. The decision whether to explore the contralateral adrenal and the retroperitoneal as well as the peritoneal cavity in order to detect any ectopic pheochromocytomas is important for the surgical strategy. In order to enable systematic exploration, the transabdominal approach is recommended (Atuk 1983;

Cryer 1985; Manger et al. 1985; Sever et al. 1980). However, it must be taken into consideration that: (a) some 90% of pheochromocytomas are situated intra-adrenally in adults (50% in children); (b) the precision of the preoperative localization technique is high with CT, MR, and above all metaiodobenzylguanidine (MIBG)–overall accuracy is 96%–98% (Shapiro et al. 1985; Cullen et al. 1985); (c) small ectopic foci are very difficult to find by simple palpation; and, (d) extensive palpation throughout the abdominal cavity may lead to iatrogenic lesions of intra-abdominal organs (spleen: Cullen et al. 1985). At our hospital, we therefore prefer the subcostal or thoracoabdominal approach route in adults with known tumor location. In the case of a tumor exclusively producing norepinephrine, in children, or in patients whose the MIBG and/or CT findings give rise to suspicion of another, extra-adrenal location, exploration from the front is indicated. The surgical strategy in every case is: sufficiently broad approach, good overview, no manipulation or compression of the tumor, management of the vessels step by step. In general, a central procedure is applied, oriented on the vena cava and the aorta. The dissection begins in the region of the renovascular pedicle with ligation of the suprarenal artery as well as the suprarenal vein on the left. The dissection is then continued along the vena cava and aorta with ligation of the vessels as appropriate and, finally, severance of the cranial and lateral connections. Intraoperative difficulties include the administration of phentolamine (possibly sodium nitroprusside), indicated during tumor dissection in hypertension. In hypotensive crises after removal of the tumor, catecholamines are without effect. Here, administration of angiotensin is indicated. Lidocaine is administered if perioperative extrasystole are observed.

Special Cases. In case of bilateral pheochromocytomas (multiple endocrine neoplasia, or MEN, IIa/IIb), we have so far regarded bilateral total adrenalectomy as indicated. If remnants of adrenal cortical tissue are left behind to avoid life-long dependence on steroids (Ram and Engelman 1979) there is risk of local recurrence (Irvine et al. 1983). Jahnsson et al. (1988) recommend bilateral removal of the adrenals in MEN IIb syndrome; in MEN IIa, unilateral resection of the tumor focus may be justified. Transplantation of adrenal cortical tissue in the case of bilateral adrenalectomy has been proposed, but the results are not yet convincing. In adults, extra-adrenal pheochromocytomas have been described at the neck, in the thorax, in the bladder, and perivesically. These are frequently multiple tumors with the corresponding symptomatology. Nowadays MIBG permits exact localization of such tumors. They are resected in accordance with the conventional rules of surgery; however, the patient must be informed that multiple tumor involvement is possible, that recurrent tumors may occur, and that a second or even a third operation may become necessary.

Surgical Mortality. Whereas 30 years ago mortality was 30% and over, lethal complications are regarded as infrequent today; Remine et al. reported 4/138 cases in 1974 and Van Heerden et al. 4/106 cases in 1982 (3.8%). In our own patients, we have not observed any deaths in 34 consecutive operations.

Long-Term Results. In the case of benign pheochromocytomas, long-term results are good. In a series of 91 cases reported by Van Heerden et al. (1982), 95% of the patients with paroxysmal hypertension and 67% of those with chronic hypertension became normotensive. Causes of persistent hypertension include (rarely) secondary tumor, intraoperative complications, essential hypertension, and acquired renovascular alterations. Follow-up observations are recomended every 6–12 months over 10–15 years and are continued throughout life (Scott and Halter 1984), above all in familial occurrence. Most secondary tumors occur within 1–2 years, but some not until 10–14 years have elapsed (Sparagamba 1988).

Aldosterone-Producing Adenoma

A few brief comments can be made regarding the surgical treatment of aldosterone-producing adenoma. The operation consists of total resection of the ipsilateral adrenal. The approach from dorsal is less stressful and has a lower morbidity because of the possibility of postoperative intestinal paralysis. Two objectives can be achieved with preoperative spironolactone treatment (Aldacton, 3 mg/kg body weight over 1–4 weeks). On the one hand, the potassium deficit can be compensated, the hypertension can be improved preoperatively, and the intraoperative complications in the form of arrhythmias and intestinal pareses can be reduced. On the other hand, after such treatment, operative resection of the adenoma may result in blood pressure normalization (Pagny et al. 1987).

Surgical Treatment in Cushing's Syndrome

The adrenal containing the tumor is to be resected totally in Cushing's syndrome with adrenal adenoma. While in small tumors the approach is from dorsal, we approach all tumors over 8 cm in diameter from subcostal or thoracoabdominal. Intraoperative and postoperative substitution is necessary. We follow the scheme of Labhart (1971) with cortisone substitution by infusion before induction of anesthesia and peroral administration of cortisone acetate on the 3rd postoperative day (4×25 mg daily) with slow dose reduction. The dosage depends on postoperative complications and the general state of the patient; with a raised stress level, as in the presence of fever and complications, higher substitution doses are given. Adrenal surgery in Cushing's syndrome is subject to an increased rate of postoperative complications, such as wound infections and delayed wound healing, thromboembolism, postoperative hematoma, and atelectases. Intensive surveillance of the patients is essential. Malignant tumors of the adrenal cortex are relatively rare and are generally diagnosed late, when they are already in the phase of local invasion or dissemination. In Cohn's series, only 30% of tumors were restricted to the adrenals. The remaining tumors were already growing invasively. The surgical strategy consists of en bloc resection, possibly partial resection of adjacent organs, and selective excision of metastases in the liver and lungs. Large adrenal carcinomas with invasion as well as malignant pheochromocytomas constitute a major challenge to the surgeon (Sigel et al. 1987).

References

Atuk NO (1983) Pheochromocytoma: diagnosis, localization and treatment. Hosp Pract 36: 187–202

Cohn K, Brennan M (1986) Adrenocortical carcinoma. Surgery 100: 1170–1177

Cryer PE (1985) Phaeochromocytoma. Clin Endocrinol Metab 14: 203

Cullen ML, Staren ED, Straus MD, et al. (1985). Pheochromocytoma: operative strategy. Surgery 98: 927

Edis AJ, Grant CS, Egdahl RH (1984) Manual of endocrine surgery, 2nd edn. Springer, Berlin Heidelberg New York Tokyo

Goldfien A (1981) Phaeochromocytoma. Clin Endocrinol Metab 10: 607

Harris RB, DelaRoca RR (1984) Pheochromocytoma: a medical review. Heart Lung 13: 73

Hoffmann JC, Weiner SN, Koenigsberg M, Morehouse HT, Smith T (1983) Pheochromocytoma: invasion of the inferior vena cava: sonographic evaluation. Radiology 149: 793

Hull CJ (1986) Phaeochromocytoma. Diagnosis, preoperative preparation and anaesthetic management. Br J Anaesth 58: 1453

Irvine GL, Fishman LM, Sher JA (1983) Familial pheochromocytoma. Surgery 94: 938

Jansson S, Tisell LE, Fjalling M, Lindberg S, Jacobsson L, Zachrisson BF (1988). Early diagnosis of and surgical strategy for adrenal medullary disease in Men II gene carriers. Surgery 103: 11

Labhart A (1971) Klinik de inneren Sekretion, 2nd edn. Springer, Berlin Heidelberg New York

Manger W., Gifford R., (1977) Pheochromocytoma. Springer, Berlin Heidelberg New York Tokyo

Manger WM, Gifford RW, Hoffman BB (1985) Pheochromocytoma: a clinical and experimental overview. Curr Probl Cancer 9: 3

Mayor G (1984) Die Chirurgie der Nebennieren. Springer, Berlin Heidelberg New York Tokyo

Pagny JY, Chatellier G, Duclos JM, Plouin PF, Corvol P, Menard J (1987) Résultats du traitement chirurgical des adenomes de Conn. Arch Mal Coeur 80: 992

Ram CVS, Engelman K (1979) Pheochromocytoma—recognition and management. Curr Probl Cardiol 5–37

Remine WH, Chong GC, Van Heerden JA, Sheps SG, Harrison EG, (1974) Current management of pheochromocytoma. Ann Surg 179: 740

Scott HW, Halter SA (1984) Oncologic aspects of pheochromocytoma: the importance of follow-up. Surgery 96: 1061.

Sever PS, Roberts JC, Snell ME (1980) Phaeochromocytoma. Clin Endocrinol Metab 9: 543

Shapiro B, Copp JE, Sisson JC, Eyre PL, Wallis J, Beierwaltes WH (1985) Iodine-131 metaiodobenzylguanidine for the locating of suspected pheochromocytoma: experience in 400 cases. J Nucl Med 26: 576

Sigel A, Weissmueller J, Hohenberger W (1987) Topik, Morphologie und Operation der Nebennieren-Malinome. In: Ackermann R(ed) Verhandlungsbericht der Deutshen Gesellschaft für Urologie, vol 39. Springer, Berlin Heidelberg New York Tokyo

Sparagamba M (1988). Late recurrence of benign pheochromocytomas: the necessity for long term followup. J Surg Oncol 37: 140

Van Heerden JA, Sheps SG, Hamberger B, Sheedy PF, Poston JG, Remine WH (1982). Pheochromocytoma: current status and changing trends. Surgery 91: 367

Molecular Biology of the Male Endocrine System

H.-U. Schweikert

Abteilung für Innere Medizin, Universität Bonn, 5300 Bonn, FRG

The testis produces sperm and steroid hormones which regulate male sexual life. Both functions are under feedback control by the hypothalamic-pituitary system; in this respect, the testis has biosynthetic and regulatory features similar to those of the ovary.

Testosterone Synthesis

Testosterone, the principal secretory product of the testis, is synthesized in the Leydig cells from cholesterol (Fig. 1). Cholesterol can either be synthesized de novo in the Leydig cell or be derived from plasma lipoproteins, mainly low-density lipoprotein. Five enzymes are required to convert cholesterol to testosterone (Eik-Nes 1975). In testosterone synthesis, the conversion of cholesterol to pregnenolone by the 20, 22 desmolase, which is regulated by the luteinizing hormone (LH) of the pituitary, is the rate limiting reaction. Once secreted, testosterone is transported in the plasma bound to protein, either to albumin or to a specific high-affinity, low-capacity protein, i.e., sexual steroid binding globulin (Dunn et al 1987). The bound fraction is in dynamic equilibrium with the free or unbound fraction which then can actually enter target cells.

Having entered target tissues, testosterone either exerts its physiological effects directly or serves as a circulating precursor or prohormone for the formation of two other types of metabolites which mediate many of the physiological processes involved in androgen action. On the one hand, testosterone can be converted by the enzyme 5α-reductase to 5α-dihydrotestosterone, the active androgen in many target tissues. On the other hand, circulating androgens can be aromatized in peripheral tissues of both sexes to form estrogen. Estradiol can synergize or oppose the action of androgens, depending on the particular tissue. Both reactions, 5α-reduction and aromatization, are irreversible under physiological conditions; furthermore, 5α-reduced androgens cannot be converted to estrogen. Thus, the physiological effects of testosterone are the result of the combined effects of testosterone itself and its active androgen and estrogen metabolites (Wilson 1975).

Recent Results in Cancer Research. Vol. 118
© Springer-Verlag Berlin–Heidelberg 1990

In young men the average daily production of testosterone and androstenedione is about 6 and 3 mg, respectively (MacDonald et al. 1979). Of the average total estradiol production rate of 45 μg/day, approximately 35% is derived from circulating testosterone and 50% from the interconversion of the weak estrogen estrone, and only about 15% originates from the testes. On the other hand, all of the estrogen produced daily, which averages about 66 μg, is derived from the aromatization of the circulating precursors, androstenedione and testosterone, in peripheral tissues. In some instances, the 5α-reduced and estrogenic metabolites exert local effects in the tissue in which they are formed, and in others they reenter the circulation and can act as circulating hormones. Circulating dihydrotestosterone is formed principally in androgen target tissues whereas estrogen formation takes place in a variety of tissues, the principal one of which is adipose tissue. The overall rate of peripheral aromatization increases with body weight and age (Siiteri and MacDonald 1973).

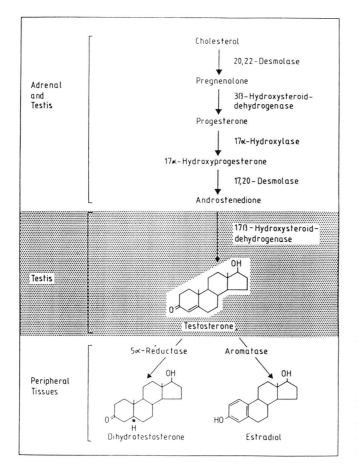

Fig. 1. Pathway of testosterone synthesis in the human testis and conversion of testosterone to the two major active metabolites of testosterone in peripheral tissues, 5α-dihydrotestosterone and estradiol

Regulation of Testosterone Synthesis

Testosterone secretion is regulated by the interaction of hypothalamic and pituitary hormones (Fig. 2). The hypothalamus is anatomically connected to the pituitary both by a portal vascular system and by neurons. The portal vascular vessels provide a system for releasing hormones from the brain to the pituitary. The peptidergic neurons in the preoptic and mediobasal region of the hypothalamus secrete luteinizing hormone releasing hormone (LH-RH) also called gonadotropin-releasing hormone. LH-RH synthesis itself is modulated by neurons from other regions of the brain which terminate at the sites of LH-RH synthesis and can influence synthesis and release of the hormone by means of catecholaminergic, dopaminergic, and endorphin-related mechanisms. LH-RH then interacts with high-affinity cell surface receptor sites on the plasma membrane of pituitary gonadotropin-secreting cells, stimulating the release of both LH and follicle-stimulating hormone (FSH) by a calcium-dependent mechanism. The secretion of

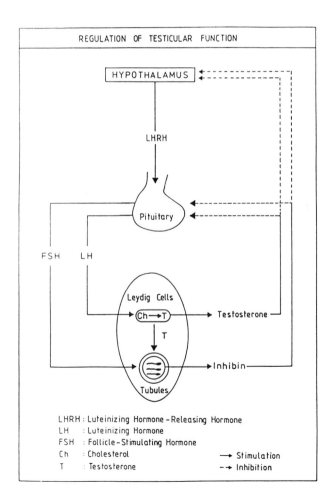

Fig. 2. Hypothalamic – pituitary – testicular axis. Schematic diagram indicating the feedback relationship of the testicular hormones testosterone and inhibin on the secretion of hypothalamic-pituitary hormones

LH-RH into the hypophyseal portal system is episodic; the episodic release of LH-RH results in the episodic release of LH and FSH. The secretory pulses of LH in adult men occur at a frequency of 8–14 pulses per day (Santen and Bardin 1973). LH interacts with specific high-affinity cell surface receptors on the plasma membrane of Leydig cells which eventually leads to testosterone synthesis and secretion (Dufau and Catt 1978).

The epithelium of the seminiferous tubules is the primary site of FSH action (Means et al. 1976; Wahlström et al. 1983). In Sertoli cells, FSH stimulates cyclic AMP formation which then stimulates messenger RNA and protein synthesis, including that for the androgen-binding protein and the aromatase enzyme complex that converts testosterone to estradiol (Dorrington et al. 1972; Dorrington and Armstrong 1975). FSH is also involved in the regulation of testosterone production by increasing the number of LH receptors on Leydig cells at the time of sexual maturation. The rate of LH secretion is controlled by the negative feedback of testosterone on both pituitary and hypothalamic centers. Testosterone or its metabolites appear to act on the central nervous system to slow down the rate of LH-RH formation or secretion and thus decrease pituitary LH episodic release (Matsumoto and Bremner 1984). The negative feedback inhibition of testicular hormones on FSH secretion is less well understood. Serum FSH concentrations increase selectively in proportion to the loss of germinal elements in the testes. Inhibin, a protein inhibitor of FSH is found in the testes, semen, and also in cultured Sertoli cells (Verhoeven and Franchimont 1982). This substance seems to exert a negative feedback action on pituitary FSH secretion.

The Action of Steroid Hormones

Steroid hormones have a multitude of effects at all different levels of cell function and organization. However, a large body of information has accumulated which suggests that different steroid hormones act via similar pathways to produce the same general effects, namely, induction of messenger RNA and protein synthesis (O'Malley 1984; Walters 1985). Steroid hormones enter most cells by diffusion, but in some cases active uptake may be involved. In cells sensitive to the hormone, i.e., the target cells, the steroid binds to specific proteins with a high affinity for the steroid, i.e., the receptor (Fig. 3) Receptors are found in both the cytoplasm and the nucleus of the cell. The binding of the steroid to an unoccupied receptor ultimately results in the formation of an activated or transformed receptor-steroid complex that has a high affinity for nuclear binding sites. In the past it was thought that the receptor is transformed exclusively in the cytoplasm; however, it now appears that this process occurs primarily in the nucleus. This is obviously the case for estrogen, whereas the androgen receptor is still thought to be transformed in the cytoplasm. The binding of the steroid receptor complex to acceptor sites in the nucleus results in de novo messenger RNA synthesis, translation into specific proteins, that modifies or alters cell function, growth, or differentiation.

Once the steroid-acceptor complex has interacted with acceptor sites, it undergoes reactions that are still poorly defined but result in the re-establishment of

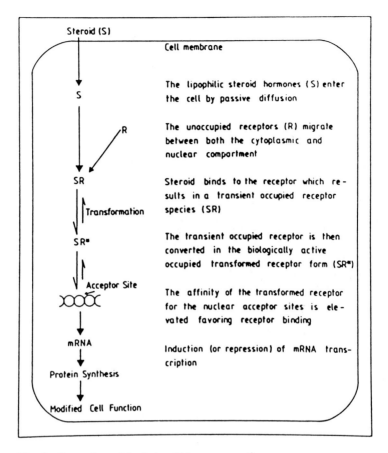

Fig. 3. General model of steroid hormone action

unoccupied receptors and the elimination of the steroid from the cell. The steroid may be metabolized to a derivate that does not bind tightly to the receptor and thus diffuses out of the cell.

The Action of Androgens

Androgens act at the cellular level in a manner similar to other steroid hormones; testosterone enters the target cell probably by passive diffusion and combines with a receptor. However, in some target tissues, notably the prostate, testosterone can be converted to dihydrotestosterone by the enzyme 5α-reductase. Testosterone or dihydrotestosterone is then bound to the androgen receptor protein. The hormone-receptor complex is transformed to the DNA-binding state and in this form attaches to nuclear acceptor sites and then induces mRNA synthesis. Based on studies of the androgen metabolism in animals and on investigations of single gene mutations that impair androgen action, it is now clear that the testosterone-

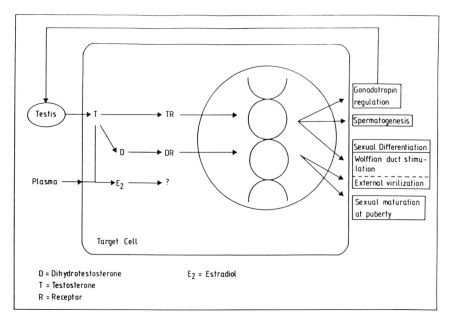

Fig. 4. Current concept of androgen action

receptor complex regulates gonadotropin secretion, spermatogenesis, and virilization of the wolffian ducts during embryogenesis, whereas the dihydrotestoster-
one-receptor complex is responsible for external virilization during embryogenesis
including development of the prostate and, after the onset of puberty, for the
development and maintenance of male secondary sex characteristics (Fig. 4; Wilson 1975).

Androgen receptors are present in highest concentrations in the accessory
glands of male reproduction, such as the prostate, which depend on androgens for
their growth and function but also in other testosterone responsive tissues (Wilson
and French 1976). Whether the presence of androgen receptors can identify a tissue
as androgen sensitive or insensitive is not yet resolved, but it is generally true that
androgen receptors are present in higher concentrations in tissues which respond
to androgens (Menon et al. 1978). In the rat the androgen receptor appears to be
the same molecule in different tissues: an 8–9 S receptor is found in buffers of low
ionic strength, and this molecule is converted to a 4.5–5 S form at buffer-salt
concentrations above 0.1 M (Lea et al. 1979; Wilson and French 1976). The
androgen receptor of human prostate and genital skin fibroblasts also sediments in
low-salt sucrose gradients as an 8–9 S molecule (Fig. 5; Schweikert et al. 1987;
Wilbert et al. 1983). Based on studies in humans and mice on androgen-resistant
mutants, it is thought that a single androgen receptor binds both testosterone and
dihydrotestosterone. However, the affinity of the androgen receptor from human
prostate and from genital skin fibroblasts for dihydrotestosterone is several times
higher than for testosterone (Breiner et al. 1986; Wilbert et al. 1983).

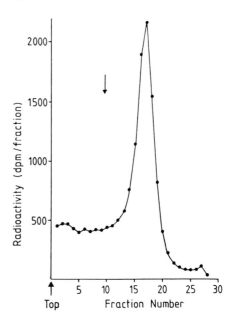

Fig. 5. Binding of dihydrotestosterone to human androgen receptor. Depicted are the results of an experiment in which cytosol from genital skin fibroblasts was incubated with [³H] dihydrotestosterone for 3 h at 0°C. Unbound ligand was removed with dextran-coated charcoal. The sample was then layered on top of a 5%–20% sucrose density gradient and centrifuged at 100 000 g for 1 h. When fractions of the sucrose gradient solutions were assayed for radioactivity, an 8-S peak of dihydrotesto-sterone binding was found. The *vertical arrow* at fraction 9 indicates the peak of a [¹⁴C] albumin marker which sediments at 4.6 S. (Adapted from Schweikert et al. 1987)

It is now known that the androgen receptor belongs to a family of nuclear hormone receptors that probably evolved from a common ancestral gene. Androgen receptors, like other steroid receptor molecules, are composed of an aminoterminal region, a central DNA-binding domain, and a carboxyterminal ligand-binding region (Chang et al. 1988; Lubahn et al. 1988; Trapman et al. 1988). Recently, human androgen receptor complementary DNA has been cloned, and the androgen receptor gene has been localized on the X chromosome (Lubahn et al. 1988)

References

Breiner M, Romalo G, Schweikert HU (1986) Inhibition of androgen receptor binding by natural and synthetic steroids in cultured human genital skin fibroblasts. Klin Wochenschr 64: 732–737

Chang C, Kokontis J, Liao S (1988) Molecular cloning of human and rat complementary DNA encoding androgen receptors. Science 240: 324–326

Dorrington JH, Armstrong DT (1975) Follicle-stimulating hormone stimulates estradiol-17β synthesis in cultured Sertoli cells. Proc Natl Acad Sci USA 72: 2677–2681

Dorrington JH, Vernon RG, Fritz IB (1972) The effect of gonadotropin on the 3′5′ cyclic-AMP levels of seminiferous tubules. Biochem Biophys Res Commun 46: 1523–1528

Dufau ML, Catt KJ (1978) Gonadotropin receptors and regulation of steroidogenesis in the testis and ovary. Vitam Horm 36: 461–592

Dunn JF, Nisula BC, Rodbard D (1981) Transport of steroid hormones: binding of 21 endogenous steroids to both testosterone-binding globulin and corticosteroid-binding globulin in human plasma. J Clin Endocrinol Metab 53: 58–68

Eik-Nes KB (1975) Biosynthesis and secretion of testicular steroids. In : Hamilton DW, Greep RO (eds) Handbook of physiology, sect 7: Endocrinology, vol V: male reproductive system. Williams and Wilkins, Baltimore, pp 95–116

Lea OA, Wilkin EM, French FS (1979) Characterization of different forms of the androgen receptor. Endocrinology 105: 1350–1360

Lubahn D, Joseph DR, Sullivan PM, Willard HF, French FS, Wilson EM (1988) Cloning of human androgen receptor complementary DNA and localization to the X chromosome. Science 240: 327–330

MacDonald PC, Madden JD, Brenner PF, Wilson JD, Siiteri PK (1979) Origin of estrogen in normal men and in women with testicular feminization. J Clin Endocrinol Metab 49: 905–916

Siiteri PK, MacDonald PC (1973) Role of extraglandular estrogen in human endocrinology. In: Greep RO, Astwood EB (eds) Handbook of physiology, sect 7: Endocrinology, vol II: female reproductive system, part I. Williams and Wilkins, Baltimore, pp 615–629

Matsumoto AM, Bremner WJ (1984) Modulation of pulsatile gonadotropin secretion by testosterone in man. J Clin Endocrinol Metab 58: 609–614

Means AR, Fakunding JL, Huckins C (1976) Follicle-stimulating hormone, the Sertoli cell, and spermatogenesis. Rec Prog Horm Res 32: 477–527

Menon M, Tananis CE, Hicks LL, Hawkins EF, McLoughlin MG, Walsh PC (1978) Characterization of the binding of a potent synthetic androgen, methyltrienolone, to human tissues. J Clin Invest 61: 150–162

O'Malley BW (1984) Steroid hormone action in eucaryotic cells. J Clin Invest 74: 307–312

Santen RJ, Bardin CW (1973) Episodic luteinizing hormone secretion in man: pulse analysis, clinical interpretation, physiologic mechanisms. J Clin Invest 52: 2617–2628

Schweikert HU, Weißbach L, Stangenberg C, Leyendecker G, Kley KH, Griffin JE, Wilson JD (1987) Clinical and endocrinological characterization of two subjects with qualitative abnormalities of the androgen receptor. Horm Res 25: 72-79

Trapman J, Klaassen P, Kuiper GGJM, van der Korput JAGM, Faber PW, van Rooij HCJ, van Kessel AG, Voorhorst MM, Mulder E, Brinkmann AO (1988) Cloning, structure and expression of a cDNA encoding the human androgen receptor. Biochem Biophys Res Commun 153: 241–248

Verhoeven G, Franchimont P (1982) Androgens promote the secretion of follicle stimulating hormone inhibiting factor "inhibin" by Sertoli cell-enriched cultures. Ann NY Acad Sci 383: 507–508

Wahlström T, Huhtaniemi I, Hovatta O, Seppälä M (1983) Localization of luteinizing hormone, follicle-stimulating hormone, prolactin, and their receptors in human and rat testis using immunohistochemistry and radioreceptor assay. J Clin Endocrinol Metab 57: 825–830

Walters MR (1985) Steroid hormone receptors and the nucleus. Endocr Rev 6: 512–543

Wilbert DM, Griffin JE, Wilson JD (1983) Characterization of the cytosol androgen receptor of the human prostate. J Clin Endocrinol Metab 56: 113–120

Wilson JD (1975) Metabolism of testicular androgens. In: Greep RO, Astwood EB (eds) Handbook of physiology, sect 7: endocrinology, vol V: male reproductive system. Willams and Wilkins, Baltimore, pp 491–508

Wilson EM, French FS (1976) Binding properties of androgen receptors: evidence for identical receptors in rat testes, epididymis, and prostate. J Biol Chem 251: 5620–5629

Development of Hormone Refractory Tumors:
Adaption Versus Clonal Selection

H. Schulze[1] and J.T. Isaacs[2]

[1] Urologische Abteilung, Marienhospital, Universität Bochum, 4690 Herne, FRG
[2] Department of Urology, The Johns Hopkins University School of Medicine,
  Baltimore, MD, USA

One of the most common characteristics of cancers is their ability to develop resistance to chemotherapy and/or hormonal manipulation to which they were initially responsive (Skipper et al. 1978; Goldie and Coldman 1979, Isaacs 1982b; Ling 1982). For example, there is an initial response rate of prostatic cancer patients to androgen ablation of about 70%–80%. However, essentially all of these patients eventually relapse to an androgen-independent state in which further antiandrogen therapy is no longer effective. Following relapse, all further attempts to ablate the low level of non-testicular androgens remaining following castration, estrogen or luteinzing hormone releasing hormone (LH-RH) analogue therapy by means of hypophysectomy, adrenalectomy, or administration of direct-acting antiandrogens have proven unsuccessful in stopping the continuous tumor growth in this androgen-independent state (Scott et al. 1980; Schulze et al. 1987).

This nearly universal development of resistance by cancers to a wide spectrum of therapeutic modalities is rather unusual when one realizes that normal tissues do not develop similar resistance to the toxic effects of these therapies with continuous exposure. Hence the propensity of prostatic cancer to develop resistance to androgen ablation therapy is in direct contrast to the normal prostate. The normal prostate chronically requires androgen to maintain its normal function and cell number. Following castration, the normal prostate rapidly involutes with a more than 80% reduction in total epithelial cell number (Lesser and Bruchovsky 1973). The involuted normal prostate can, however, be fully restored simply by treatment with exogenous androgen. Once fully restored, the prostate reinvolutes if the treatment with exogenous androgen is discontinued. By alternating treatment of castrated hosts with exogenous androgen followed by a period of no treatment, the normal prostate can be made to go through a cyclic process of restoration and involution. Even if this process of androgen treatment followed by a period of no treatment is cyclically continued many times, the normal prostate always responds with restoration-involution, demonstrating that it does not become resistant to androgens (Sandford et al. 1984; Isaacs 1987). This demonstrates that there is a fundamental difference between the normal and the malignant prostate with regard to the ability to develop resistance to androgen withdrawal.

As stated above nearly all men with metastatic prostatic cancer treated with surgical or chemically induced castration have an initially often dramatic, beneficial response to such androgen withdrawal therapy (Scott et al. 1980; Leuprolide Study Group 1984). Although this initial response is of substantial palliative value, nearly all treated patients eventually relapse to an androgen-insensitive state and succumb to the progression of the cancer, unless they die of intercurrent disease first; cures are rare (Scott et al. 1980; Menon and Walsh 1979). Because of this nearly universal relapse phenomenon, the annual death rate from prostatic cancer has not decreased at all over the nearly 50 years since androgen withdrawal has become standard therapy (Devesa et al. 1978). Over the past five decades, the apparently safe androgen withdrawal therapy has tended to disguise the fact that metastatic prostatic cancer is still a fatal disease for which no therapy is available that effectively increases survival (Lepor et al. 1982).

What is the mechanism for this relapse phenomenon in which an initially androgen-responsive prostatic cancer progresses after androgen ablation to an androgen-resistant state? The answer to this question is fundamental since, depending on the mechanism, it may or may not be possible to prevent the development of such androgen resistance. The importance of such a possibility is that once resistance to androgen withdrawal has occurred, any possibility of curing the patient with hormone therapy alone is lost.

One reason for the relapse after androgen withdrawal may be that prostatic cancers may initially be composed of tumor cells that are homogeneous, at least with regard to their dependence on androgenic stimulation for maintenance and continuous growth (i.e., androgen-dependent cancer cells). After castration, most of these dependent cells stop proliferating and die, thus producing an initial positive response to androgen suppression. Some of these androgen-dependent cells, however, randomly adapt under environmental pressure to become androgen independent. These androgen-independent cells, once formed, proliferate without requiring androgenic stimulation and thus repopulate the tumor, producing a relapse after castration. For this to occur, the changing host environmental conditions after castration are assumed to be critically involved in inducing the adaptive transformation of an initially androgen-dependent tumor cell to an androgen-independent tumor cell. Hence this process is called the environmental adaption model.

In contrast to this model, where the changing androgen environment after castration is assumed to play a direct inductive part, is an alternative explanation that the part played by the changing androgen environment after castration is only indirect. It is possible that initially prostatic cancers are heterogeneous, being composed of preexisting clones of androgen-dependent and androgen-independent tumor cells. The androgen-independent cancer cells may be of two types: cells which are neither dependent on nor sensitive to androgenic stimulation for their growth (i.e., androgen-independent insensitive cells) or cells which grow faster in the presence of adequate androgen levels but which can still grow continuously even when no androgen is present (i.e., androgen-independent sensitive cells; Isaacs 1982a). Regardless of whether the androgen-independent cells present were insensitive or sensitive, castration in such a context would result in the death of only the androgen-dependent cells without stopping the continuous growth of the androgen-independent cells. Although this clinically would produce an initially positive response, these independent cells would continue to proliferate after castration. Even if these androgen-independent cells initially represented only a small fraction of the starting tumor, their continuous growth would eventually not only completely replace any tumor loss due to the death of the androgen-dependent cells, but progressively reexpand the tumor, producing a relapse. Thus, in this environmental selection model there is a selective outgrowth during therapy of preexisting hormone-independent cells present within an initially heterogeneously hormone-sensitive tumor population.

Regardless of whether environmental adaption of selection is the mechanism for relapse after androgen withdrawal therapy, clones of androgen-independent prostatic cancer cells eventually grow and kill the patient. The importance of resolving whether adaption or clonal selection is the mechanism responsible for relapse lies in the fact that the optimal therapy for prostatic cancer is very different depending on which one it is.

If the environmental adaption model is the mechanism for the relapse after standard androgen ablation therapy, then it is possible that the present forms of androgen withdrawal may not be ideal for the treatment of prostatic cancer. This is because, although the standard forms of surgical or chemically induced castration lower the serum testosterone level by over 90%, they do not completely eliminate all potential serum androgens. Since low levels of nontesticular (e.g., adrenal) androgens are left after castration, this treatment induces only a partial androgen withdrawal. This has led some investigators to suggest that a more complete form of androgen withdrawal, in which the very low levels of nontesticular serum androgen that remain after castration are neutralized by simultaneous treatment with a direct-acting antiandrogen, might be more effective than castration alone (Guiliani et al. 1980; Labrie et al. 1985). Because of the known production of androgens by the adrenal cortex, different approaches to deplete the adrenal androgen level either in the serum or in the prostatic tissue after orchiectomy or estrogen treatment in cases of recurrent prostatic cancer were performed over the past four decades. A summation of reported experiences with hypophysectomy, surgical or medical adrenalectomy, or administration of different antiandrogens showed for each of these treatments a transient objective response rate of 5.6%–7.2% (Schulze et al. 1987). And although nearly all reported series have a number of patients who exhibit a prolonged response and survival time, the overall survival data are not significantly improved over what one would expect from the natural history of prostatic cancer (Thompson et al. 1974).

Recently Labrie and coworkers (1985) claimed that it would be most important to start administration of an antiandrogen at the same time as surgical or medical castration. This group asserts that "99% of prostatic tumors, even at the stage of metastases are still androgen-sensitive. Instead of being present at the beginning of treatment, most androgen-insensitive cells develop when tumor cells are exposed to the low androgen milieu provided by the adrenal androgens." Since once these androgen-independent prostatic cancer cells develop, the patients become incurable by any type of hormonal therapy, Labrie et al. have postulated that by combining antiandrogens with castration (either surgical or chemical), it might be possible to kill all of the androgen-dependent prostatic cancer cells before they can progress to become androgen-independent cancer cells. In support to this hypothesis Labrie et al. (1987) have reported data from a nonrandomized clinical trial that men with previously untreated metastatic prostatic cancer given an LH-RH analog plus an antiandrogen have an over 300% decreased death rate during the first 2 years of treatment compared to reported data of other clinical trials using castration alone (i.e., partial androgen withdrawal). However, in the meantime preliminary results of prospective randomized clinical trials by other groups have been published which raise doubt that by complete androgen blockade significant therapeutic advantages can be obtained beyond castration in terms of response and survival rates (Crawford et al. 1988. Schroeder et al. 1987; Schulze et al. 1988).

Although the theoretical basis for complete androgen blockade is scientifically reasonable, there are several major clinical observations which do not support the critical assumptions upon which this theory is based. First, although the adrenals do supply steroids to the blood, which theoretically could act as androgen, no one has actually demonstrated that in humans these adrenal androgen precursors have major effects upon prostatic cell growth. Indeed, Oesterling et al. (1986) have demonstrated by both histological and morphometrical criteria that adrenal androgens alone do not have a stimulatory effect on the normal human prostate and are not capable of supporting prostatic growth.

Second, when prostatic cancers become clinically manifest, they are rarely phenotypically homogeneous with regard to the clones of cancer cells comprising individual tumors. For example, it has been demonstrated in clinically manifest prostatic cancers removed surgically from previously untreated patients, that prostatic carcinoma is multifocal in origin (Byar et al. 1972; Hayashi et al. 1987) and is at least 60% histologically heterogeneous, being composed of a mixture of several different cancer cell types of widely varying differentiation (admixture of glandular, cribriform and anaplastic morphology within the same cancer) (Kastendieck 1980). Similar cellular heterogeneity in individual cancers, even before hormone therapy was initiated, was demonstrated by immunocytochemical methods to examine the cellular distribution of prostatic specific acid phosphatase (Mostofi and Sesterbenn 1981), prostatic specific antigen (Viola et al. 1986), carcinoembryonic antigen (Viola et al. 1986) and p21 Harvey-*ras* oncogene protein (Viola et al. 1986). These results clearly show that prostatic cancer cell heterogeneity may occur early in the course of the disease, and that there is no requirement for a reduction in serum androgen level.

This has led several investigators to suggest that the major reason that androgen withdrawal therapy is not curative is not due to an inadequate decrease in the systemic level of androgen after therapy but to the fact that prostatic cancers are heterogeneously composed of clones of both androgen-dependent and androgen-independent cancer cells before hormone therapy is begun (Prout et al. 1976; Sinha et al. 1977; Smolev et al. 1977; Isaacs and Coffey 1981). If this is correct, then treatment of such a heterogeneous prostatic cancer with androgen withdrawal alone would kill only the androgen-dependent clones of cancer cells without stopping the continuous clonal growth of the preexisting androgen-independent prostatic cancer cells, no matter how complete this androgen withdrawal therapy might be.

In order to get a better understanding of the tumor biology of prostatic cancer many animal studies have been undertaken. However, spontaneous adenocarcinoma of the prostate has rarely been reported among nonhuman mammals. In a bibliographic survey of reports of prostatic carcinomas among laboratory animals published between 1900 and 1977, Riverson and Silverman (1979) found no cases in mice, one case in the rhesus monkey, and two cases in Syrian golden hamsters. Of the common laboratory animals, certain strains of aged rats appear to have the highest incidence of prostatic cancer. The transplantable Dunning (1963) and Pollard (1980) rat prostatic adenocarcinoms developed spontaneously in a small number of aged rats of Copenhagen and Lobound Wistar strains, respectively. A high incidence of spontaneous prostatic carcinoma has been reported only in rats of the ACI/seg strain (Shain et al. 1975, 1977; Ward et al. 1980).

Prostatic tumors among domestic animals are most frequently found in dogs. The incidence of prostatic carcinoma among dogs 6 years old or over has been reported to be approximately 5% (Lear and Ling 1968). Metastases occur among dogs with prostatic carcinoma and bone metastases are not rare (Durham et al. 1986).

Interpretation of the incidence data among laboratory animals must include consideration of the following factors. Prostatic cancer is a disease of older animals. Therefore, the prostates of the animals in question must be examined near the end of the natural life span. In addition, not all older animals are autopsied, and the prostate may not be examined thoroughly in every case. Although it appears likely that the incidence of prostatic cancer is underestimated, this tumor clearly occurs less frequently among laboratory animals than among humans. This low incidence has limited efforts to study this cancer under controlled conditions among laboratory animals.

One of the best characterized models of spontaneous prostatic adenocarcinomas among laboratory rats are the Dunning tumors (Isaacs et al. 1986). First described by Dunning in 1963 as arising from the dorsolateral prostate of an aged Copenhagen rat, in the meantime following serial in vivo passages of the original R3327 tumor, sublines with differing biological characteristics were obtained and carefully characterized (Isaacs et al. 1986). This parent Dunning tumor, termed R3327-H was shown to be a slow-growing, androgen-sensitive, well-differentiated adenocarcinoma having both the high-affinity androgen-specific receptor and the ability via 5α-reductase to metabolize testosterone to dihydrotestosterone (Voigt and Dunning 1974; Voigt et al. 1975). The Dunning tumor has been shown to be an important model for human prostatic cancer since it mimics many of the properties of the human disease (Isaacs et al. 1978). One of its important similarities is its response to androgen ablation. If intact male rats bearing an exponentially slow-growing H tumor are castrated, the tumor appears to stop growing for about 50–60 days. This initial response to castration is inevitably followed by a subsequent relapse in which the tumor again starts to grow. In this regard, the H tumor mimics very closely the clinical situation in metastatic human prostatic cancer, where the initial response to androgen ablation therapy is also almost universally followed by a subsequent relapse that is resistant to hormonal control. The relapse of the H tumor to androgen ablation has been demonstrated to be dependent upon the initial heterogeneity of the H tumor. By fluctuation analysis Isaacs and Coffey (1981) could show that the tumor is composed of a mixture of preexisting clones of both androgen-dependent and androgen-independent tumor cells.

The fluctuation analysis was based on the technique originally developed by Hakansson and Troupe (1974). If the H tumor is initially heterogeneous, being composed of substantial areas of androgen-dependent and androgen-independent tumor cells small trocar pieces of identical size taken at random from the tumor should have the same total number of tumor cells composed, however, of widely fluctuating rations of androgen-dependent and -independent cells. If allowed to grow in intact animals, all such trocar inoculua should grow to produce tumors of 1 cm^3 volume with essentially identical times (i.e., small fluctuation in time) since the total number of starting cells in each case is identical, and under such conditions both androgen-dependent and -independent cells grow equally well. In direct contrast to the consistency in intact rates, the time required for trocar pieces to grow to 1 cm^3 in castrate rats should require widely fluctuating times if the original H tumor is heterogeneous, since each trocar piece would have varying starting numbers of androgen-independent cells. If the H tumor is not heterogeneous but is instead homogeneously composed of androgen-dependent cells and castration actively induces the random development of androgen-independent cells from the initially dependent tumor cells, then individual trocar pieces of identical cell numbers inoculated into castrate male rats should each have the same frequency of this induction, and thus the time required to grow to 1 cm^3 in castrates should be very similar for all trocar pieces. Therefore, the fluctuation in the time required for individual trocar pieces to grow to 1 cm^3 in castrate rats can be used to differentiate whether the relapse of the H tumor to hormonal therapy is due to adaption or clonal selection.

The results obtained in this study (Isaacs and Coffey 1981) revealed that the fluctuation for the intact animals was very small. This was expected since under these intact conditions both androgen-dependent and -independent cells grow equally well, and thus any variation in the relative proportion of either cell type does not matter, only the total number of cells inoculated, which was identical for all intact animals. In direct contrast, the fluctuation for the castrate rats was not identical and revealed a huge standard deviation of the mean. These results clearly demonstrate that the H tumor is heterogeneously androgen sensitive even before androgen ablation therapy is begun. The relapse of the H tumor to hormonal therapy thus involves a process of clonal selection brought about by androgen ablation therapy of a preexisting population of androgen-independent tumor cells present within the initially heterogeneous androgen-sensitive H tumor.

Using the serial transplantable Dunning R3327 system of rat prostatic cancers, it has been possible to demonstrate consistently that androgen-dependent prostatic cancer cells can randomly give rise to completely androgen-independent cancer cells even when the original androgen-dependent cancer cells are grown in an intact (i.e., noncastrated) male host (Isaacs et al. 1982). This progression to the androgen-independent state has been shown to involve genetic instability since definitive changes in the genetic make-up of the prostatic cancer cells have been demonstrated (Wake et al. 1982). In addition, the development of increased growth rate, metastatic ability, and hormonal independence by different sublines of the R3327-H tumor is accompanied by chromosomal alterations (Wake et al. 1982) The development of metastatic capacity in anaplastic sublines is associated with complex chromosomal rearrangements and chromosome loss from tetraploidy. The androgen-insensitive sublines display a preferential association of abnormalities involving chromosome 4. Thus tumor progression in this model of prostatic cancer is accompanied by increased chromosomal abnormalities, although there was no consistent correlation of a specific alteration with a particular phenotypic shift (Wake et al. 1982)

In conclusion, the results obtained with the Dunning tumor model suggest that the process of genetic instability coupled to clonal selection is at least one mechanism for the change in tumor phenotype characteristically associated with tumor progression (Isaacs et al. 1982).

The Dunning tumor model shares a restriction common to all animal models of human cancer: results obtained with animal tumors must be extrapolated to the human disease with caution (Ware 1987). In addition, the anatomical differences between the human prostate and the rat prostate (McNeal 1983; Jesik et al. 1982) have been cited by several investigators as a source of uncertainty in comparing the pathobiology of prostatic carcinomas of rats and men. However, the Dunning tumor model provides a fascinating and useful system for the study of different portions of prostatic tumor progression from the initiated cell to the metastatic progeny.

The results obtained by the Dunning tumor model are consistent with the clinical findings that patients die of their prostatic cancer due to androgen-independent cell clones, no matter how complete the androgen ablation. It is important to realize that the approach of controlling prostatic cancer growth simply by deprivation of androgens alone kills only the androgen-dependent cells. In order to increase the effectiveness of treatment of prostatic cancer, androgen ablation must by combined with therapies targeted specifically at controlling androgen-sensitive and androgen-independent cancer cells. Using such a combined approach, it should be possible to affect the growth of all populations of malignant cells within the prostatic cancer (i.e., androgen-dependent, -sensitive, and -independent) and thus increase the effectiveness of the combined therapy above that obtained with hormonal treatment alone. Indeed, in the Dunning tumor model, such combinational therapy early in the course of the disease does produce substantial increase in survival above that produced by hormonal therapy alone (Isaacs 1984).

References

Byar DP, Mostofi FK (1972) Carcinoma of the prostate: prognostic evaluation of certain pathological features in 208 radical prostatectomies, examined by the step section technique. Cancer 30: 5–13

Crawford ED, MeLeod D, Dorr A, Spaulding J, Benson R, Eisenberger M, Blumenstein B (1988) Treatment of newly diagnosed stage D2 prostate cancer with leuprolide and flutamide or leuprolide alone, phase III, intergroup study 0036. J Urol 139: 339A

Devesa SS, Silverman DT (1978) Cancer incidence and morbidity trends in the United States: 1935–1974. J. Natl Cancer Inst. 60: 545–571

Dunning WF (1963) Prostate cancer in the rat. NCI Monogr 12: 351–369

Durham, SK, Dietze, AE (1986) Prostatic adenocarcinoma with and without metastasis to bone in dogs. J Am Vet Assoc 12: 1432–1436

Giuliani L, Pescatore D, Giberti C, Martorana G, Natta G (1980) Treatment of advanced prostatic carcinoma with cyproterone acetate and orchiectomy. 5 year follow-up. Eur Urol 6: 145–148

Goldie GH, Coldman AJ (1979) A mathematical model formulating the drug sensitivity of tumors to their spontaneous metastatic rate. Cancer Treat Rep 63: 1727

Hakansson L, Troupe C (1974) On the presence within tumors of clones that differ in sensitivity to cytostatic drugs. Acta Pathol. Microbiol. Scand (A) 82: 32

Hayashi T, Taki Y, Ikai K, Hiura M, Kiriyama T, Shizuki K (1987) Latent and clinically manifest prostatic carcinoma. Prostate 10: 275–279

Isaacs JT (1982a) Hormonally responsive versus unresponsive progression of prostatic cancer to antiandrogen therapy as studied with the Dunning R – 3327 – AT and -G rat adenocarcinomas. Cancer Res 42: 5010 – 5014

Isaacs JT (1982b) Cellular factors in the development of resistance to hormonal therapy. In: Bruchovsky N, Goldie JH (eds) Drug and hormone resistance in neoplasia, vol I. CRC, Boca Raton, pp 139–156

Isaacs JT (1984) The timing of androgen ablation therapy and/or chemotherapy in the treatment of prostatic cancer. Prostate 5: 1–18

Isaacs JT (1987) Control of cell proliferation and cell death in the normal and neoplastic prostate: a stem cell model. In: Rodgers CH, Coffey DS, Cunha G, Grayhack JT, Hinman F, Forton R (eds) benign prostatic hyperplasia, vol 2. NIH publication 87–2881. NIH, Bethesda, pp 85–94

Isaacs JT, Coffey DS (1984) Adaptation vs. selection as the mechanism responsible for the relapse of prostatic cancer to androgen ablation as studied in the Dunning R – 3327 – H adenocarcinoma. Cancer Res 41: 5070–5075

Isaacs JT, Heston, WDW, Weissman, RM Coffey, DS (1978) Animal models of the hormon-sensitive and -insensitive prostatic adenocarcinomas: Dunning R-3327-H, R-3327-HI, and $-3327-AT. Cancer Res 38: 4353–4359

Isaacs JT, Wake N, Coffey DS, Sandberg AA (1982) Genetic instability coupled to clonal selection as a mechanism for tumor progression in the Duning R 3327 rat prostatic adenocarcinoma system. Cancer Res 42: 2353–2361

Isaacs, JT, Issacs WB, Feitz WFJ Scheres J. (1986) Establishment and characterization of seven Dunning rat prostatic cancer cell lines and their use in delveloping methods for predicting metastatic abilities of prostatic cancers. Prostate 9: 261–281.

Jesik CJ, Holland JM, Lee C (1982) An anatomic and histologic study of the rat prostate. Prostate 3 : 81–97

Kastendieck H (1980) Correlation between atypical primary hyperplasia and carcinoma of the prostate. Histologic studies on 180 total prostatectomies due to manifest carcinoma. Path Res Pract 169: 366–387

Labrie F, Dupont A, Belanger A (1985) Complete androgen blockade for the treatment of prostate cancer. In: Devita VT Hellman S, Rosenberg S (eds) Important advances in oncology. Lippincott, Philadelphia, pp 193–217

Labrie F, Dupont A, Belanger A, Emond J, Monfette G (1987) flutamide in combination with castration (surgical or medical) is the standard treatment in advanced prostate cancer. J Drug Dev 1 (suppl 1)34–51:

Lepor H, Ross A, Walsh PC (1982) The influence of hormonal therapy on survival of men with advanced prostatic cancer– J Urol 128: 335– 340

Lesser B, Bruchovsky N (1973) the effects of testosterone, 5α-dihydrotestosterone, and adenosine 3', 5'-monophosphate on cell proliferation and differentiation in rat prostate. Biochim. Biophys. Acta 308: 426–437

Leuprolide Study Group (1984) Leuprolide versus diethylstilbestrol for metastatic prostatic cancer. N Engl J Med 311: 1281–1286

Ling V (1982) Genetic basis of drug resistance in mammalian cells. In: Bruchovsky N, Goldie JH (eds) Drug and hormone resistance in neoplasia, vol I. CRC, Boca Raton, pp 1–19

McNeal JE (1983) Monographs in urology. In: Stamey TA (ed) Custom Princeton, vol 4, pp 3–33

Menon M, Walsh PC (1979) Hormonal therapy for prostatic cancer. In: Murphy GP (ed) Prostatic cancer. PSG, Littleton,MA, pp 175–200

Mostofi FK, Sesterhenn J (1981) The role of prostatic acid phosphatase in histological diagnosis of carcinoma of the prostate. Proceedings of the seventy-sixth annual meeting of the American Urological Association, Boston, Abstract 42

Oesterling JE, Epstein JI, Walsh PC (1986) The inability of adrenal androgens ot stimulate the adult human prostate: an autopsy evaluation of men with hypogonadotropic hypogonadism and panhypopituitarism. J Urol 136: 1030–1034

Pollard M (1980) The Pollard tumors. In: Murphy GP (ed) Models for Prostate cancer. Liss, New York, pp 293–302

Prout GR, Leiman B, Daly JJ, MacLoughlin RA, Griffin PP, Young HH (1976) Endocrine changes after diethylstilbestrol therapy. Urology 7: 148–155

Rivenson A, Silverman J (1979) The prostatic carcinoma in laboratory animals. Invest Urol 16: 468–478

Sandford NL, Searle JW, Kerr JFR (1984) Successive waves of apoptosis in the rat prostate after regulated withdrawal of testosterone stimulation. Pathology 16: 406–410

Schroeder FH, Klijn JG, de Jong FH (1987) Metastatic cancer of the prostate managed with buserelin versus buserelin plus cyproterone acetate. J Urol 137: 912–918

Schulze H, Isaacs, JT, Coffey DS (1987) A critical review of the concept of total androgen ablation in the treatment of prostate cancer. In: Murphy GP et al. (eds) Prostate cancer. Part A. Prog Clin Biol Res 243: 1–19

Schulze H, Kaldenhoff H, Senge T, Westfälische Prostata-Karzinom study group (1988) Evaluation of total versus partial androgen blockade in the treatment of advanced protatic cancer. Urol Int 43: 193–1

Scott, WW, Menon M Walsh PC (1980) Hormonal therapy of prostatic cancer. Cancer 45: 1929–1936

Shain SA, McCullough B, Segaloff A (1975) Spontaneous adenocarcinoma of the ventral prostate of the aged AXC rats. J Natl Cancer Inst 55: 177–180

Shain SA, McCullough B, Nitchuk M, Boesel RW (1977) Prostatic carcinogenesis in the AXC rat. Oncology 34: 114

Sinha AA, Blackard, CE, Seal USA (1977) A critical analysis of tumor morphology and hormone treatments in the untreated and estrogen-treated responsive and refractory human prostatic carcinoma. Cancer 40: 2836–2850

Skipper HE, Schabel FM, Lloyd MM (1978) Selection and overgrowth of specifically and permanently drug-resistant tumor cells. Exp Ther Kinetics 15: 207–217

Smolev JK, Heston WD, Scott WW, Coffey DS (1977) Characterization of the Dunning R – 3327 – H prostatic adenocarcinoma. An appropriate animal model for prostatic cancer. Cancer Treat Rep 61: 273–287

Thompson JB, Greenberg E, Pazianos A, Pearson OH (1974) Hypophysectomy in metastatic prostate cancer. NY State J Med 74: 1006–1008

Viola MV, Fromowitz F, Oravez MS, Deb S., Finket G, Lundy J, Harel P, Thor A, Schlom J (1986) Expression of ras oncogene p21 in prostatic cancer. Engl. J Med 314: 133–137

Voigt W, Dunning WF (1974) In vivo metabolism of testosterone–^{3}H in R – 3327, an androgen–sensitive rat prostatic adenocarcinoma. Cancer Res 34: 1447–1450

Voigt W, Feldman, M, Dunning WF (1975) 5α-Dihydrotestosterone binding proteins and androgen sensitivity in prostatic cancers of copenhagen rats. Cancer Res 35: 1840–1846

Wake N, Isaacs JT, Sandberg AA (1982) Chromosomal changes associated with progression of the Dunning R-3327 rat prostatic adenocarcinoma system. Cancer Res 42: 4131–4142

Ward JM, Reznik G, Stinson SF, Lattatuda CP, Longfellow DG, Cameron TP (1980) Histogenesis and morphology of naturally occuring prostatic carcinoma in the ACI/segHapBR rat. Lab Invest 43: 517–522

Ware JL (1987) Prostate tumor progression and metastasis. Biochim. Biophys. Acta 907: 279–298

Antiandrogenic Substances in the Management of Prostatic Cancer

F.H. Schröder

Department of Urology, Erasmus University, P.O. Box 1738,
3000 DR Rotterdam, The Netherlands

Introduction

Antiandrogens are substances which counteract the effect of exogenous or endogenous hormones at target cells independently of feedback mechanisms. Because of the difficulty in ruling out activity exerted due to the influence on feedback mechanisms, antihormones are usually tested under experimental conditions allowing the exclusion of feedback. In the example of antiandrogens this means that an antiandrogen is a substance which counteracts the effect of exogenous androgens in castrated animals. Antiandrogens probably exert their action at the target cell level by competing with androgens for receptor binding sites and by inhibiting the translocation of the hormone receptor complex into the nucleus (Neri 1977; Brinkmann et al. 1983).

Many substances with antiandrogenic activity have been synthesized. Most of these substances belong either to the steroidal or to the nonsteroidal antiandrogens. Examples of steroidal antiandrogens are cyproterone acetate (CPA), cyproterone, megestrol acetate (MGA), and medroxyprogesterone acetate (MPA). Nonsteroidal antiandrogens are: flutamide and hydroxyflutamide, the active metabolite of flutamide and anandron, a substance that is closely related to flutamide. The structural formulas of cyproterone acetate and flutamide are indicated in Fig. 1. Some antiandrogens, mainly the steroidal ones, besides being antiandrogens also have antigonadotropic properties; these are lacking in nonsteroidal antiandrogens.

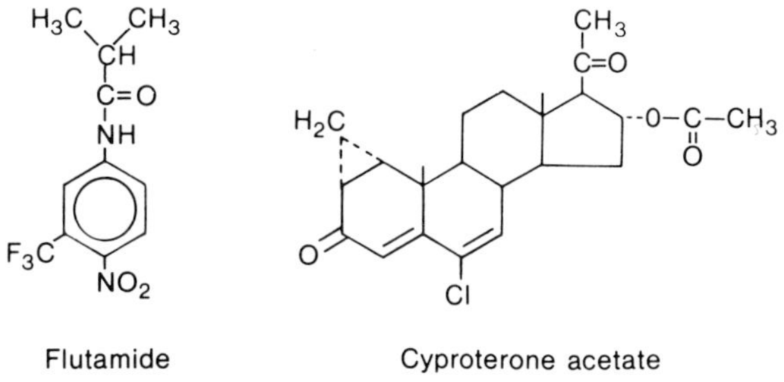

Fig. 1. Structural formulas of cyproterone acetate and flutamide, examples of steroidal and nonsteroidal antiandrogens

Flutamide

Cyproterone acetate

Recent Results in Cancer Research. Vol. 118
© Springer-Verlag Berlin·Heidelberg 1990

For this reason this latter group is also termed "pure" antiandrogens. However, there are also steroidal "pure" antiandrogens which do not have gestagenic or antigonadotropic activity (e.g., cyproterone).

Endocrine Effects of Antiandrogens

Target cells for antiandrogens are all androgen-dependent cells in which androgen action is mediated by the androgen receptor. This is also the case for the cells in the diencephalon which are involved in the regulation of luteinizing hormone releasing hormone (LH-RH) secretion. On this system androgens and estrogens act in such a way that a decrease in the plasma levels of these steroid hormones leads, to an increase in LH-RH and subsequently luteinizing hormone (LH) secretion. So called "pure" antiandrogens of the flutamide type block this system and lead to an increase in LH-RH and LH secretion. This subsequently causes an increase in testosterone production and secretion by Leydig's cells. This relationships is depicted in Fig. 2. CPA, a substance which besides having antiandrogenic activity also acts as an antigonadotropin, inhibits the LH secretion which would normally result from its antiandrogenic action. Consequently the use of flutamide and CPA results, in different effects on the concentration of plasma hormone levels related to this system in intact humans, as studied by knuth et al. (1984). Flutamide given over a period of 2 weeks leads to a significant rise in plasma testosterone, dihydrotestosterone (DHT), and estradiol (E_2). This is accompanied by an elevation in LH and follicle-stimulating hormone (FSH). No changes in serum prolactin are observed. The rise of these plasma hormone levels is the result of the inhibition of the negative feedback of steroids in the hypothalamic region on the release of LH-RH.

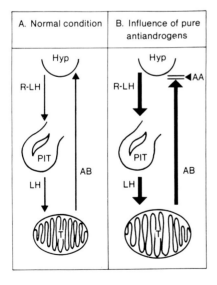

Fig. 2. Hypothalamic effects of the antiandrogens flutamide and cyproterone acetate. (From Neumann et al. 1984). *LH*, luteinizing hormone; *Hyp*, hypothalamus; *PIT*, pituitary; *R-LH*, lH-Releasing hormone; *T*, testes; *AB*, androgen blood level; *AA*, antiandrogenic activity

The effect of CPA on the same parameters is different. CPA leads to a reduction in plasma testosterone, DHT, and E_2. Plasma levels of LH and FSH are also reduced. The response of gonadotropins to exogenous LH-RH is decreased. Prolactin remains unaffected. This is the result of the antigonadotropic effect of CPA; the antiandrogenic action of CPA does not become visible in these parameters.

Antiandrogenic Effectiveness of Antiandrogens of the Flutamide and Cyproterone Acetate Type

As already mentioned, antiandrogens and their antiandrogenic effectiveness can best be studied in vivo in systems in which the regulation of androgens by feedback mechanisms is excluded. The classical model is the castrated rat substituted by exogenous androgens. Ventral prostate and seminal vesicle weights respond proportionally to androgenic depletion and repletion of the animals. Neri et al. (1972) and El Etreby et al. (1987) among others have studied the two substances in this system comparatively. The effect of antiandrogens is dose dependent within a wide range. Flutamide is clearly a stronger antiandrogen than CPA. This difference disappears if doses of 10 and 100 mg of either substance per kilogram body weight of the animals are used. With both substances reduction of seminal vesicle and ventral prostate weight to castration levels can be achieved. This is not the case for the gestagen antiandrogen (MGA), as reported by El Eltreby et al. (1987).

It can be concluded that pure antiandrogens act only at the androgen target cell level, which leads to an increase in plasma testosterone levels in intact rats and human males. With constant dosage of the antiandrogen plasma testosterone levels stabilize at a certain level. At this moment it is not known whether the increased amount of androgens is effectively counteracted by the antiandrogens at the target cell level. Considering the mechanism of action of the pure antiandrogens, this seems unlikely. Studies of tissue concentrations of androgens, especially of the DHT in prostatic nuclei, would be important to elucidate at this point, but unfortunately these have not been carried out. It will also be useful to see whether human benign prostatic hyperplasia (BPH) involutes with the regular recommended dosage of 750 mg flutamide per day, and, if such involution occurs, whether it persists without increasing the dosage of flutamide as plasma testosterone rises. In combination with castration, an LH-RH agonist or other castrating principles flutamide effectively counteracts the remaining adrenal androgens at target cells.

With CPA the problem of rising plasma androgen levels does not exist because of the antigonadotropic effect of this drug. In experimental studies CPA was shown to be more effective in excluding testosterone action in the intact rat (El Etreby et al. 1987), and used at proper dosage levels it should be effective in counteracting adrenal androgens after castration or under LH-RH agonist use. It has been shown by klijn et al. (1985) that CPA suppresses prostatic acid phosphatase, a marker for the total mass of marker-producing prostatic cancer cells during the initial phase of stimulation of plasma testosterone with the use of an LH-RH agonist.

Androgenic Effects of Antiandrogens

It has been claimed by Poyet and Labrie (1985) that CPA is androgenic and therefore not suited for the treatment of prostatic cancer. This claim was based on findings obtained by the application of CPA during the regression phase of the ventral prostate of the rat after castration. These authors showed a significant inhibition of prostatic regression by CPA and MGA but not by flutamide. If flutamide is given simultaneously with MGA and CPA, the observed inhibition of prostatic regression is inhibited. The data are significant when compared to the volumes of the ventral prostate obtained after castration during the same period of time but amount to only less than 10% of the volume of the intact prostate, as shown by El Etreby et al. (1987). The results of a reproduction of this experiment by El Etreby et al. (1987) are shown in Fig. 3. The involution of the prostate is an active process requiring an increase in prostatic catabolic activities, which in intact rats is normally inhibited by androgens. However, not only low dosages of androgens but also agents known to inhibit protein and RNA synthesis such as

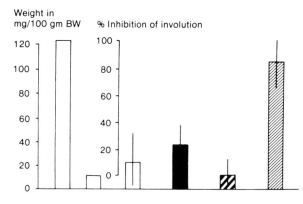

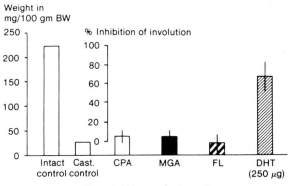

Fig. 3. Effects of cyproterone acetate (*CPA*), megestrol acetate (*MGA*), and flutamide (*FL*) on ventral prostate and seminal vesicle weights on the regression phase of these organs during the 3 weeks following castration. Organ weights in intact animals after castration and after stimulation with dihydrotestosterone (*DHT*) are used for comparison. The differences of inhibition seen for equal doses of CPA, MGA, and FL after 3 weeks are not significant. (El Etreby et al. 1987)

Table 1. Effect of Cyproterone acetate (CPA) in immature orchiectomized rats treated by subcutaneous injections for 7 days. (From Neri et al. 1967)

Daily treatment	Relative organ weights (mg/100 g bodyweight)	
	Seminal vesicles	Ventral prostate
Control	4.5 ± 0.3	7.7 ± 0.9
Testosterone 100 mg	34.9 ± 5.1	53.6 ± 6.1
CPA 100 mg/kg	8.6 ± 0.7	11.1 ± 1.8
20 mg/kg	6.0 ± 0.4	8.1 ± 0.8
10 mg/kg	4.1 ± 0.3	7.5 ± 0.7
1 mg/kg	4.6 ± 0.3	7.5 ± 0.7

Control, castrated at age 3–4 weeks.

actinomycin B and cyclohexamide can prevent the rapid rate prostatic cell death, as shown by Isaacs (1984). For this reason it is possible that this effect of CPA of inhibiting the complete involution of the prostate may not be related to the androgenicity but rather to a direct or direct inhibitory effect of CPA on prostatic catabolic activities.

Neri et al. (1967, 1972) have extensively compared biological effects of various dosages of flutamide and CPA. Table 1 shows some of their data relating to the effect of CPA on the ventral prostate and the seminal vesicles in immature castrated rats. It can be seen that in extremely high dosages a stimulation of the weight of these organs occurs which amounts to ± 10% of organ weights under physiological and exogenous stimulation by androgens. This effect disappears with the 10- and 20-mg doses per kilogram body weight which would normally be used to achieve an effect of CPA on androgen-dependent organs in the rat.

In contrast to these findings in the rat, there is no evidence in other animal species, for example, in the dog, which was extensively studied, that CPA may have any androgenic activities especially on the prostate gland. Histologically and regarding prostate weights the effect of CPA in the dog is indentical to that of castration (Tunn et al. 1979). Also in other sensitive systems, such as the viriliz-ation studies carried out in fetal female mice exposed to androgens in utero (Neumann 1984), no androgenic activity of CPA could be shown.

Clinical Use of Antiandrogens

Considering the differences in the mechanisms of actions of the two types of antiandrogens, pure and endocrine active, different clinical effects may be expected if these drugs are used in intact males. If used in conjunction with castration, LH-RH agonists or other treatment principles resulting in castration levels of plasma testosterone an identical effect of the two substances may be expected in counter-acting the remaining androgenic activity from adrenal androgens. The latter approach, which has been termed "total androgen suppression" or "total androgen blockade," has in recent years been promoted by Labrie and his coworkers (1983, 1985). It was claimed that total androgen blockade would produce clinical results in the management of metastatic prostatic cancer which are far superior to those obtained by castration or other standard forms of treatment. This claim has stimulated a large effort of clinical and basic research directed at confirming or rejecting the hypothesis of Labrie et al. At this time enough evidence has accumulated to define the precise role of total androgen suppression in the management of prostatic cancer. A review these recent developments is given below.

Total Androgen Suppression

It has been shown by several authors that the level of DHT in human prostatic tissue decreases after castration. Data by Bélanger and coworkers (1986), which are summarized in Table 2, show that testosterone and the DHT concentrations in human prostatic carcinoma tissue can be further suppressed by means of castration with the addition of flutamide. The possibility that the remaining androgen concentrations in the prostatic tissue after castration are still capable of stimulating growth of prostatic carcinoma cells is the theoretical basis for the clinical application of the concept of total androgen blockade. Arguments for and against the biological effectiveness of such androgen concentrations have recently been reviewed by Schröder and van Steenbrugge (1988). Data by van Steenbrugge et al. (1987) obtained with the use of the hormone-dependent human prostatic carcinoma tissue line transplantable in nude mice PC 82 however, show, clearly that the cut-off point for stimulation by DHT is in the range of 13–15 pmol/g tissue. These figures are just below the normal level for DHT found in this particular system. It is evident that experimental data cannot resolve the important question as to whether patients would benefit from total androgen blockade more than from castration and other standard forms of treatment. The results of large clinical studies comparing these two treatment principles are available now for review.

Clinical Studies on Total Androgen Blockade

Two French studies have been reported by Brisset (1986) and Namer et al. (1987) in which castration is compared to total androgen suppression regimens. Both of

Table 2. Androgen levels in prostatic cancer tissue. (From Bélanger et al. 1986)

Treatment	n	Testosterone (ng/g)	Dihydroxy testosterone (ng/g)
Untreated	6	4.9 ± 0.3	14.6 ± 1.7
Castrated	5	3.4 ± 1.0	5.8 ± 2.0
Castrated +	3	1.6 ± 0.7	< 1.0

these studies show a difference in early response rates in favor of total androgen suppression which is not reflected in an improvement in survival rates.

Iversen et al. (1988) reported on a large Danish clinical study comparing castration alone to the use of total androgen blockade by means of Zoladex (goserelin) in combination with flutamide; 248 ml patients were recruited to this trial. Criteria recommended by the World Health Organization (WHO) and subjective criteria were used. Progression and death served as end points. Short-term observations up to 12 months indicated no difference in subjective and objective response rates. At the time of the last evaluation, reported orally in March 1988, 26 patients were in progression in the total androgen suppression arm as opposed to 34 patients in the castration arm. This difference at an average follow-up of 12 months was statistically significant. One case of acute hepatic failure was observed in the group of patients treated with flutamide.

A Canadian study reported by Fradet and coworkers (1988) compared castration plus placebo versus castration plus anandron, a pure antiandrogen, in a double-blind study of previously untreated patients with metastatic prostatic cancer; 149 patients were recruited. National prostatic cancer project criteria were used; progression and death were studied as end points. Pain relief at 3 and 6 months as well as best response were significantly better in the total androgen blockade arm. At 6 months a significant difference between the progression rates was observed in favor of the total androgen suppression arm. This difference had disappeared at 12 months. Survival curves showed a small difference in favor of the total androgen suppression, which was not statistically significant. Disturbance of visual adaptation and alcohol intolerance was seen in 30% of patiens treated by means of anandron.

Crawford et al. reported in 1988 only on the large American study initiated by the National Cancer Institute, initially conducted by the National Prostatic Cancer Project and later taken over by the Intergroup for Oncological Research (study no. 0036). In this study 352 patients with metastatic prostatic carcinoma were compared in two treatment groups utilizing the LH-RH analogue leuprolide versus leuprolide plus flutamide. The study was double-blinded for flutamide. Patients with performance WHO status 4 or 5 were excluded. At the time of entry into the study 40% of patients had pain. National prostatic cancer project criteria were used to study subjective and objective response. Progression and death served as end points. Pain was significantly improved at 1- and 4-week evaluations in favor of total androgen suppression. The same was true for PAP suppression at weeks 4 and 12. The improvement of performance showed a trend in favor of the combination arm which, however, was statistically not significant. There was no difference in best response rates between the two groups. In the total androgen blockade arm median time to progression amounted to 16.2 months as opposed to 13.6 months in the LH-RH arm; this difference of 2.6 months was statistically significant. These data are based on a report given in March 1988. Three months later in June 1988 the same authors reported orally a small but significant difference in survival which is in the same range as the difference in progression rate.

Schröder et al. (1987) reported on a Dutch study of 58 patients with metastatic prostatic carcinoma treated with buserelin alone as opposed to 13 patients treated by means of buserelin and castration. The study was prospective but not random-ized. Progression rates in the two arms of the study were identical. They amounted to 37% in the LH-RH agonist and 41.7% in the combination arm. All patients were studied exactly at the 12-month follow-up point.

Long before total androgen suppression was promoted by Labrie and his coworkers the Genitourinary Group of the European Organization for Research and Treatment of Cancer (EORTC) decided in 1979 to carry out a study which included a total androgen suppression regimen in the form of castration plus CPA 150 mg/day. This arm was included in protocol 30805 with the purpose of studying the effect of counteraction of adrenal androgens after castration by means of CPA in comparison to castration alone and to 1 mg diethystilboestrol (DES), a regimen which is known not to suppress plasma testosterone to castration levels. The study was carried out from 1980 through 1984. Preliminary results have been published by Robinson and Hetherington (1986). Response was not studied in this protocol. Progression and survival rates showed no differences between the treatment arms.

Another EORTC study of which preliminary results were reported by Denis et al. (1989) compares the effect of castration versus the antiandrogen flutamide in combination with the LH-RH agonist Zoladex in 322 previously untreated meta-static prostatic carcinoma patients. Progression and survival rates show no differ-ences at first evaluation.

With regard to total androgen suppression in the management of patients with metastatic prostatic carcinoma, there are two studied in which total androgen suppression regimens produced slight advantages in progression and survival rates (Iversen et al. 1988; Crawford et al. 1988). Although statistically significant, it is questionable whether differences in progression and survival curves, which amount to 2–3 months, have clinical significance and justify the cost and effort of using total androgen suppression regimens. In addition, there is overwhelming evidence from other studies which shows no such differences in progression and survival rates. Possibly there is an advantage in early response rates in favor of total androgen blockade especially in those patients who are seriously ill as a result of a very large metastatic mass. It has been shown beyond doubt that the addition of a pure or steroidal antiandrogen to an LH-RH analogue during the first 4 weeks of treatment can prevent the disease flair-up which may result from stimulation of malignant tumor cells during the initial rise in plasma testosterone levels. Also, CPA can prevent hot flushes occurring with castration and other endocrine treatment modalities as shown by Eaton and McGuire (1983). Experimental data suggest that to suppress the growth of human prostatic carcinoma it may not be necessary to reach castration levels of androgens in tumor tissue.

Antiandrogens as Monotherapy for Prostatic Cancer

Potential differences in the effectiveness of pure and endocrine active antiandrog-ens as monotherapy on theoretical grounds have already been discussed. No comparative study of these two types of antiandrogens is available. Also, un-fortunately no prospective randomized trial of sufficient size has been carried out to answer the question as to whether treatment with a "pure" antiandrogen as monotherapy is equally effective as standard forms of management.

Phase II studies of flutamide alone have been reported by Sogani (1979), MacFarlane and Tolley (1985), Lundgren (1987), and Lund and Rasmussen (1988). The results concerning the suppression of tumor growth and also concerning the side effects of flutamide are quite variable, and the authors come to different conclusions. Lundgren and MacFarlane and Tolley report a high incidence of nonresponse and side effects and consider flutamide not suitable for monotherapy of prostatic cancer; Sogani and Lund and Rasmussen conclude the contrary. In all groups gastrointestinal side effects are seen with variable incidence. The most serious reported side effect is acute hepatitis, such as in reversible deterioration of liver function parameters, necessitating the discontinuation of treatment. Nausea and diarrhea are other side effects encountered by these investigators. It is remarkable that virtually all patients reported to be potent and sexually active at the time of initiation of flutamide monotherapy remained potent.

Lund and Rasmussen as well as Lundgren report plasma testosterone values in their patients prior to treatment and then in 3-month intervals up to 1 year. The highest values are found after 3 months; plasma testosterone decreases and in the series of Lund and Rasmussen reaches precastration values after 12 months. In the same study the effect of flutamide alone is compared to 3 mg DES per day in 20 patients per treatment group. No differences in response and progression rates are seen. The series is too small to produce statistically or clinically significant results.

The problem of clinical effectiveness of pure antiandrogens in the management of metastatic prostatic cancer remains one of the few open questions concerning endocrine treatment of this disease. If it could be shown in a prospective randomized study that pure antiandrogens are indeed equally as effective as standard treatment, then, if cost and side effects were acceptable, because of preservation of potency preference should be given to these substances.

Regarding CPA a prospective randomized trial of the EORTC Genitourinary Group has shown that 250 mg CPA per day is equally as effective as diethyl stilbestrol (DES) 1 mg tid when progression and death rates are considered. In the same study, protocol 30761, CPA produces significantly fewer side effects compared to 3 mg DES per day. Interestingly, a third arm of this study using MPA at low dose showed significantly poor progression and survival even after correction for prognostic factors in the treatment group. The end results of this trial have been reported by Pavone et al. (1986). Treatment with CPA is usually associated with loss of potency.

Summary

Endocrine-active and pure antiandrogens have different mechanisms of action and different endocrinological effects in the intact male. With pure antiandrogens as a monotherapy an elevation of plasma testosterone occurs which probably leads to the preservation of potency, the clinical significance of which in the management of prostatic carcinoma is not known. Plasma testosterone is reduced to pretreatment levels after 12 months. Longer observations are not available. In total androgen suppression regimens both types of antiandrogens have been shown in prospective trials to be at least equally effective as standard treatment.

The clinical effectiveness of CPA alone in prostatic cancer has been shown to be equal to that of DES 1 mg tid. Sufficiently large prospective studies on flutamide alone in comparison to standard treatment have not been carried out. The use of antiandrogens is recommended during the initial 4 weeks of management of prostatic carcinoma patients with LH-RH agonists to prevent disease flare-up and to achieve higher early response rates in selective patients.

References

Bélanger A, Labrie F, Dupont A (1986) Androgen levels in prostatic tissue of patients with carcinoma of the prostatic treated with the combined therapy using an LHRH agonist and a pure antiandrogen. Eur J Cancer Clin Oncol 22: 742

Brinkmann AO, Lindh LM, Breedveld DI, Mulder E, Molen HJ, Van der (1983) Cyproterone acetate prevents translocation of the androgen receptor in the rat prostate. Mol Cell Endocrinol 32: 117–129

Brisset JM, Boccon-Gibod L, Botto H, Camey M, Cariou G, Duclos JM, Duval F, Gonties D, Jorest R, Lamy L, Le Duc A, Mouton A, Petit M, Prawerman A, Richard F, Savatovsky I, Vallancien G (1987) Anandron (RU 23908) associated to surgical castration in previously untreated stage D prostate cancer: a multicenter comparative study of two doses of the drug and of a placebo. In: Murphy GP, Khoury S, Kuss R, Chatelain C, Denis L (eds) Prostate cancer. Part A. Prog Clin 243: 411–422

Crawford ED, McLeod D, Dorr A, Spaulding J, Benson R, Eisenberger M, Blumenstein B (1988) Oral communication, International symposion on GnRH analogues in cancer and human reproduction, Geneva, Switzerland

Denis L, Carneira de Moura, Smith P, Newling D, Sylvester R, the EORTC gu-group (1989) Zoladex and flutamide versus orchidectomy: first final analysis of EORTC 30853, J urol 141 (2): 565 (Abstract) Eaton AC, McGuire N (1983) Cyproterone acetate in treatment of post-orchidectomy hot flushes. Double blind cross trial. Lancet 1336–1337

El Etreby MF, Habenicht UF, Louton T, Nishino Y. Schröder HG (1987) Effect of Cyproterone acetate in comparison to flutamide and megestrol acetate on the ventral prostate, seminal vesicle, and adrenal glands of adult male rats. Prostate 11: 361–375

Fradet Y, Béland G, Elhilali M, Laroche B, Ramsey EW, Tewari ED, Trachtenberg J, Venner PN (1988) Oral communiation, International symposion on GnRH analogues in cancer and human reproduction, Geneva, Switzerland

Isaacs JT (1984) Antagonistic effect of androgen on prostatic cell death. Prostate 5: 545–557

Iversen P, Hvidt V, Krarup T, Rasmussen F, Rose C (1988) Oral communication, International symposion on GnRH analogues in cancer and human reproduction, Geneva, Switzerland

Klijn JGM, De Voogt HJ, Schröder FH, DeJong FH (1985) Combined treatment with buserelin and cyproterone acetate in metastatic prostatic carcinoma. Lancet II: 493 (letter to the editor)

Knuth UA, Hano R, Nieschlag E (1984) Effect of Flutamide or cyproterone acetate on pituitary and testicular hormones in normal men. J Clin Endocrinol Metab 59: 963–969

Labrie F, Dupont A, Belanger A, Lacoursiere Y, Raynaud JP, Husson JM, Gareau J, Fazekas ATA, Sandow J, Monfette G, Girard JG, Emond J, Houle JG (1983) New approach in the treatment of prostate cancer: complete instead of partial withdrawal of androgens. Prostate 4: 579–594

Labrie F, Dupont A, Bélanger A, Giguere Y, Lacoursière J, Emond J, Monfette G, Bergeron V (1985) combination therapy with flutamide and castraction (LHRH agonist or orchiectomy) in advanced prostate cancer: a marked improvement in response and survival. J Steroid Biochen 23: 833–841

Lund F, Rasmussen F (1988) Flutamide versus stilboestrol in the management of advanced prostatic cancer. A controlled prospective study. Br J Urol 61: 140–142

Lundgren R (1987) Flutamide as primary treatment for metastatic prostatic cancer. Br J Urol 59: 156–158

MacFarlane JR, Tolley DA (1985) Flutamide therapy for advanced prostatic cancer: a phase II study. Br J Urol 57: 172–174

Namer M, Toubol J, Adenis L, Amiel J, Couette J, Douchez J, Droz JP, Fargeot P, Kerbrat P, Mangin P, Petiot A, Bertagna C, Francois JP (1988) Oral communication, International symposon on GnRH analogues in cancer and human reproduction, Geneva Switzerland

Neri RO (1977) Studies on the biology and mechanism of action of nonsteroidal antiandrogens. In: Martini L, Motta M (eds) Androgens and antiandrogens. Raven, New York, pp 179–89

Neri RO, Monahan MD, Meyer, JG, Afonso BA, Tabachnick IA (1967) Biological studies on an anti-androgen (SH 714). Eur J Pharmacel 1: 438–444

Neri RO, Florance K, Koziol P, Cleave S van (1972) A biological profile of a nonsteroidal antiandrogen, SCH 13521 (4'-nitro-3'-trifluoromethylisobutyranilide). Endocrinology 91: 427–37

Neumann F, Habenicht UF, Schacher A (1984) Antiandrogens and target cell response – different in vivo effects of cyproterone acetate, flutamide and cyproterone. In: McKerns W, Aakvaag A, Hansson V (eds) Regulation of target cell responsiveness, vol 2. Plenium, New York, 489–527

Pavone–Macaluso M, de Voogt HJ, Viggiano G, Barasolo E, Lardennois B, de Pauw M, Sylvester R (1986) Comparison of diethylstilbestrol, cyproterone acetate and medroxyprogesterone acetate in the treatmnt of advanced prostatic cancer: final analysis of a randomized phase III trial of the European Organization for Research on Treatment of Cancer Urological Group. J Urol 136: 624–631

Poyet P, Labrie F (1985) Comparison of the antiandrogenic/androgenic activities of flutamide cyproterone acetate and megestrol acetate. Mol Cell Endocrinol 42: 283–288

Robinson MRG, Hetherington J (1986) The EORTC studies: is there an optimal endocrine management for Ml prostatic cancer? World J Urol 4:1–5

Schröder FH, Van Steenbrugge GJ (1988) Rationale against total androgen withdrawal. Ballieres Clin Oncol 2: 621–633

Schröder FH, Lock MTWT, Chadha DR, Debruyne FMJ, Karthaus HFM, De Jong FH, klijn JGM, Matroos AW, De Voogt HJ (1987) Metastatic cancer of the prostate managed with buserelin versus buserelin plus cyproterone acetate. J Urol 137: 912–918

Sogani PC, Vagaiwala MR, Whitmore WF, Jr (1984) Experience with flutamide in patients with advanced prostatic cancer without prior endocrine therapy. Cancer 54: 744–750

Van Steenbrugge GJ, Van Dongen JJW, Reuvers PJ, De Jong FH, Schröder FH (1987) Transplantable human prostatic carcinoma (PC-82) in athymic nude mice. I. Hormone dependence and the concentration of androgens in plasma and tumor tissue. Prostate 11: 195–210

Tunn U, Senge T, Schenck B, Neumann F (1979) Biochemical and histological studies on prostates in castrated dogs after treatment with androstanediol, oestradiol and cyproterone acetate. Acta Endocrinol 91: 373–384

LH–RH Agonist Monotherapy in Patients with Carcinoma of the Prostate and Reflections on the So-called Total Androgen Blockade

G.H. Jacobi

Urologische Fachpraxis, Friedrich–Ebert–Straße 176, 4100 Duisburg 18, FRG

Shortly after it had been demonstrated that synthetic analogues of luteinizing hormone releasing hormone (LH-RH analogues or LH-RH agonists), if applied in "supraphysiological" doses and in continuous seccession, act to suppress testosterone to the castrate level, this principle of action was introduced in the so-called contrasexual therapy of metastatic carcinoma of the prostate (Jacobi et al. 1987a; Wenderoth and Jacobi 1985). The key position of LH-RH agonists lies within the framework of contrasexual measures altering the hypothalamus – pituitary – gonad axis. Meanwhile, several LH-RH agonists have been commercialized, either for pernasal (buserelin), for subcutaneous (buserelin, leuprolide, gonadorelin) or for intramuscular (gonadorelin depot) administration. Other depot forms of these analogue hormones (buserelin, goserelin) are at the present time the object of worldwide experimental and clinical studies.

Our present knowledge – based on 6 years of clinical research on patients with advanced carcinoma of the prostate – permits the conclusion that all the above-mentioned LH-RH agonists are equally effective in their castration effect, clinical potency, and low incidence of tolerable side effects. Advantages or disadvantages, if there are any, concern only the costs of treatment, the various forms of application, and the resulting different degrees of compliance.

Our institution has been engaged in intensive animal experiments and clinical trials with the LH-RH analogues buserelin (Suprefact) and gonadorelin (Decapeptyl Depot) since October 1981. A randomized therapy study has now been under way for 3 years, conducted by the European Organization of Research on the Treatment of Cancer (EORTC; de Voogt, Amsterdam; Klijn, Rotterdam).

Buserelin or Decapeptyl Depot as Monotherapy

Between October 1981 and September 1987 more than 200 patients with advanced carcinoma of the prostate were treated at the Department of Urology of the University of Mainz. The present long-term analysis of the results covers 151 patients: 122 treated with buserelin and 29 with Decapeptyl Depot. We presently

Recent Results in Cancer Research. Vol. 118
© Springer-Verlag Berlin·Heidelberg 1990

Table 1. Dosage regimens for pernasal and subcutaneous buserelin and for intramuscular Decapeptyl-Depot administration

---

Buserelin

2 × 200 µg/day s.c. 14 days	
3 × 1000 µg/day s.c. 6 days	and 3 × 4000 µg/day
3 × 500 µg/day s.c. 6 days	p.n. thereafter
3 × 300 µg/day p.n. contineously	

Decapeptyl
  D-Trp 6-LHRH 3.2 mg microencapsulated
  in 119 mg lyophilisate injected i.m. every 5
weeks

---

have 85 patients under treatment with buserelin and 22 patients under treatment with Decapeptyl Depot, with a follow-up period of at least 18 months. Table 1 shows the different dosage schemes for the two LH-RH analogues. Over the past 2 years buserelin was applied only pernasally at a continuous dose of 3×300 µg/day.

All patients had advanced cancer of the prostate with no preceding therapy. The age of the patients varied between 49 and 86 years (average, 70 years). Whereas 76 patients had carcinoma of category M_1 with distant metastases (71%), 31 patients (29%) suffered from an advanced locoregional carcinoma of the tumor category $T_3N_xM_0$. All patients showed measurable tumor lesions to evaluate an objective tumor regression by means of computerized tomography, sonography, and X-ray diagnosis. All patients were checked by repeated skeleton scans. Further controls in all patients covered such laboratory parameters as prostate-specific phosphatase and prostate-specific antigen (since 1984).

Results

Figure 1 shows the long-term testosterone curve and the behavior of basal LH and LH after stimulation with native LH-RH for the buserelin group. A short stimulation phase between days 3 and 7 of treatment – with the testosterone values rising from 4.8 ± 2.2 ng/ml to 6.5 ± 2.4 ng/ml – is followed by downregulation, which after 4 weeks leads to castrate values for serum testosterone (0.5 ng/ml). As long as treatment continues, serum testosterone remains at the castrate level. At the same time the stimulability of LH ceases in spite of the administration of 25 µg native LH-RH (inset of Fig. 1). The injection of Decapeptyl Depot at intervals of 5 weeks gives a comparable testosterone curve (Fig. 2), with stimulation-induced values from 4.5 ± 1.2 initially to 6.3 ± 1.8 ng/ml on day 2 after injection and a downregulation to castrate levels after no more than 3 weeks. The testosterone curve is parallelled by the serum LH curve (inset of Fig. 2).

Four patients asked for a continuation of medication with intramuscular injections of Decapeptyl Depot for 11–26 months (average, 18 months) after the

Buserelin

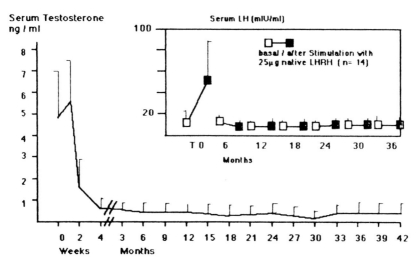

Fig. 1. Serum testosterone curve (mean values ± standard deviation) in 85 patients on a buserelin monotherapy. *Inset,* results of the LH-RH stimulation test in 14 patients. (From Jacobi 1988)

Decapeptyl

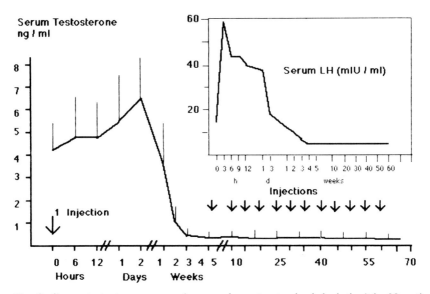

Fig. 2. Serum testosterone curve (mean values ± standard deviation) in 22 patients on Decapeptyl-Depot monotherapy. Inset, Serum LH curve in the same group of patients as in Fig.3. (From Jacobi 1988)

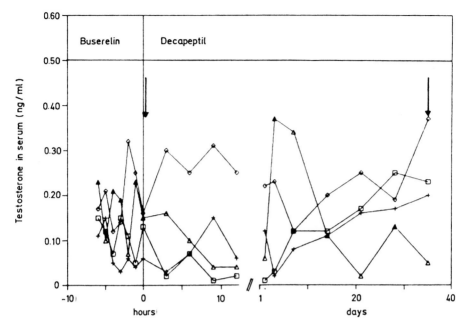

Fig. 3. Serum testosterone curves in four patients prior to and after switching from
$3 \times 300\,\mu g$ buserelin per day pernasally to injections of 3.2 mg Decapeptyl Depot
(*DTrp–6–LHRH*) i.m. once every 5 weeks; for further explanations see text. (From Jacobi
1988)

pernasal buserelin therapy. After the pernasal buserelin application the serum
testosterone level was determined at hourly intervals over 6 h, and the first
intramuscular Decapeptyl injection was given; testosterone was determined at 3–h
intervals over 12 h and then weekly. As can be seen from Fig. 3, this therapy
change did not cause a significant difference in the testoterone downregulation: the
testosterone levels remained in all patients at the castrate level (under 0.5 ng/ml).
All patients remained in the condition of objective remission.

To evaluate the clinical response to buserelin or Decapeptyl Depot therapy, we
first applied the response criteria of the EORTC and compared the data obtained
with those based on the criteria of the National Prostatic Cancer Treatment Group
(NPCTG). The clinical response was evaluated 6 months after commencement of
treatment. The patients treated with buserelin had a follow-up period of 2–4.5
years, and those treated with Decapeptyl one of 15–24 months. Table 2 shows the
response data under the EORTC criteria, whereas Table 3 gives a comparison of
the clinical response rates. The average response time (partial or complete remission) was 23 months for the buserelin treated patients and 14 months for the
Decapeptyl Depot group. The subjective response to the therapy was determined 2
months after commencement of treatment; 32 out of 40 patients with osseous
metastases reported a significant reduction in metastatic bone pain. Clinical
examples are demonstrated in Fig. 4 for a complete objective response, in Fig. 5 for
partial response, and in Fig. 6 for "no change" despite subjective improvement.

Table 2. Clinical response rates (EORTC criteria) in 107 patients (evaluated after 6 months) on monotherapy with LH-RH agonists

	Buserelin (n = 85)	Decapeptyl (n = 22)
Objective		
Partial and complete remission	54%	51%
No change	25%	33%
Progression	21%	16%
Subjective	25/31 (81%)	7/9 (78%0

Table 3. Comparison of clinical response rates in 107 patients in terms of NPCTG and EORTC criteria

NPCTG	
Partial or complete remission	53%
Stable disease	28%
Progression	19%
EORTC	
Partial or complete remission	52%
No change	30%
Progression	18%

The category "stable disease" in the NPCTG criteria is considered as a therapy success whereas that of "no change" in the EORTC criteria is considered a therapy failure.

Relapses After Buserelin

The remission rate of 54% after buserelin (Table 2) was based on a 6 month follow-up regime. However, out of the entire group of patients treated since 1981, 46 showed a relapse after a primary partial or complete remission. These patients have meanwhile been in the follow-up regime for 30–58 months, which covers the following parameters: first objective sign of secondary progression, correlation of the initial serum testosterone levels, time interval until the occurrence of progression, additional palliative therapy, survival time, time interval between occurrence of progression and death, and cause of death. The indicator lesions, which helped to objectivate the secondary progression, were osseous metastases (M_1) in 39 patients, lymph node metastases (categories N_2–N_4) in four patients, and the advanced locoregional tumor (category T_4) in three patients.

Fig. 4 a-c. Complete objective remission of pelvic lymph node metastasis after buserelin ▶ treatment (EORTC criteria). Computed tomographic scan. **a** Before treatment. **b** After 12 months. **c** After 25 months

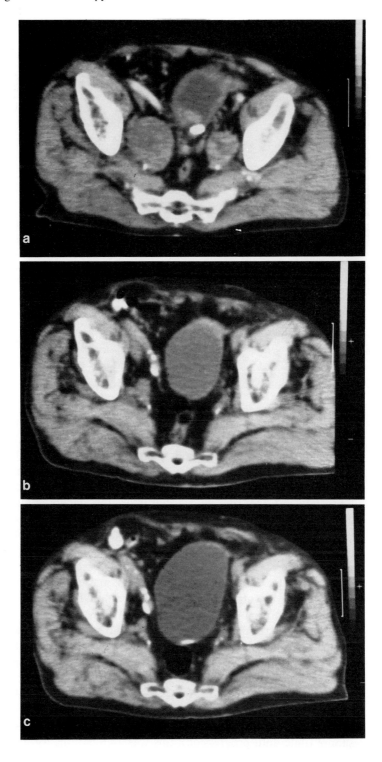

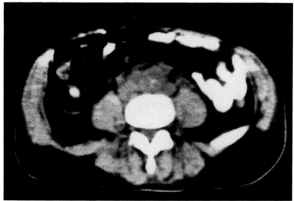

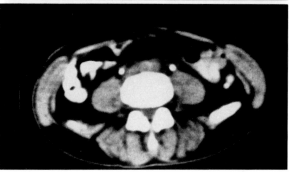

Fig. 5. Partial remission of retroperitoneal lymph node metastases after buserelin treatment (EORTC criteria). *Upper part,* before treatment with total ureteral obstruction and uremia (percutaneous nephrostomies); *lower part,* after 3 months with normal urinary flow from upper tract (ureters patent again)

In 36 patients the above-mentioned indicator lesions were the first clue of progression needing additional treatment, as compared to 10 patients in whom the progression was signaled by major pains from osseous metastases (Fig. 7). The time interval until the occurrence of progression ranged from 3 to 45 months (average, 13.6 months). Of the 32 patients (70% who died, 31 did so from cancer of the prostate and one from myocardial infarction (Jacobi et al. 1987b). The time interval from the objective secondary progression to death was 0–30 months (average, 10.5 months); the survival time ranged from 3 to 58 months (average, 27 months). At the time of the progression 36 patients, while continuing the buserelin therapy, were treated with additional palliative measures: high-dose intravenous fosfestrol therapy (Honvan, 12 g per 10 days) and/or estramustine phosphate (31 patients); local radiotherapy of painful skeleton regions (5 patients); systemic therapy with the radioisotope yttrium (9 patients).

To determine the degree to which the initial androgen balance of patients may have an impact on the long-term results of pharmacological castration by means of LH-RH agonists, we correlated the response rates to initial (pretherapy) serum testosterone, differentiating patients with normal serum testosterone levels (above 2.5 ng/ml) from those with an initial serum testosterone below this level. Of the 46 patients with a secondary relapse 14 (30.4%) had subnormal pretherapy testosterone levels, which, however, had no influence on the time interval of the clinical response (time until progression); this was 13.6 months for all 46 patients – 14.2

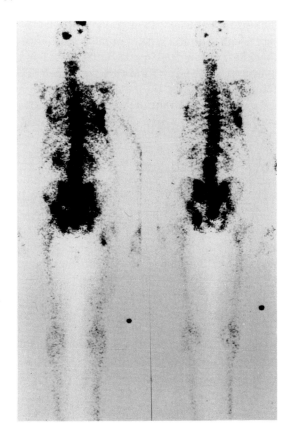

Fig. 6. So-called "no change" response according to EORTC criteria despite subjective improvement (relief of metastatic bone pain) and reduction of bone lesions in size and number. Bone scan before (*left*) and 6 months after treatment with Decapeptyl Depot (*right*)

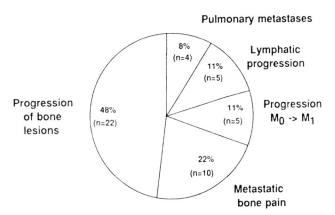

Fig. 7. First sign of relapse in 46 patients on buserelin monotherapy after a primary partial or complete remission; the ten patients with pain from osseous metastases had skeletal metastases already initially and were free from pain during the objective remission phase. (From Jacobi 1988)

months for patients with an initially normal testosterone level and 12.5 months for those with an initially subnormal testosterone level. This result is in contrast to that of a study by Hickey et al. (1986) based on heterogeneous material as far as the contrasexual therapy forms are concerned. These authors observed no objective tumor regression in any of the patients with an initial serum testosterone under 2.0 ng/ml, although the pretherapy testosterone levels were not significantly different in the groups with a clinical response or a therapy failure.

Total Androgen Blockade

The rationale for additional suppression of the residual androgens after orchiectomy or a contrasexual therapy with LH-RH agonists (testosterone lower than 0.5 ng/ml) at the target organ is presented in the hypothesis by Labrie et al. (1986), according to which adrenal androgens accumulate in prostate cancer as dihydrotestosterone thus stimulating the further growth of the carcinoma. Furthermore, an additional testosterone- dependent proliferation of carcinoma of the prostate is supposed to set in during the initial stimulation phase of LH-RH agonist therapy (Figs. 1, 2).

Dealing with this problem lies at the center of an EORTC protocol (30843), which was initiated in 1984 (Fig. 8). Patients with an untreated carcinoma of the prostate with distant metastases were randomly distributed to three therapy groups:

1. Bilateral orchiectomy as a so-called reference therapy.
2. Buserelin for pharmacological castration, combined with the antiandrogen cyproterone acetate over the first 2 weeks of therapy, followed by buserelin monotherapy. This treatment arm has the purpose of suppressing the testosterone stimulation phase of the first 2 weeks by the action of the antiandrogen.
3. Buserelin plus cyproterone acetate as a continuous combined therapy (so-called total androgen blockade). This treatment arm has the purpose of determinating the clinical impact of the residual adrenal androgens (after castration) neutralized by the antiandrogen in the cancer cell.

The daily doses in this study were 3×400 µg buserelin (Suprefact) pernasally and 3×50 mg cyproterone acetate (Androcur) orally.

We have treated 23 patients according to this protocol, whose testosterone curves are compared in Fig. 9 to an earlier group of patients on buserelin monotherapy. If the contrasexual therapy is initiated with buserelin plus cyproterone acetate, the antiandrogen causes no significant change in the testosterone stimulation phase, as compared to the buserelin monotherapy. There occurs, however, a faster downregulation of testosterone with the fall to the castrate level being advanced by about 1 week. This observation is essentially identical with the results obtained by Klijn et al. (1985) on a similar series.

But if the two therapy components of the total androgen blockade (LH-RH agonist plus antiandrogens) set in with a time lag between them, the testosterone

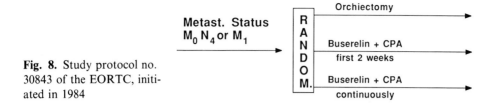

Fig. 8. Study protocol no. 30843 of the EORTC, initiated in 1984

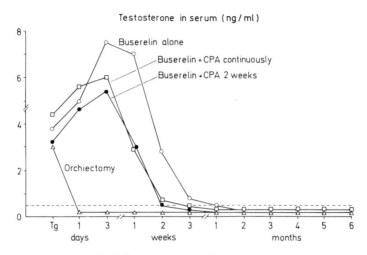

Fig. 9. Serum testosterone curves of the following groups of patients: 64 patients with a buserelin monotherapy (historical control group), 8 patients with buserelin plus cyproterone acetate (*CPA*) continuously, 8 patients with buserelin plus CPA over 2 weeks, and 7 patients with bilateral orchiectomy. (From Jacobi, 1988)

stimulation phase of the LH-RH agonists can be modulated. Svensson et al. (1986) gave their prostate cancer patients a 15-day pretreatment with cyproterone acetate thus achieving a significant diminution in serum testosterone and an intracellular blockade of the action of androgens. The following additional therapy with the LH-RH agonist Zoladex (goserelin) did produce a transitory testosterone stimulation with a peak on day 4, but the testosterone levels failed to reach the pretherapy range. The castrate level for testosterone was reached 2 weeks after the first Zoladex Depot implantation and was maintained after the second implantation 4 weeks later – in spite of the discontinuation of cyproterone acetate. Boccon-Gibod et al. (1986) obtained almost identical results in a 7-day therapeutic premedication phase with cyproterone acetate and a subsequent additional therapy with the LH-RH agonist buserelin, as did Urwin et al. (1986) with cyproterone acetate plus Zoladex.

Habenicht et al. (1986) investigated this phenomenon in detail in young healthy volunteers. These authors demonstrated the LH-RH agonist-induced testosterone suppression of stimulation with a premedicated antiandrogen in the same group of volunteers. These were treated first with buserelin (3×500 µg s.c. per day) over 7 days, during which time the testosterone stimulation occurred. After a 28-day wash-out phase the subjects received first a 5-day cyproterone acetate mono-therapy (3×50 mg per day orally), which caused a significant fall in testosterone values, but one which did not reach the castrate level. During the subsequent additional therapy with the abovementioned dose of buserelin over 7 days the testosterone stimulation was significantly weakened, with the testosterone levels reaching only the pretherapeutic range. By this combined therapy the castrate level for serum testosterone was reached after no more than 9 days, i.e., 2 weeks in advance of that with buserelin monotherapy. This confirms that premedication with cyproterone acetate over several days suppresses the testosterone stimulation phase in a subsequent therapy with LH-RH agonists thus preventing the possible clinical effects of cancer proliferation.

Another effect of the combined therapy can be derived from the afore-mentioned EORTC study at a time when clinical reference data are not yet available. The frequency rates for the sometimes annoying hot flushes in patients on monotherapy with buserelin, as far as they are communicated in the literature, vary between 50% and 68%. In the above study this rate could – with the additionally administered cyproterone acetate – be reduced to 12%–24%. In the group of orchiectomized patients hot flushes occurred in 13%.

Hot flushes after bilateral orchiectomy or during an LH-RH agonist therapy are the result of the excessive fall in peripheral androgen concentration. The attempt centrally to produce a counterregulation leads to an increased release of noradrenaline, which in turn is responsible for a disturbed thermoregulation. It has been shown in several studies that cyproterone acetate – with its centrally in-hibitory antigonadotrophic component – causes a significant suppression of hot flushes in orchiectomized patients (Eaton and Mc Guire 1983; Gingell 1984; Moon 1985). Whereas Claes et al. (1986) also suppressed LH-RH agonist-induced hot flushes with cyproterone acetate, this same effect was not achieved with the pure antiandrogen flutamide, which lacks an antigonadotrophic effect (Labrie et al. 1986).

Clinical data are not yet available from randomized studies with a long follow-up period, which might confirm the advantage of the complete androgen blockade over castration produced by surgery or drugs alone and, consequently, back the results obtained by Labrie et al. (1986) Schroeder et al. (1987), at least, found identical progression rates in two separate prospective studies with buserelin alone and buserelin plus cyproterone acetate. Very recently Crawford et al. (1989) have reported on a controlled randomized trial demonstrating a longer progression-free survival and an increase in the median length of survival for patients treated with leuprolide plus flutamide as compared to leuprolide monotreatment.

References

Baccon-Gibod L, Laudat MH, Dugue MA, Steg A (1986) Cyproterone acetate lead-in prevents initial rise of serum testosterone induced by luteinizing hormone-releasing hormone analogs in the treatment of metastatic carcinoma of the prostate. Eur Urol 12: 400–402

Claes H, Vandenbussche L, Vereecken RL (1986) Treatment of advanced carcinoma of the prostate by LHRH agonists. 7th Congress Eur Assoc Urol, Budapest. Abstract 1016

Crawford ED, Eisenberger MA, McLeod DG, Spanlding JT, Benson R, Dorr FA, Blumenstain BA, Davis MA, Goodman PJ (1989) A controlled trial of leuprolide with and without flutamide in prostatic carcinoma. New Engl J Med 321: 419–424

Eaton AC, Mc Guire N (1983) Cyproterone acetate in treatment of post-orchidectomy hot flushes, double-blind cross-over trial. Lancet 8363: 1336–1337

Gingell, JC (1984) Does orchiectomy cause excessive sweating? Br Med J 288: 6418

Habenicht UF, Witthaus, E, Neumann F. (1986) Antiandrogene und LH-RH-Agonisten; Endokrinologie in der initialphase ihrer Anwendung. Aktuel Urol 17: 10–16

Hickey D, Todd B, Soloway, MS (1986) Pre-treatment testosterone levels: significance in androgen deprivation therapy. J Urol 136: 1038–1040

Jacobi GH (1988) Endocrine management of prostatic cancer. In: Klosterhalfen H (ed) New developments in biosciences, vol 4. de Gruyter, Berlin, PP 127–137

Jacobi, GH, Wenderoth, UK, Ehrenthal W, von Wallenberg H, Spindler, H-W, Engelmann U, Hohenfellner R (1987a) Endocrine and clinical evaluation of 107 patients with advanced prostatic carcinoma under long term pernasal buserelin or intramuscular decapeptyl depot treatment. In: Klijn JGM et al. (eds). Hormonal manipulation of cancer. Raven, New York, pp. 235–248

Jacobi GH, Wenderoth UK, von Wallenberg H, Gatto M. (1987b) Progression and death following luteinizing hormone releasing hormone analogue monotreatment in advanced prostatic carcinoma. 82nd Annual meeting American Urological Association Anaheim. Abstract no 609, p 256 A

Klijn JGM, De Voogt HJ, Schröder FH, De Jong FH. (1985) Combined treatment with buserelin and cyproterone acetate in metastatic prostatic carcinoma. Lancet 8453: 493

Labrie F, Dupont A, Bélanger A, St Arnaud R, Giguère M, Lacourcière, Y, Emond J, Monfette, G (1986) Treatment of prostatic cancer with gonadotropin-releasing hormone agonists. Endocr Rev 7: 67–74

Moon TD (1985) Cyproterone acetat for treatment of hot flashes after orchiectomy. J Urol 134: 155–156

Schroeder FH, Lock MTWT, Chadha Dev R, Debruyne FMJ, Karthaus HFM, De Jong FH, Klijn JGM, Matroos AW, De Voogt, HJ. (1987) Metastatic cancer of the prostate managed by buserelin (HOE 766) versus buserelin plus cyproterone acetate (CPA). J Urol 137: 912–918

Svensson M, Varenhorst E, Kagedal B. (1986) Initial administration of cyproterone acetate (CPA) to prevent the rise of testosterone concentration during treatment with an LH-RH agonist in prostatic cancer. Anticancer Res 6: 379

Urwin, GH, Williams JL, Kanis JA (1986) Antiandrogens attenuate testosterone "flare" following Zoladex depot LHRH analogue in patients with prostatic cancer. 7th Congress Eur Assoc Urol, Budapest. Abstract no 216

Wenderoth UK, Jacobi GH (1985) Langzeitergebnisse mit dem Gn-RH-Analogon Buserelin (Suprefact[R]) bei der Behandlung des fortgeschrittenen Prostatakarzinoms seit 1981. Aktuel Urol 16: 58–63

New Developments in Biological Markers in Prostate Cancer

J.E. Pontes

Cleveland Clinic Foundation, 9500 Euclid Avenue, Cleveland, OH 44106, USA

Introduction

The use of biological markers in the diagnosis and follow-up of patients with prostate cancer was pioneered by the work of Gutman et al. in 1936. In the intervening 50 years refinements in techniques and in the understanding of the physiological function of these normally occurring enzymes and proteins have enabled us to understand the potential and the problems associated with the use of these markers in clinical medicine. A review of biological markers in the prostate published previously by me (Pontes 1983) gave an extensive analysis of the value of specific and nonspecific markers in prostate cancer.

In this chapter I discuss the present status of both prostatic specific markers – prostatic acid phosphatase (PAP) and prostatic-specific antigen (PSA).

Prostatic Acid Phosphatase

Earlier assays for the measurement of PAP used enzymatic analysis based on the action of this phosphoesterase upon different substrates, and this has given rise to the different assays used. (Pontes 1983). In the 1970s, several immunochemical assays were developed based on the immunological, specificity of PAP. Today most assays in clinical use are either radioimmunoassays (RIA) or enzymoimmuno-assays (EIA). Although these assays are more sensitive and more specific than the presently used enzymatic methods, it is clear that they cannot be used for screening of the general population, and because phosphosterases are widely present in many organs, despite the specificity of PAP, a certain small percentage of cross-reactivity occasionally exists. Because the development of PAP assays happened during a long period of time, and methodologies appeared slowly, important biological information such as the half-life of PAP and the relationship of tumor volume to PAP levels was never properly addressed. Indeed, until recently there was only one article that addressed the half-life of PAP, which demonstrated two exponential curves of decay of this enzyme (Vihko et al. 1982). In that article, the second exponential curve was probably due to methodological problems since no true half-life was ever estimated (Vihko et al. 1982).

Recently we studied the half-life of PAP in six patients undergoing radical prostatectomy (Pontes et al., to be published). The average half-life of PAP in these patients was 7.2 h with a SE of $\pm$ 0.7 h (Pontes et al., to be published). Although we continued to detect variable levels of PAP in long-term follow-up of these patients, this could attributable either to background "noise" due to the assays or to cross-reacting phosphoesterase from different sources.

Prostatic-Specific Antigen

Since the characterization of PSA by Wang in 1979 several assays for determining PSA have become available. Two assays are presently widely used in the United States – the Yang RIA (Liedtke and Batjer 1984) and the Tanden monoclonal immunoradiometric assay (Chan et al. 1986). Using each one of these assays, Stamey et al. (1987) and Oesterling et al. (1987) have done extensive clinical studies on PSA. In these studies, the half-life of PSA was calculated at 2.2 days and 3.15 days, respectively (Stamey et al. 1987; Oesterling et al. 1987). The discrepancies observed among the two studies have been addressed recently by us (Pontes et al., to be Published) our results are similar to those published by Stamey et al. (1987). Data published from these studies on the relationship between tumor volume and the level of PSA and on the relationship to the level of PSA in identifying early carcinoma of the prostate reveal that there is a significant overlap between levels in benign prostatic hyperplasia and early carcinoma, and that there is no direct relationship between the volume of tumor and levels of PSA (Stamey et al. 1987; Oesterling et al. 1987). However, it is clear that after radical prostatectomy PSA is the best indicator for recurrent disease.

Material and Methods

Our studies comprised two groups of patients. In the first group, six patients undergoing radical prostatectomy had multiple sequential serum samples following removal of the prostate for calculation of the half-life of PAP and PSA (Pontes et al., to be published). The second group consisted of 30 patients who underwent radical prostatectomy, and in whom samples of PAP and PSA were obtained before and after surgery in an attempt to correlate the preoperative levels with the stage of the disease. PAP was measured using the PAP-EIA reagent (Abbott Laboratory Diagnostic Division, North Chicago IL 60064). The method is solid-phase EIA based on the "sandwich" principle. For the half-life studies of PSA the Yang RIA technique was used (Yang Laboratory, 1401 149th Place NE, Bellevue WA 98067). For the remaining studies the Tanden-R monoclonal radiometric assay was used (Hybritech Inc., 11095 Torreyanna Rd, San Diego, CA 92126).

Results

The half-live of PAP and PSA were found to be 7.25 ± 0.7 h and 45.5 ± 4.4 h, respectively (Pontes et al., to be published). In two patients, despite the return to normal of PAP levels, PSA continued to be elevated. Both patients developed metastatic prostatic carcinoma within 6 months of radical prostatectomy (Pontes et al., to be Published).

The comparison between preradical prostatectomy PAP and PSA levels and pathological staging is shown in Tables 1 and 2. Prior to surgery, 22 patients had normal PAP values while only 18 patients had normal PSA values. There was no good correlation between the values of either marker and the extent of the disease although levels of PSA above 40 ng/ml were associated either with seminal vesical invasion or with metastatic lymph nodes. Two patients demonstrated elevation of PAP levels with normal PSA while six patients had elevated PSA with normal PAP. Postoperatively, detectable levels of PAP continued to be found in every patient while the majority of patients had PSA levels which were undetectable.

Discussion

Recent developments in the biology of PAP and PSA have allowed us to understand better the pathophysiology of the production of each marker and the utilization of these markers in clinical medicine (Pontes et al., to be published; Stamey et al. 1987; Oesterling et al. 1987). There is evidence in these recent studies that PSA is significantly more sensitive than PAP. It is evident also that PSA is a powerful indicator of recurrent disease following radical prostatectomy (Stamey et

Table 1. Relationship of preoperative PAP level and pathology ($n = 30$)

	PAP < 3 ng/ml	PAP > 3 ng/ml
Intraprostatic and microscopic capsular invasion	11	4
Capsular perforation	3	1
Seminal vesical involvement	6	1
Positive pelvic lymph nodes	2	2

Table 2. Relationship of preoperative PSA level and pathology ($n = 30$)

	PSA < 10 ng/ml	PSA 10–40 ng/ml	PSA > 40 ng/ml
Intraprostatic and microscopic capsular invasion	12	3	0
Capsular perforation	2	3	0
Seminal vesical involvement	2	1	1
Positive pelvic lymph nodes	2	1	3

al. 1987; Oesterling et al. 1987). However, it is clear that neither marker can be utilized in the detection of early prostatic carcinoma of the prostate since there is significant overlap between PSA levels in the early stage of prostatic carcinoma and those in benign prostatic hyperplasia. A clear-cut relationship between volume of tumor and level of PSA cannot be found probably because of the heterogeneous production of PSA by the tumor. In general, however, there is a progressive increase in both PAP and PSA with the stages of the disease.

These studies have improved our understanding of the production of these markers in prostatic cancer and allow us to utilize these tests clinically in a wise fashion.

References

Chan DW, Bruzek D, Rock R, Waldron C (1986) evaluation of a monoclonal immunora-diometric assay for prostate-specific antigen. Clin Chem 32: 1125, Abstr 373

Gutman E, Sproul E, Gutman A (1936) Significance of increased phosphatase activity of bone at the site of osteoplastic metastases secondary to carcinoma of the prostate gland. Am J Cancer 28: 485

Liedtke RJ, Batjer JD (1984) Measurement of prostate-specific antigen by radioimmuno-assay. Clin Chem 30: 649–652

Oesterling JE, Chan DW, Epstein JI, Kimball AW, Bruzek DJ, Rock RC, Brendler CB Walsh PC (1987) Prostate specific antigen in the preoperative and postoperative evalu-ation of localized prostatic cancer treated with radical prostatectomy. J Urol 139: 766

Pontes JE (1983) Bological markers in prostate cancer. J Urol 130: 1037

Pontes JE, Jabalameli P, Montie J, Foemmel R, Howard PD, Boyett J (to be published), Disappearance rate of biological markers following radical prostatectomy — prognostic implications. Urology (to be published)

Stamey TA, Yang N, Hay AR, McNeal JE, Freiha F, Redwine E (1987) Prostate specific antigen as a serum marker for adenocarcinoma of the prostate. N Engl J Med 317: 909

Vihko PM, Schroeder FH, Lukkarinen O, Vihko R (1982) Secretion into and elimination from blood circulation of prostate specific acid phosphatase, measured by radioimmuno-assay. J Urol 128: 202

Aspects of Endocrine-Active and Endocrine-Related Tumors of the Female Genital Tract

Endocrine and Clinical Aspects of New Compounds for Treatment of Hormone-Related Cancer in Gynecology

H. von Matthiessen and W. Distler

Universitäts-Frauenklinik, Moorenstraße 5,4000 Düsseldorf, FRG

In recent years new compounds and new principles have been introduced for endocrine treatment in gynecologic oncology. These have led to a remarkable expansion in the range of therapeutic modalities, for example, in the treatment of breast cancer. Traditionally, endocrine therapy was divided into additive procedures (administration of hormones) and ablative procedures (oophorectomy, adrenalectomy, hypophysectomy). The following new approaches to the treatment of hormone-related cancer have now become of interest: (a) blockade of adrenal steroidogenesis and conversion of androgens to estrogens in extraglandular tissue by aromatase inhibitors; (b) Gonadal suppression in premenopausal women with gonadotropin-releasing hormone (GnRH) analogues; and (c) the use of tamoxifen-derivatives in the antiestrogen treatment of breast cancer.

Aromatase Inhibitors

The aromatase inhibitor aminoglutethimide (AG) is now well recognized as an effective compound for treating advanced breast cancer in postmenopausal patients. Rates of complete or partial remission that have been reported range from 14% to 49% (average, 34%), as a review of 14 studies on a total of 1211 patients shows (von Matthiessen 1985). These results were reached with a dose of 250 mg AG q.i.d. combined with 40 mg hydrocortisone. A comparable effect of AG could be seen even with a dose of 250 mg b.i.d. in combination with hydrocortisone (Stuart-Harris et al. 1984; Bonneterre et al. 1985; Illiger et al. 1985) or without cortisone replacement (Höffken et al. 1987).

AG inhibits the biosynthesis of adrenal and extra-adrenal C_{19} steroids and the peripheral conversion of androgens to estrogens. Thus AG decreases the serum levels of estrone, estradiol, androstendione, aldosterone, dehydroepiandrosterone, and urinary-free cortisol. The change in the steroid milieu may be responsible for some side effects, e.g., lethargy (33%), skin rash (23%), and nausea (15%). To reduce side effects and to obtain more specific aromatase inhibition a number of compounds have been evaluated, of which the C_{19} 3–ketosteroids have proven to be the most active. The best aromatase inhibitors were found to be androstene-3,6, 17-trione, 1,4,6-androstatriene-3,17-dione, and 4-hydroxyandrostendione-3,17-dione (4-OHA; Brodie 1982).

Early clinical trials with 4-OHA (Coombes et al. 1987; Dowsett et al. 1987) were undertaken to optimize dose and route of administration and to evaluate its antineoplastic effect. Coombes et al. (1987) compared the following dosages: 500 mg weekly i.m.; 250 mg every 2 weeks i.m.; and 500 mg p.o. daily. They demonstrated similar response rates for each group of patients (17/51, 33%; 9/25, 36%; 8/24, 33%) and concluded that 4-OHA is an effective endocrine agent for the treatment of postmenopausal patients with breast cancer. Side effects were less severe than with AG and were not found in more than 10% of patients in the orally treated group: lethargy 2.5%, skin rash 1.6%, and nausea 1.6%.

GnRH Analogues

The pulsatile secretion of GnRH from the hypothalamus causes the release of the gonadotropic hormones luteinizing hormone (LH) and follicle-stimulating hormone (FSH) from the pituitary. In women the cyclic release of estradiol and progesterone from the ovaries is regulated by LH and FSH. Estrogens and progesterone stimulate and maintain secondary sexual characteristics as well as normal functioning of sexual organs such as the uterus and mammary glands.

Administration of GnRH in a precise pulsatile pattern can restore cyclic secretion of the gonadotropins in women with hypothalamic amenorrhea. However, when administered chronically, GnRH or its analogues inhibit pituitary gonadotropin secretion (Sandow et al. 1976). In the latter way the pituitary-ovarian axis can be "dissected" in a nonsurgical and fully reversible fashion. The realization of a medical gonadectomy forms the basis for the application of GnRH analogues in various hormone-dependent cancer models.

To date the mechanism of action of GnRH analogues in suppressing pituitary LH and FSH secretion has not been completely elucidated. However, it is established that GnRH analogues cause desensitization of the gonadotroph (Sandow et al. 1978). The down-regulation of GnRH receptors is probably part of this phenomenon, and there is evidence that uncoupling of the GnRH receptor from the post-receptor mechanisms is of importance for the desensitization (Adams et al. 1986).

Since the isolation, identification, and synthesis of GnRH in 1971, a large number of agonist analogues have been synthesized. The various chemical approaches include (a) replacement of the C-terminal Gly-NH$_2$ residue by an ethylamide or an azaglycinamide residue and (b) substitution of Gly^6 by more bulky hydrophobic or hydrophilic residues. These have led to agonist analogues which are 100–200 times more potent than GnRH (Dutta 1988). Some of these analogues, e.g., buserelin (Suprefact), tryptorelin, histrelin, leuprolide, lutrelin, nafarelin, gonadorelin (DecaPeptyl), and goserelin (Zoladex), have been investigated for their physiologic and therapeutic properties.

Potent GnRH antagonists have also now become available (Dutta 1988). unlike the agonists, which contain only one or two structural changes in the parent peptide, potent antagonists have been obtained only by substituting at least four of the original amino acid residues. Although significant progress has been made in terms of increased potency, none of the antagonists has yet reached an advanced stage of development comparable to that of agonists. A large majority of the potent antagonists have been shown to release histamine in various test systems. The development of GnRH antagonists with low histamine-releasing potency is in progress (Karten et al. 1988).

The potential use of GnRH analogues for treatment of endocrine-dependent cancer was first suggested by DeSombre et al. (1976) and Johnson et al. (1976) on the basis of investigations in animals. In female rats GnRH antagonists led to regression of mammary tumors in the dimethylbenzanthracene-induced rat tumor model. Almost the first report on treatment of advanced breast cancer in premenopausal patients with buserelin was published by Klijn and de Jong (1982). There after several studies on treatment of metastatic breast cancer were published (Table 1).

By way of preliminary conclusion from these studies it can be stated that: (a) GnRH analogues reach the same response rates (30%–40%) in advanced breast cancer as the other additive or ablative hormonal procedures, (b) their efficacy is restricted to premenopausal patients, and (c) the response rates seem to be related to the receptor status.

Side effects of GnRH analogues are limited to the symptoms of estrogen deficiency. From 22 patients treated with goserelin 14 had moderate and 6 severe

Table 1. Studies on the treatment of metastatic breast cancer with GnRH analogues

Reference	*n* PAT	MS (#)	Compound	Dosage/Route	Response
Harris et al. (1987)	23	Prem	Goserelin	3.6 mg s.c. monthly	RR + PR : 1/23
Hoffken et al. (1986)	15	Prem	Buserelin	1 mg t.i.d. s.c. day 1–7 then 3 × 0.8 mg i.n. or 2 × 0.3 mg s.c./day	CR PR NC P 3 4 –8–
Klijn et al. (1985)	31	Prem	Buserelin	3 mg i.v. day 1–7 then (a) 3 × 0.4 mg i.n., (b) 2 × 1 mg s.c./day	a) CR + PR 4/12 b) CR PR NC P 2 3 --10-
Kaufmann (1988)	22	Prem	Goserelin	3.6 mg s.c. monthly	--10-- 8
Nicholson et al. (1987)	27	Prem	Goserelin	0.5–1 mg s.c. daily	--14-- 3 2
	26	Prem	Goserelin	3.6 mg s.c. monthly	
Wander et al. (1987)	10	Prem	Goserelin	3.6 mg s.c. monthly	1 4 2
	6	Postm	Goserelin	3.6 mg s.c. monthly	- - 6

MS, menopausal status; CR, complete remission; Pr, partial remission; NC, no change; P, progression of disease; Prem, premenopausal; Postm, postmenopausal.

hot flushes; 13 had a weight increase and 5 a loss of weight. One severe and one mild depression were recognized (Kaufmann et al. 1988). Nicholson et al. (1987) reported that all patients treated with GnRH developed amenorrhea within 2 months of the beginning of therapy. However, some women experienced some spottings after 2 months of goserelin treatment.

Whereas buserelin had to be given at first two to four times daily subcutaneously or intranasally, depot preparations with slow release over 4 weeks are now available for goserelin and buserelin.

Tamoxifen Derivatives

Although used as an antiestrogen, the intrinsic estrogenic activity of tamoxifen exerts unwanted side effects, for example tumor flare. In addition, tamoxifen and its metabolites possess long biological half-lives of 7–14 days (Furr and Jordan 1984). Therefore it would be of advantage to have compounds without intrinsic estrogenic activity, improved antiestrogenic activity, and a rapid elimination rate. The advantage of rapid resorption and fast elimination on the part of tamoxifen derivatives is seen with the intermittent therapy in expecting retardation of tumor cell resistance to the drug. Furthermore, the toxic effect of tamoxifen to induce hepatocellular carinoma in animals was not noticed with droloxifene in comparative investigations (Rattel et al. 1987). Some of the tamoxifen derivatives are under intensive preclinical and clinical investigation, for example, toremifen is being tested in phase III, zindoxifen in phase I, and droloxifene in phases I and II studies.

Therefore clinical data on tamoxifen derivatives are rare at present. Breitbach et al. (1987) reported on 14 patients treated with droloxifene in a phase I/II study; six of these were evaluated for tumor response. There was one complete and one partial remission, three with stable disease, and one progression. Ahlemann et al. (1987) observed in a phase II study on ten patients with intermittent treatment (100 mg droloxifene every 2nd or 3rd day) three complete and four partial remissions, one no change, and three progressions of disease; side effects were limited to hot flushes in some cases. Stamm et al. (1987) described in three patients evaluated for efficacy of treatment (20 mg daily) one stable disease and two remissions without any serious side effects.

References

Adams TE, Cumming S, Adam BM (1986) Gonadotropin-releasing hormone (GnRH) receptor dynamics and gonadotrope responsiveness during and after continuous GnRH stimulation. Biol Reprod 35: 881

Ahlemann LM, Heil M, Staab HJ (1987) Droloxifene: 3rd International intermittent therapy in metastatic breast cancer. Congress on hormones and cancer, Hamburg, Nov 6. Abstract C–030

Bonneterre J, Coppens H, Mauriac L (1985) Aminoglutethimide in advanced breast cancer: clinical results of a French multicenter randomized trial comparing 500 mg and 1 gr/day. Eur J Cancer Clin Oncol 21: 1153

Breitbach GP, Möbius V, Bastert G, Kreienberg R, Huber HJ, Staab HJ (1987) Droloxifene: efficacy and endocrine effects in treatment of breast cancer. 3rd International congress on hormones and cancer, Hamburg, Nov 6. Abstract C–031

Brodie AMH (1982) Overview of recent development of aromatase inhibitors. Cancer Res (Suppl) 42: 3312

Coombes RC, Goss PE, Dowsett M, Hutchinson G, Cunningham D, Jarman M, Brodie AMH (1987) 4-Hydroxyandrostendione treatment for postmenopausal patients with advanced breast cancer. Tumor Diagn Ther 8: 271

De sombre ER, Johnson ES, White WF (1976) Regression of rat mammary tumors effected by a gonadoliberin analog. Cancer Res 36: 3830

Dowsett M, Goss PE, Powles TJ, Hutchinson G, Brodie AMH, Jeffcoate SL, Coombes RC (1987) Use of the aromatase inhibitor 4-hydroxyandrostendione in postmenopausal breast cancer: optimization of therapeutic dose and route. Cancer Res 47: 1957

Dutta AS (1988) GnRH analogues in cancer and human reproduction. Gynecol. Endocrinol (Suppl) 1: 12

Furr BJA, Jordan VC (1984) The pharmacology and clinical use of tamoxifen. Pharmacol Ther 25: 127

Harris AL, Cantwell BMJ, Carmichael J, Farndon J, Wilson R, Dowsett M (1987) Use of LH-RH agonist Zoladex in postmenopausal breast cancer. 3rd International congress on hormones and cancer, Hamburg, Nov 6. Abstract C–034

Höffken K, Miller AA, Miller B (1986) Niedrigdosierte Aminoglutethimid-Therapie ohne Cortisolsubstitution beim metastasierten Mammakarzinom in der Postmenopause. Med Klin 81: 638

Höffken K, Miller B, Fischer P, Becher R, Scheulen ME, Miller AA, Callies R, Schmidt CG (1986): Buserelin in the treatment of postmenopausal breast cancer. Eur J Cancer Clin Oncol 22: 746

Illiger HJ, Caffier H, Cortierer H, Eggeling B, Hartlapp J, Hartwich G, Kaetlitz E, Katz R, Klasen H, Mayer AC, Preiss J, Rieche K, Wellens W (1987) Aminoglutethimid beim fortgeschrittenen Mammakarzinom: Sind 500 mg pro Tag genug? Tumor Diagn Ther 8: 187

Johnson ES, Seely JH, White WF (1976) Endocrine-dependent rat Mammary tumour regression: use of a gonadotropin releasing hormone analog. Science 194: 329

Karten MJ, Hook WA Siraganian RP (1988) The evolution of GnRH antagonists with low histamine releasing potency. Gynecol Endocrinol (Suppl) 1: 17

Kaufmann M, Schmid H, Kiesel L, Schachner-Wünschmann E (1988) Zoladex as GnRH agonist depot in premenopausal patients with metastatic breast cancer. Gynecol Endocrinol (Suppl) 1: 133

Klijn JGM, de Jong FH (1982) Treatment with a luteinizing hormone-releasing analogue (buserelin) in premenopausal patients with metastatic breast cancer. Lancet 1: 1213

Klijn JGM, De Jong FH, Lamberts SWJ, Blankenstein MA (1985) LHRH-agonist treatment in clinical and experimental human breast caner. J Steroid Biochem 23 (5b): 867

Nicholson RI, Walker KJ, Turkes A, Dyas J, Gotting KE, Plowman PN, Williams MR, Elston CW, Blamey RW (1987) The British experience with the LH-RH agonist Zoladex in the treatment of breast cancer. In: Klijn GM et al. (eds) Hormonal manipulations of cancer: peptides growth factors, and new (anti) steroidal agents. Raven, New York, p 331

Rattel B, Löser R, Dahme EG, Liehn HD, Seibel K (1987) Comparative toxicology of droloxifene (3–OH tamoxifen) and tamoxifen; hepatocellular carcinomas induced by tamoxifen. Biannial international breast cancer research conference, Miami, 1–5 March. Abstract F–18

Sandow J, v. Rechenberg W, Koenig W, Hahn M (1976) Physiological studies with highly active analogues of LH-RH chem 100: 537

Sandow J, v. Rechenberg W, Koenig W, Jerzabek G, Stoll W (1978) Pituitary gonadotropin inhibition by a highly active analog of luteinizing hormone-releasing hormone. Fertil Steril 30: 205

Stamm H, Roth R, Almendral A, Staab HJ, Heil M (1987) Tolerance and efficacy of the antiestrogen droloxifene in patients with advanced breast cancer. 3rd International congress on hormones and cancer, Hamburg, Nov 6 Abstract C–029

Stuart-Harris R, Dowsett M, Bozek T (1984) Low dose aminoglute-thimide in treatment of advanced breast cancer. Lancet ii: 604

Wander, HE, Kleeberg, UR (1988) Zoladex – synthetic GnRH analog in the treatment of pre- and postmenopausal advanced breast cancer. Gynecol. Endocrinol. (Suppl) 1: 137

Williams MR, Walker KJ, Turkes A, Blamey RW, Nicholson RI (1986) The use of an LH-RH agonist (ICI 118630, Zoladex) in advanced breast cancer. Br J Cancer 53: 629

von Matthiessen H (1985) Experimentelle und klinische Untersuchungen zur individuellen medikamentösen Therapie des metasierten Mammakarzinoms. Dissertation, Faculty of Medicine, University of Düsseldorf

Basic and Clinical Relevance of Hormonal Influence in Breast Cancer

K.Pollow[1], H.-J. Grill[1], R. Kreienberg[1], G. Hoffmann[2], T. Beck[1],
K. Schmidt-Gollwitzer[3], and B. Manz[1]

[1]Abteilung für Experimentelle Endokrinologie, Frauenklinik,
 Johannes-Gutenberg-Universität, Langenbeckstraße 1, 6500 Mainz, FRG
[2]St. Josefs-Hospital, Salusstraße 15, 6200 Wiesbaden, FRG
[3]Schering AG, Müllerstraße, 1000 Berlin, FRG

Introduction

In the Federal Republic of Germany breast cancer has a leading place among malignant tumors in women. Genital and breast cancers account for 32% of all female deaths from malignant neoplasias. The distribution of types of cancer is as follows: breast 52%, uterine cervix 9%, corpus uteri 4.5%, adnexae 19%, and other sex organs 15.5% (Maas and Sachs 1972; Schmidt-Matthiesen 1975, Vorherr 1980). Besides general epidemiological factors such as geographical distribution, dietary factors, age distribution, familial disposition, and socioeconomic influences, possible hormonal components are discussed in connection with the etiology of breast cancer (Fischedick and Lux 1977; Henderson et al. 1974; Lilienfeld 1963, Maass et al. 1970; MacMahon et al. 1973; De Waard 1969; Wynder et al. 1960; Waterhouse et al. 1976; Anderson 1974; Carroll et al. 1968; Thijssen 1968; Lewison 1976; Centers for Disease Control Cancer and Steroid Hormone Study 1983; Thomas 1984; Ketcham and Sindelar 1975). For example, an early menarche or a late menopause leads to an increased incidence of breast cancer, bilateral ovariectomy before the 40th year of life reduces the risk of breast cancer, and childlessness is regarded as a risk factor for breast cancer.

In connection with advances in the field of molecular biology made in recent decades, considerations of the etiology of breast cancer at the level of endocrine regulation are concentrated today on the receptors, the molecular response partners of hormones in the target cell (Pollow 1983; King 1976; Clark and Peck 1979; Jensen and DeSombre 1972; Baulieu et al. 1975; Baxter and Funder 1979; Edelman 1975; Katzenellenbogen 1980). On the basis of the notion that the presence of a certain receptor species in the cell very probably indicates its responsiveness to the concordant hormone (e.g., estradiol receptor–estradiol), whereas the absence of the receptor precludes this possibility, investigations have been carried out on breast cancer during the past two decades with the aim of establishing a possible connection between the receptor content and the potential success of hormone therapy. Correlations between the estrogen receptor content and the degree of remission after endocrine therapy in breast cancer in women

Recent Results in Cancer Research. Vol. 118
© Springer-Verlag Berlin·Heidelberg 1990

show that about 56% of all estrogen receptor-positive tumors react to ablative or additive endocrine therapy measures with an objective remission, whereas the receptor-negative carcinomas have only a small chance (about 6%) of responding to endocrine therapy with objective remission (McGuire et al. 1975; Maass and Jonat 1979).

We report here on our own investigations with regard to comparative biochemical analysis of steroid hormone receptors in breast cancer and human uterus, the current spectrum of techniques for identification of steroid hormone receptors, hormonal influences in breast cancer concentrated on the pituitary, ovary, adrenal cortex and thyroid, as well as the clinical relevance in the light of our own therapy studies.

Hormonal Influences in Breast Cancer

In 40 patients with confirmed breast cancer, 26 with mastopathy, 14 with genital carcinoma, 12 with benign genital diseases, and 48 healthy women as control population, various serum hormone levels were measured, and a combined pituitary function test was performed. The main interest was attached to hormones which influence prolactin secretion. Compared to the control population, on average the group of breast cancers showed the highest basal prolactin level (PRL_0) but without the normal range being exceeded (Table 1). Compared to the women with benign genital diseases and the normal group, PRL_0 was indeed raised to a statistically significant extent ($p < 0.0001$). The prolactin measurements 15 min after thyrotropin-releasing hormone (TRH) injection also showed the highest values for the group of breast cancer patients. These were also raised to a statistically significant extent compared to the patients with benign genital diseases ($p = 0.0022$) and the normal population ($p < 0.0001$). The same applies to the 30 min values determined after TRH injection and the TRH-inducible pituitary prolaction reserve Δ-PRL. The following causes must be discussed: ectopic prolactin production in the tumor itself, simultaneously existing microprolactinomas, nonspecific rise by a mechanical stimulation of the breast via the mamillary reflex, manifestation of a nonspecific stress situation in advanced disease, but also the influence of other hormones (above all estrogens) since the release of prolactin is closely linked to the pattern of release of estrogens and the thyroid hormones, since TRH not only stimulates the pituitary thyrotropin but also releases prolactin (Malar key et al. 1963; Turkington 1971; Rees et al. 1974; von Werder et al. 1977; Kolodny et al. 1972; Noel et al. 1974; Guthrie 1982; Kucera et al. 1983; Vekemans et al. 1977; Judd et al. 1978; von Werder and Rjosk 1979).

In the present investigation, significant differences in the estradiol serum and estrone serum concentrations could not be established between breast cancer patients and the control populations. Furthermore, the serum levels for growth hormone, 17α-hydroxyprogesterone, testosterone, and DHEA sulfate as well as for the gonadotropins were in the normal range in all patient groups investigated.

The results for the thyroid parameters are summarized in Table 2. Triiodothyronine (T_3) was lowered to a statistically significant extent ($p < 0.0001$) in the group

Table 1. Prolactin (PRL) before and after TRH stimulation and human growth hormones (HGH) in the serum of the overall population

Serum hormones		Breast cancer (n = 40)		Benign breast diseases (n = 26)		Gynecologic tumors (n = 15)		Benign gynecologic diseases (n = 12)		Control group (n = 48)	
		x̄	SD	x̄	SD	x̄	SD	x̄	SD	x̄	SD
PRL_0	mg/ml	11.0	5.8	8.5	3.6	9.3	7.2	6.3	1.7	6.0	1.9
PRL_{15}	mg/ml	54.6	23.3	46.0	16.0	48.3	20.8	33.3	11.1	26.7	8.5
PRL_{30}	mg/ml	43.3	20.2	36.3	13.5	40.4	21.5	28.2	9.1	20.6	7.3
ΔPRL	mg/ml	43.6	22.0	37.5	14.3	39.1	18.1	27.1	10.6	20.7	7.5
HGH	ng/ml	0.97	1.14	1.08	2.4	0.93	0.90	0.82	0.39	1.01	0.79

Table 2. Thyroid parameters in the serum of the overall population

Serum hormones		Breast cancer (n = 40)		Benign breast diseases (n = 26)		Gynecologic tumors (n = 15)		Benign gynecologic diseases (n = 12)		Control group (n = 48)	
		x̄	SD	x̄	SD	x̄	SD	x̄	SD	x̄	SD
T_4	μg/dl	8.9	1.9	7.7	1.4	7.3	1.5	7.6	2.5	8.8	1.9
FT_4	ng/dl	1.13	0.25	1.18	0.20	1.08	0.20	1.20	0.46	1.28	0.31
T_3	ng/dl	103.1	24.2	113.5	19.6	102.6	25.6	116.0	19.9	127.6	23.3
rT_3	pg/dl	313.8	115.0	202.5	65.6	279.0	98.1	190.3	50.0	180.8	66.9
TSH_O	μU/ml	2.5	0.9	2.3	1.1	2.5	2.2	2.8	1.5	2.4	0.6
TSH_3	μU/ml	8.2	5.2	10.3	6.4	14.6	23.6	12.7	11.3	7.5	3.9
ΔTSH	μU/ml	5.8	4.7	7.9	5.8	12.4	21.9	9.9	10.0	5.2	3.6
T_3 index		1.02	0.11	0.95	0.11	1.03	0.18	0.93	0.11	1.0	0.08
TBG	μg/ml	19.6	3.5	17.7	2.3	20.0	4.5	18.6	2.1	20.3	2.8

of patients with breast cancer and the group of genital cancers compared to the remaining control groups. On the other hand, the serum levels for rT_3 were higher to a statistically significant extent ($p < 0.0001$) than in the reference groups in the group of breast cancer patients. When the average T_3 and rT_3 values of the patients with breast cancer are related to the individual criteria of the pTMN classification, it becomes evident that the T_3 values decrease in the higher stages of malignancy, whereas the rT_3 values rise. This is especially evident when the early cases are compared with the advanced breast cancers. The thyroid parameters total thyroxin (T_4), free thyroxin (FT_4), TSH_o, TSH_{30}, δ-TSH, T_3, and thyroxin-binding globulin (TBG) did not show any differences between the individual patient groups.

Correlations between disorders of thyroid function and breast cancer have been known for a long time. An increased occurrence of hypothyroidism in breast cancer patients has been observed. In the present investigation, there was a history of thyroid disease in 23% of the breast cancer patients. This incidence was markedly higher than that of the reference population and higher than the average incidence in the general population. The lowering of T_3 is not to be assessed as a manifestation of a T_3 hypothyroidism but is to be interpreted as a low-T_3 syndrome and thus corresponds to the typical hormone pattern in many extra-thyroid diseases, such as severe consumptive general diseases, lung cancer, and malnutrition. These are probably secondary alterations of peripheral T_4 metabolism in which the conversion to rT_3 is favored (Adami et al. 1978; Rose and Davis 1978, 1979; Hesch 1981; Chopra et al. 1975; Meinhold 1977).

Steroid Hormone Receptor Status in Breast Cancer and Its Clinical Significance

In 439 patients with breast cancer, the estradiol and progesterone receptor content was quantified simultaneously in the carcinoma tissue. For the estradiol receptor, there is a skewed distribution in the correlation analysis between the age of the breast cancer patient and the receptor content of the primary tumor with values from nonmeasurable to 3995 fmol/mg protein (Fig. 1). In the overall population of all breast cancer patients, the proportion of estradiol receptor-negative tumors was 44.4%. In postmenopausal women, the estradiol receptor content was on average four times higher compared to premenopausal patients.

The average progesterone receptor content in the overall population of all breast cancer patients was 309 fmol/mg protein, and the proportion of receptor-negative tumors was 48.3% (Fig. 2). Neither difference between premenopausal and postmenopausal tumors with regard to their content of progesterone receptors nor an age dependence of this parameter could be established.

When the combined receptor status in breast cancer is correlated with the histological grading according to Bloom and Richardson (1957) as well as the nuclear and cellular polymorphism and the rate of mitosis, the following picture results (Table 3): an increase in degree of malignancy leads to a decrease in the proportion of estradiol receptor-positive tumors. On the other hand, the qualitative progesterone receptor status does not display any alterations between the

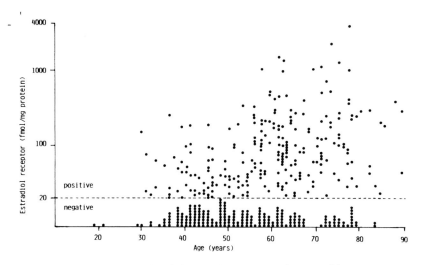

Fig. 1. Correlation analysis of the relation between the age of breast cancer patients and the content of estradiol receptors in the primary tumor

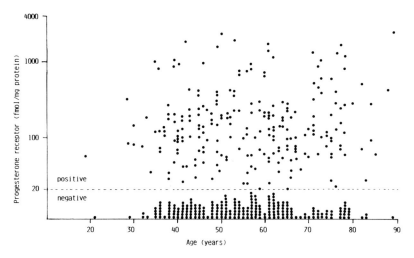

Fig. 2. Correlation analysis of the relation between the age of breast cancer patients and the content of progesterone receptors in the primary tumor

individual stages of malignancy. In consideration of the degree of differentiation of the cells, no differences can be detected between mature and dedifferentiated tumors with regard to the estrogen receptor finding. In nuclear and cellular polymorphism, a higher percentage of estradiol receptor-positive tumors is observed in the isomorphic tumors than in the polymorphic tumors. The progesterone receptor status does not reveal any differences in this histological criterion. With regard to the degree of mitosis, a marked decrease in the estrogen receptor-positive findings is shown with increasing cell division. In accordance

Table 3. Receptor status of primary breast cancers in relation to the grading according to Bloom and Richardson (1957) as well as the evaluation according to differentiation, polymorphism, and rate of mitosis

	n	Estradiol receptor		Progesterone receptor	
		+	−	+	−
Grade					
I	14	10	4	8	6
II	27	17	10	14	13
III	15	9	6	8	7
Differentiation					
Well differentiated	31	19	12	13	18
Undifferentiated	43	28	15	23	20
Polymorphism					
Isomorphic	39	26	13	20	19
Polymorphic	17	10	7	9	8
Rate of mitosis					
Maximum 1/HPF	23	17	6	15	8
2/HPF	27	17	10	13	14
≥ 3/HPF	6	2	4	1	5

with the grading, the ratio of positive to negative findings decreased from 2.8 to 1.7 to 0.5. A similar tendency, although less pronounced, is also shown with regard to the progesterone receptor evaluation. With regard to the qualitative distribution of the steroid hormone receptors in relation to the proportion of accompanying stroma in the carcinoma tissue, the following picture is shown: in the high-stroma breast cancers, steroid hormone receptors could be demonstrated very much more frequently than in the low-stroma tumors. The ratio of the estradiol-receptor positive to estradiol receptor-negative findings decreased from 0.4 in the low-stroma to 2.7 in the moderately high-stroma carcinoma tissues to 3.6 in the high-stroma carcinoma tissues. In the case of the progesterone receptor, these ratios were 0.6, 1.2, and 1.6, respectively.

In the context of a controlled therapy study, the objective results of treatment were determined after high-dose medroxyprogesterone acetate (MPA) therapy in advanced, metastasizing breast cancers in relation to the receptor status measured in the primary tumor. In the study, 108 metastasizing breast cancers which had been pretreated with chemotherapy or with tamoxifen were included and treated with 1000 mg MPA per os in the context of a third-line therapy.

Under the therapy, the MPA serum level (above all in terms of the safety of medication intake) was measured. The result of therapy is shown in Table 4. The response rate was 58%, including full and partial remissions and those with no change of the disease; in 42% there was progression of tumor growth. When the results of therapy are considered in relation to the receptor status (Table 5), it is shown that (a) the receptor-positive tumors respond better to a high-dose MPA

Table 4. Success of high-dose MPA therapy in advanced breast cancer

Results	n	%	Duration of remission	
Complete remission	7	6	Median:	74 weeks
			Range:	58–148 weeks
Partial remission	15	13	Median:	42 weeks
			Range:	21–108 weeks
No change	44	39	Median:	23 weeks
			Range:	13–61 weeks
Progression	47	42		

Table 5. Relationship between clinical response on 3-month high-dose MPA treatment and receptor status

Receptor status	Complete remission/partial remission + no change ($n = 66$)
ER+/PR+	41 (62%)
ER+/PR−	9 (14%)
ER−/PR+	14 (21%)
ER−/PR−	2 (3%)
ER (+)	
< 100 fmol/mg protein	23
≧ 100 fmol/mg protein	27
PR (−)	
< 100 fmol/mg protein	17
≧ 100 fmol/mg protein	38

ER, Estrogen receptor; PR, progesterone receptor.

therapy than the group with the receptor-negative tumors, and (b) that within the group of receptor-positive tumors, the tumors with receptor concentrations over 100 fmol/mg protein display the most favorable results of therapy, a result which confirms the therapeutic results of other study groups (Wander et al. 1983; Kreienberg et al. 1985; Blossey et al. 1982a, b, 1984; Salimtschik et al. 1980; Jonat et al. 1984; Tamassia 1986; Mahlke et al 1985; Izuo et al. 1982; Pollow et al. 1984; Possinger et al. 1985; Grill et al. 1985a).

Different Techniques for Receptor Determination

Ligand-Binding Assays

Various methods have been described for detecting and quantifying steroid hormone receptors in tumor tissue. Most of these are protein-binding assays designed to measure the ability of a tumor cytosol to bind and retain specifically radioactively labeled steroids (Toft and Gorski 1966; Jensen 1971; Korenman and Dukes 1970; Jungblut et al. 1972; Wagner and Jungblut 1976; Wrange et al. 1976; Erdos et al. 1970; Godefroi and Brooks 1973; Chamness and McGuire 1979; Press and Greene 1984). In general, the procedure of protein-binding assays for steroid receptor quantification in the cytoplasm of target cells is as follows: a cytosol–a soluble supernatant of the tissue homogenate–is prepared and incubated with increasing concentrations of radioactively labeled steroid under conditions that saturate the steroid receptor (total binding). In a parallel set of test tubes, a 100- to 200-fold excess of nonradioactive competitor steroid is incubated together with the labeled steroid in order to determine the amount of binding to nonreceptor proteins (nonspecific binding).

After reaching equilibrium, the labeled hormone receptor complex is separated from the unbound ligand using dextran-coated charcoal, and the protein-bound radioactivity is determined. Specific binding is calculated by subtracting the amount of nonspecific binding from total binding. When corrections for nonspecific binding are made at each concentration of labeled hormone used in the titration, the data obtained from the amount of hormone bound at each dose can then be analyzed with Scatchard's (1949) method by plotting specifically bound/free versus specific binding, as demonstrated in Fig. 3. The dissociation constant (K_d) is identical with the reciprocal value of the slope of the regression line, and the number of binding sites corresponds to the intercept of the abscissa.

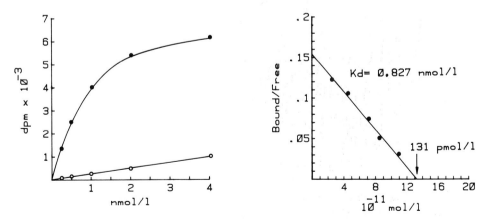

Fig. 3. Titration and Scatchard plot analyses of estradiol receptor (*right panel*) in mammary carcinoma cytosol using ^{125}I-labeled estradiol (*left panel*) as radioactive ligand

The inclusion of an appropriate unlabeled competitor for the receptor-specific hormone in such a titration assay permits easy determination of the number of true, competitive binding sites.

Detection and assay of these cytoplasmic receptors have not been without difficulties, since natural hormones such as estradiol or progesterone are often also tightly bound by other proteins located within in the cell or present due to serum contamination such as that by corticosteroid-binding globulin (CBG) or sex hormone binding globulin (SHBG). Furthermore, natural hormones are often metabolized under in vitro experimental conditions even at 0°C.

To avoid these problems arising from the use of natural steroids, potent synthetic hormones without these disadvantages have been introduced to receptor determination in the past few years. These synthetic steroids have been selected on the basis of their lack of binding to serum proteins, their resistance to degradation under in vitro incubation conditions, their specificity for the respective receptor, the slow dissociation rate from the receptor protein, and the possibility of labeling them at a high molar specific activity.

For estrogen receptor assays, the tritium-labeled estradiol and the synthetic estrogen R2858 (Moxestrol) are commonly used as radioligand. Except for estradiol, R2858 does not bind specifically to serum proteins and is totally specific for the estrogen receptor (Table 6). Furthermore, this synthetic estrogen is metabolically stable under the in vitro conditions of receptor assay.

Recently, the successful synthesis of radioiodinated $[^{125}I]$ 16α-iodoestradiol was reported by Hochberg (Hochberg 1979; Hochberg and Rosner 1980). This new ligand for estrogen receptor determination has similar binding characteristics to the estrogen receptor as the commonly used tritium-labeled estradiol but does not bind to serum proteins (Table 7). Furthermore, this radioiodinated ligand has several other advantageous features: high specific molar activity (theoretically up to 2000 Ci/mmol), minor problems with radioactive waste due to its short half-life, and an extreme metabolic stability, especially against 17β-hydroxysteroid dehydrogenase, under the in vitro conditions of estrogen receptor assay. For progesterone receptor measurement, synthetic progestins such as R5020 (Raynaud 1977) or Org2058 – rather than progesterone itself – are generally used. These synthetic hormones – unlike progesterone itself – do not bind to CBG (Table 8). The synthetic progestins therefore reduce the extent of nonspecific binding. Other reasons for the use of synthetic progestins are that they have a lower rate of dissociation from progesterone receptor than progesterone itself, and that they are characterized by a high metabolic stability. However, none of these synthetic progestins are totally specific to the progestin receptor. R5020 competes to 9.0% for labeled dexamethasone binding to rat liver glucocorticoid receptor; Org2058 competes only to 1.4%.

The successful synthesis of an iodinated estrogen by Hochberg (Hochberg 1979; Hochberg and Rosner 1980) has stimulated us in the past 3 years to search for a progestin analog. Iodinated steroids are certainly more sensitive ligands for detection of steroid receptors with all the advantages of a γ-emitting label. For this purpose, we investigated the (Z)-and (E)-17α-(2-iodovinyl) derivatives of 19-nortestosterone synthesized by Schering, West Berlin (Fig. 4).

Table 6. In vitro relative binding affinity (%) for specific steroid receptors and competition for specific serum binding

	Estrogen receptor	Progesterone receptor	Androgen receptor	Glucocorticoid receptor	Mineralocorticoid receptor	Corticosteroid-binding globulin	Sex hormone binding globulin
Estradiol	100	1.2	4.2	0.4	0.2	<0.1	70
Moxestrol	100	<0.1	<0.1	<0.1	<0.1	<0.1	<0.1

Table 7. In vitro relative binding affinity (%) for human estrogen receptor and competition for sex hormone binding globulin

	Estrogen receptor	Sex hormone binding globulin
Estradiol	100	70
Diethylstilbestrol	120	<0.1
16β-Bromoestradiol	1	68
16α-Iodoestradiol	100	1
Dihydrotestosterone	<0.1	100

Table 8. In vitro relative binding affinity (%) for specific steroid receptors and competition for specific serum binding

	Estrogen receptor	Progesterone receptor	Androgen receptor	Glucocorticoid receptor	Mineralocorticoid receptor	Corticosteroid-binding globulin	Sex hormone binding globulin
R5020	<0.1	100	2.8	9	0.3	<0.01	<0.01
Org2058	<0.1	350	1.4	1.4	0.1	<0.01	<0.01
Progesterone	<0.1	40	4.8	0.3	7.5	100	<0.01

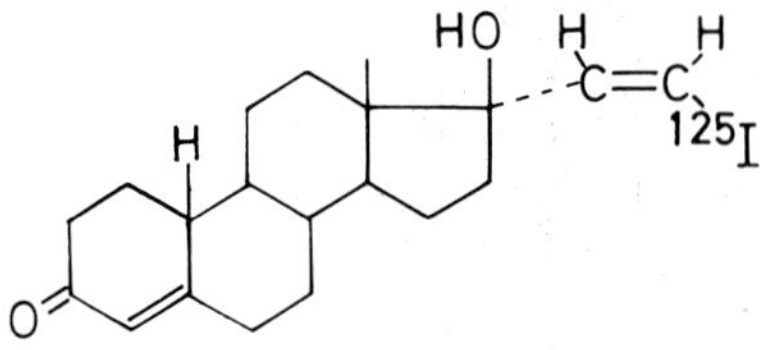

206   K. Pollow et al.

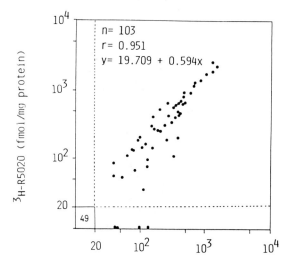

Fig. 4. Structure of $[^{125}I](Z)$-17α-(2-iodovinyl)-nortestosterone (SH-D510)

Fig. 5. Quantification of progesterone receptor in 103 samples of human mammary tumor cytosol using $[^{3}H]R5020$ and $[^{125}I](Z)$-17α-(2-iodovinyl)-nortestosterone as radioactive ligands

Table 9. In vitro relative binding affinity (%) for specific steroid receptors and competition for specific serum binding

Receptor	Reference steroid	RBA (%)	
		Iodovinylnortestosterone	R5020
Progesterone	R5020	900	100
Glucocorticoid	Dexamethasone	4	9
Estrogen	Estradiol	<0.01	<0.1
Androgen	Dihydrotestosterone	9	2.8
Serum proteins			
SHBG	Dihydrotestosterone	0.9	<0.01
CBG	Cortisol	<0.01	<0.01

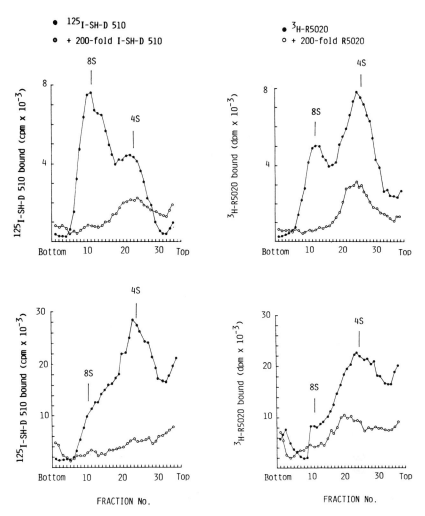

Fig. 6. Sucrose density gradient analysis of [³H]R5020 and [¹²⁵I](Z)-17α-(iodovinyl)-nortestosterone protein complexes on 5%–20% linear sucrose density gradients under low (*upper panels*) and high (*lower panels*) salt conditions

The relative binding affinities calculated according to Korenman and Dukes (1970) are summarized in Table 9. The relative binding affinity (RBA) for the progestin receptor was 900% for the (Z)-17α-(2-iodovinyl) derivative compared to R5020 (100%). RBA values were lowered by a factor of about 8 for the isomer, halogenated in the (E)-configuration; the RBA value was 110%. Binding to estrogen receptor and to CBG was negligible; binding to glucocorticoid receptor and SHBG was below 5%. As all steroids investigated are 19-nor derivatives; binding to androgen receptor should be expected but was found to be 9%.

In 103 progestin receptor-positive human mammary tumor cytosols the progestin receptor concentrations were determined in parallel with [¹²⁵I] (Z)-17α-(2-

iodovinyl)-nortestosterone $\pm$ 200-fold R5020 and [^{3}H]R5020 $\pm$ 200-fold R5020 using a five-point saturation assay with Scatchard plot analysis of the binding data. The mean K_d values were 0.5 $\pm$ 0.35 × 10^{-9}M for [^{125}I] (Z)-17α-(2-iodovinyl)-nortestosterone and 1.05 $\pm$ 0.87 × 10^{-9}M for [^{3}H]R5020. The correlation coefficient (r) between the two radioactive ligands was 0.951 (Fig. 5).

On linear 5%–20% sucrose density gradients human uterine cytosols were preincubated with [^{125}I](Z)-17α-(2-iodovinyl)-nortestosterone $\pm$ 200-fold cold (Z)-17α-(2-iodovinyl)-nortestosterone and [^{3}H]R5020 $\pm$ 200-fold R5020 centrifuged. Under low-salt conditions (PEN buffer) for both ligands 8S and 4-S forms of progestin receptor could be demonstrated (Fig. 6). In the presence of 0.4 M KCl (high salt) only the 4S form was detectable for both ligands.

Dual-Labeling Assay for Simultaneous Determination of Estrogen and Progesterone Receptors

Recently, we have reported criteria for a dual-labeling assay for simultaneous determination of estrogen receptor and progesterone receptors in one and the same set of tubes using [^{125}I]16α-iodo-3,17β-estradiol and [^{3}H]R5020 or [^{3}H]Org2058, respectively (for details, see Grill et al. 1982, 1983, 1984, 1985b). The accuracy of this assay system depends strongly on the counting technique. It should be stressed that the quench curves must be carefully established and controlled, and the scintillation counter well calibrated. The counter must also be able to store four quench curves so that the spillover of iodine 125 and tritium can be calculated and subtracted. The advantages of this assay system should be discussed briefly: (a) costs and working expenditure can be significantly reduced; (b) the amount of radioactive waste (counting vials and cocktail) is diminished by half; and (c) the amount of tissue necessary for a valid 4- to 6-point titration analysis is reduced by half. This enables the investigator to quantify estrogen receptors and progesterone receptors, for example in lymph nodes, needle biopsies, and cell cultures.

Density Gradient Centrifugation

Another highly effective and widely used method for steroid hormone receptor analyses in the cytoplasmic fraction of target tissues is sucrose density centrifugation (see Fig. 6). This technique demonstrates the 8S molecular form of both the estrogen and progestin receptors. McGuire et al. (1979) found that from a quantitative standpoint the sucrose density centrifugation and the dextran-coated charcoal assays yielded remarkably similar results. The disadvantage of the sucrose density gradient technique is the major limitation in the number of samples that can be processed using horizontal swinging buckets and the lack the K_a value that is inherent in the dextran-coated charcoal assay with scatchard analysis—giving good information about ligand receptor interaction.

Immunoassay Procedures for Estrogen Receptor Determination

Recently, Abbott introduced immunoassay procedures on the basis of monoclonal antibodies against estrogen receptors for the quantification and visualization of estrogen receptors of human origin (Heubner et al. 1986; Beck et al. 1986; Jonat et al. 1985; Köhler and Bässler 1986; Reiner et al. 1986; Remmele and Stegner 1987). Since most clinical derive from to the biochemical ligand-binding assay, a new method must show strict correlation with classically determined receptor concentrations. Our data obtained by determination of estrogen receptor levels in 82 mammary carcinomas show a quite good correlation between both techniques ($r = 0.706$).

The number of estrogen receptor-positive tumors (cutoff level > 20 fmol/mg protein) was lower with dextran-coated charcoal assay (58.5%) than with the estrogen receptor enzymoimmunoassay (ER-EIA; 86.6%). It was found that in 11 cases in which the result of the ligand-binding assay was negative, the ER-EIA result was positive. Therefore, no tumor samples determined as positive by Scatchard analysis were classified as negative by ER-EIA. The slope of the regression line was found to be 1.9. This can only mean that estrogen receptor content measured immunologically is higher than measured with our routine ligand-binding assay. One reason for this phenomenon could be that the antibody recognizes not only estrogen receptors but also the estradiol-occupied estrogen receptors, which possibly are not measurable with the binding assay at 4°C incubation temperature. This would result in an underestimation of the actual receptor levels with the biochemical assay. Another explanation could be that in the biochemical assay only receptor molecules which are able to bind steroid can be detected, whereas with the ER-EIA also precursors of the estrogen receptor or somehow altered molecules, which are not able to bind steroid, are still detectable. Our investigations concerning heat inactivation of cytosol suggest that the latter is rather unlikely, since the ER-EIA behaves like the biochemical assay. Heat treatment of cytosol leads to a complete loss of receptors. In other words, both techniques are strongly dependent on uninterrupted cooling from the operation theater to the receptor laboratory to guarantee the stability of the receptor protein.

Classification of estrogen receptor immunocytochemical assay (ER-ICA) results with an immunocytochemical score was established including the intensity of staining, the percentage of the immunoperoxidase-stained cancer cell nuclei within the sample of tissue, and the relation of tumor cells to connective tissue (Remmele and Stegner 1987). In 231 out of 299 cases (77.2%) the immunocytochemical results correlated well with those of the ligand-binding assay (cutoff level > 20 fmol/mg protein). A discrepancy between the results of ER-ICA and those of the binding assay was observed in 22.8% of all cases: 55 tumors were specifically stained by ER-ICA but revealed a receptor concentration below 20 fmol/mg protein, and 13 cases with an estrogen receptor level more than 20 fmol/mg protein where ER-ICA was negative.

In conclusion, immunocytological analysis is a useful supplement to the quantitative assay as described by other investigators (Heubner et al. 1986; Beck et

Table 10. Comparison of in vitro relative binding affinity for specific progesterone receptor (reference steroid R5020) of normal human uterus and mammary cancer tissue

Competitor steroid	RBA (%)	
	Human uterus	Mammary cancer tissue
Progesterone	33	45
R5020	100	100
Org2058	350	250
Levonorgestrel	150	210
Medroxyprogesterone acetate	115	130
Cyproterone acetate	80	85
Megestrol acetate	100	110
Gestodene	85	200
Dexamethasone	0.1	0.1
Cortisol	0.1	0.1
Estradiol	0.8	0.8
Testosterone	0.9	1.1
Dihydrotestosterone	0.8	0.7

al. 1986; Jonat et al. 1985; Köhler and Bässler 1986; Reiner et al 1986; Remmele and Stegner 1987). The method provides information about heterogeneity and distribution as well as a semiquantitative evaluation of estrogen receptors in frozen tissue samples of target tissues. Furthermore, the assay is nearly independent of the quantity of tissue or cytological samples.

Comparative Biochemical Characterization of Progesterone Receptors from Breast Cancer Tissue and Human Uterus

Analysis of Competition

Determination of the specificty of binding between a radioligand and the receptor is carried out in competitive binding studies. For this purpose, a constant concentration of radioactively labeled ligand receptors is incubated in the presence of rising concentrations of unlabeled competitors under saturation conditions. In order for the potency of competition of various competitors to become quantifiable, and thus comparable, the results are related to the concentration of the competitor which can displace 50% of the radioligand binding. This value is designated as the RBA value. Table 10 summarizes the results of the comparative RBA analysis of the progesterone receptors from the human uterus and breast cancer tissue. The progesterone receptors from the two tissues display analogous behavior toward a broad spectrum of synthetic and natural competitor steroids.

Chromatography Methods

Anion exchange chromatography (e.g., DEAE cellulose), the molecular sieve method, and isoelectric focusing are methods which have been established for years in the characterization and purification of steroid hormone receptors (O'Malley and McGuire 1968; Smith et al. 1981; Grandics et al. 1982; Wrange et al. 1976, 1978; Schrader et al. 1977). However, for the preparative imaging of progesterone receptors (highly labile macromolecules which only occur in very tiny concentrations in the target tissue), these separation techniques have proved to be problematical, because they are very time consuming and thus automatically entail

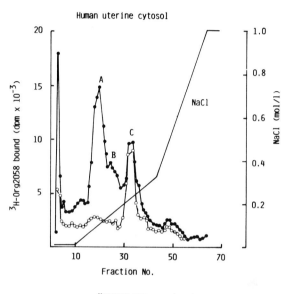

Human uterine cytosol

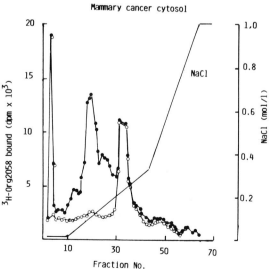

Mammary cancer cytosol

Fig. 7. FPLC anion exchange chromatography (mono-Q) of native, [³H]Org2058-labeled cytosol from human uterus and breast cancer. Cytosol was incubated with 32 nmol/l [³H]Org2058 with (○) or without (●) a 200-fold molar excess of Org2058 at 4°C for 16 h; 500-μl aliquots were then applied to the column and eluted over an NaCl gradient

the danger of proteolytic degradation of the receptor proteins. This is manifested above all in the only small yields in purification of these receptors from cell homogenates (Schrader et al. 1977; Lessey et al. 1983). The adaptation of this separation method which is by now is classical in protein chemistry, to the modern fast protein liquid chromatography (FPLC) technique which requires only little time is reported below in the context of the characterization and purification of progesterone receptors.

FPLC Anion Exchange Chromatography (Mono-Q). In Fig. 7, typical elution profiles over a mono-Q anion exchange column are shown after chromatography of the cytosols from human uterus and breast cancer tissue incubated with

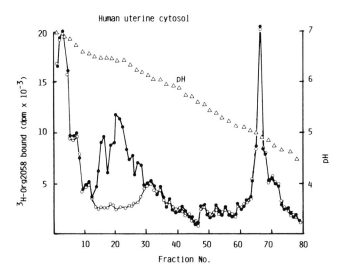

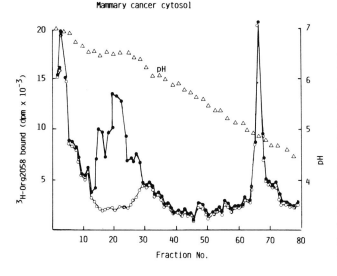

Fig. 8. FPLC chromatofocusing (mono-P) of native, [³H]Org2058-labeled cytosol from human uterus or breast cancer. Cytosol was incubated for 16 h at 4°C with 32 nmol/l [³H]Org2058 with (○) or without (●) a 200-fold molar excess of Org2058; 500-μl aliquots were then applied to the column and eluted with polybuffer 74

[³H]Org2058 under saturation conditions. Specifically bound [³H]Org2058 eluted both for uterus and breast cancer tissue in two peaks (A and B) at salt concentrations of 0.075 and 014 mol/1 NaCl, respectively. This radioactivity (peak C) eluting at 0.2 mol/1 NaCl, which could not be displaced by a 200-fold molar excess of Org2058, showed identical elution behavior to that of serum albumin (detection of albumin contamination by specific immunoprecipitation by means of LC Partigen plates, Behringwerke, Marburg, FRG).

FPLC Chromatofocusing (Mono-P) Figure 8 shows typical elution profiles after chromatofocusing of the cytosols from uterine and breast cancer tissue labeled with [³H]Org2058. A heterogeneous pattern of specific binding of [³H]Org2058 could be verified in the pH range 6.2–6.5 for both tissues. It is unclear to what extent the peaks of specific binding eluting in this pH range are identical with intact receptor molecules or their subunits of the polymer-structured progesterone receptor (O'Malley and McGuire 1968; Sherman et al. 1976) or only constitute degradation products of this receptor which are still capable of binding.

Purification of the Progesterone Receptor from Breast Cancer Tissue

A basic precondition for successful purification of labile progesterone receptors is a highly specific, but at the same time rapid technique based on affinity chromatography preventing the degradation of receptor protein by endogenous proteases. The affinity gel should fulfill the following requirements:

1. The ligand bound to the affinity matrix must interact in a highly specific way with the binding site on the progestrone receptor.
2. The basic matrix of the affinity gel coupling the ligands must react largely inertly to proteins in order to keep the foreign protein contamination of the enriching receptor protein low.
3. The linkage of the ligand to the gel matrix must take place via stable, covalent binding which insures that the ligand is not split off under the conditions of incubation of the affinity gel with receptor-carrying cytosol.

Org2058 was used as ligand for the synthesis of the affinity gel for purification of progesterone receptors (see Heubner et al. 1985 for details). Org2058 is characterized by a high affinity to the progesterone receptor, lower affinity to the glucocorticosteroid receptor, and lack of binding to CBG (Table 11). In addition, Org2058 forms stable complexes with the progesterone receptor. These properties characterize Org2058 as an ideal ligand for the preparation of an affinity gel for purification of progesterone receptors. The Scatchard plot analyses presented in Fig. 9 show that no receptor can be demonstrated in the cytosol after 16 h of incubation of breast cancer cytosol with the affinity gel. Proteolytic degradation of the receptor could be largely ruled out, since only a maximum of 5%–10% of the progesterone receptor is lost from breast cancer cytosol within 24 h at 4°C under identical conditions of incubation.

In the elution of the progesterone receptor bound via ligand to the affinity gel, two different strategies can be followed: (a) the specific elution by exchange with a

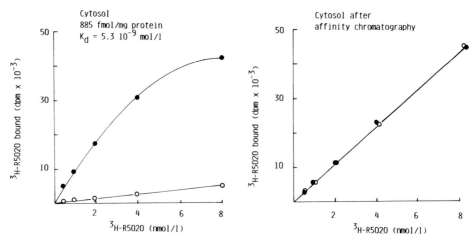

Fig. 9. Quantification of the cytoplasmic progesterone receptor before and after affinity chromatography by Scatchard plot analysis. Aliquots (0.1 ml) of the cytosol were incubated with rising concentrations (1–32 nmol/l) of [³H]R5020 with (○) or without (●) a 200-fold molar excess of R5020 at 4°C for 16 h. Free steroid was separated by dextran-coated charcoal treatment

Table 11. Relative binding activities of various steroids compared to the binding of [³H]R5020 on the uterine progesterone receptor, [³H]dexamethasone on the glucocorticoid receptor from the rat liver of adrenalectomized animals and [³H]cortisol on CBG from pregnancy serum diluted 1:20

Ligand	RBA (%)		
	Progesterone receptor	Glucocorticoid receptor	Corticosteroid-binding globulin
Org2058	350	1.4	<0.01
Desoxycorticosterone	5	8.0	96
R5020	100	9.0	<0.01
Progesterone	40	0.3	100
Dexamethasone	ND	100	ND

ND, not measured.

high-affinity ligand binding at the receptor (e.g., Org2058) and (b) the detachment of the progesterone receptor by salt extraction. Both methods are beset with problems. The first method entails the danger that the silica gel used as a basic matrix has steroid hormone binding properties per se, so that the current supply of steroids which is necessary to elute the receptor quantitatively can only be calculated with difficulty. The problem of salt elution consists above all in the fact that the receptor loses its capacity to bind specific ligands owing to salt-induced conformational changes.

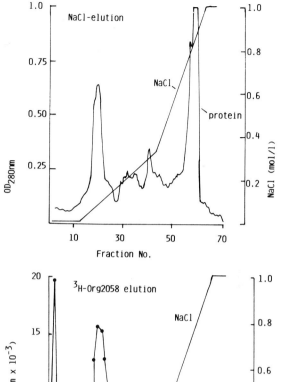

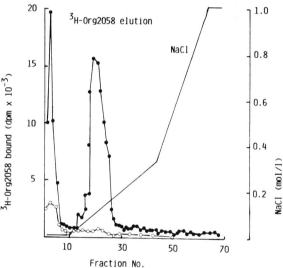

Fig. 10. FPLC anion exchange chromatography (mono-Q) of the eluate containing progesterone receptors after affinity chromatography of breast cancer cytosol. After incubation of the affinity gel with cytosol, elution was carried out either with NaCl or with [³H]Org2058 with (○) or without (●) a 200-fold molar excess of Org2058. After separation of the affinity gel by centrifugation, the respective supernatant was transferred to the mono-Q and eluted via an NaCl gradient

Figure 10 (top) shows a representative protein profile after anionic exchange chromatography (mono-Q) of the proteins detached from the affinity gel by salt extraction. Since a recharging of the progesterone receptors eluted from the affinity gel with salt was not possible with [³H]Org2058, only the protein pattern arising is shown in the figure. A prominent main protein peak which elutes with 0.075 mol/1 NaCl and thus corresponds to the specifically binding peak A in Fig. 7 is demonstrable. The protein peak eluting at high salt concentration is not identical with albumin. Figure 10 (below) shows the corresponding result when a progesterone receptor bound to affinity gel is eluted with [³H]Org2058. The protein profile arising is essentially identical with that obtained after salt extraction. The specific

Table 12. Purification of progesterone receptor from human mammary cancer cytosol by combination of affinity chromatography and FPLC anion exchange chromatography

Steps of Purification	Volume (ml)	Protein (mg)	Receptor (ng)	Receptor Concentration (ng/mg)	Recovery (%)	Purification (n-fold)
Cytosol	175	735	68 441	93.1	100	1
Eluate after affinity chromatography 0.075 mol/l NaCl	8	0.8	63 778	79 723	93	856
eluate after mono-Q chromatography	2.5	0.0734	60 555	825 000	88.5	8861

All calculations are based on an assumed mean molecular weight of 100 000 for the progesterone receptor.

radioactivity peak (suppressable by a 200-fold molar excess of Org2058) elutes at 0.075 mol/l NaCl and thus shows identical elution behavior to the progesterone receptor of native cytosol labelled with [^{3}H]Org2058 (Heubner et al. 1984).

Table 12 summarizes the results of the individual purification steps. After two chromatography steps, the yield of progesterone receptor protein is 86% in an 8861-fold enrichment. If it is assumed that not more than 0.01%–0.015% receptor protein is present in the target cell in relation to the total cellular protein, more

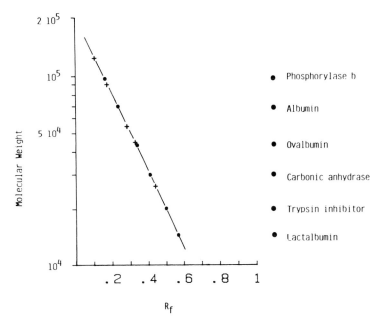

Fig. 11. SDS gel electrophoresis of the progesterone receptor protein enriched after affinity chromatography over mono Q. The fractions 18–25 from Fig. 10 were incubated in 500 μl buffer (10 mmol/l Tris/HCl, 1 mmol/l EDTA, 1% SDS, 5% beta-mercaptoethanol, 15% glycerol, pH 8.0) for 5 min at 100°C after desalting and freeze-drying; 20-μl aliquots were then electropherographed on a shallow gel (collecting gel: 4% polyacrylamide; separating gel: 12.6% polyacrylamide). The proteins were stained and fixed in water/ethanol/acetic acid (v/v/v; 5/5/1) under addition of 2% Coomassie blue. *Crosses* on the calibration curve specify the respective position of the protein bands

than 90% purification of the progesterone receptor has been achieved with the two-step purification procedure presented. To appraise the degree of purity of the protein fraction (0.075 mol/l NaCl eluate) obtained in the last purification step via anion exchange chromatography, this was subjected to sodium dodecyl sulfate gel electrophoresis (Fig. 11). A heterogeneous pattern of five Coomassie blue-stainable protein bands with molecular weights 121 000, 89 000, 53 000, 43 000, and 27 000 is shown.

Since the native conformation of the progesterone receptor remains unknown even today, but on the other hand proteins of various molecular weights with gestagen-binding properties have been described after receptor purification by numerous authors (Smith et al. 1981), the result found here is not surprising. The spectrum of gestagen-binders described so far ranges from high molecular weight polymers via monomers to low molecular weight fragments of the progesterone receptor formed by protease degradation. The latter are regarded as the gestagen-binding core and are designated as meroreceptors.

Detection of Antiprogesterone Receptor Antibodies

The progesterone receptor that we purified in the two-step technique was applied to rabbits for induction of polyclonal antibodies. After the third boosting, immunoglobulins could be demonstrated which interacted specifically with the cytoplasmic progesterone receptor. In accordance with the results of gel chromatographic separation of native, [^{3}H]Org2058-labeled cytosol, the cytosolic progesterone receptor eluted in the 27-Å region when it was mixed with preimmune serum (Fig. 12). On the other hand, after incubation of the same cytosol fraction labeled with [^{3}H]Org2058 in the presence of immune serum which was obtained from the induction experiments, a shift of the radioactivity into the molecular weight range over 300 000 was to be observed in consequence of the complexing of the antiprogesterone receptor antibodies with the [^{3}H]Org2058-labeled receptors. An analogous result could be achieved by means of density gradient centrifugation (Fig. 13). These findings are a major indication that progesterone receptors are indeed enriched with the purification procedure presented.

To summarize, the modern FPLC technique – in combination with effective column materials for anion exchange and gel chromatography as well as for chromatofocusing – adapted to the special problems of protein separation, is

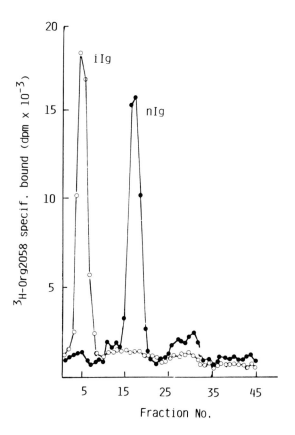

Fig. 12. Detection of the antiprogesterone receptor antibody by FPLC gel chromatography. *nIg*, preimmune serum; *iIg*, antiprogesterone receptor antibody

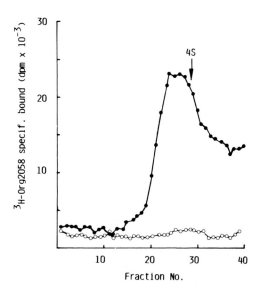

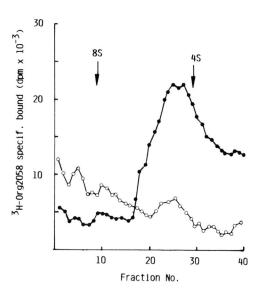

Fig. 13. Detection of the anti-progesterone receptor antibody by sucrose density gradient centrifugation. *Upper panel,* sedimentation profile of the [³H]Org2058-labeled progesterone receptor with (○) or without (●) a 200-fold molar excess of Org2058 from breast cancer cytosol in the presence of 0.4 mol/l KCl. *Lower panel,* sedimentation profiles after incubation of breast cancer cytosol with [³H]Org2058 in the presence of preimmune serum or antiprogesterone-receptor antibodies

superior to conventional chromatography techniques which are mostly elaborate and time consuming in methodological terms. This is the case at least in the field of analysis and preparative visualization of steroid hormone receptor proteins referred to. Furthermore, the chromatographic comparison as well as the competition analysis demonstrate in an exemplary way the similarity in the molecular structure of these progesterone receptors in the cytosol of normal uterus as well as breast cancer tissue. This is to be considered at least as a distinct indication that the progesterone receptor of one species is synthesized independently of the organ, and that no major structural modifications are introduced by a neoplastic transformation.

References

Adami HO, Rimsten A, Thoren L, Vegelius J, Wide L (1978) Thyroid disease and function in breast cancer patients and non-hospitalized controls evaluated by determination of TSH, T_3, rT_3 T_4 levels in serum. Acta Chir Scand 144: 89–97

Anderson DE (1974) Genetic study of breast cancer: identification of a high risk group. Cancer 34: 1090–1097

Baulieu EE, Atger M, Best-Belpomme M, Corvol P, Courvalin JL, Mester J, Milgrom E, Robel P, Rochefort H, Catalogne D (1975) Steroid hormone receptors. Vitam Horm 33: 649–736

Baxter JD, Funder JW (1979) Hormone receptors. N Engl J Med 301: 1149–1161

Beck T, Pollow K, Heubner A (1986) Monoklonale Antikörper zum immunhistochemischen Nachweis des Östrogenrezeptor-Status am Gewebeschnitt primärer Mammakarzinome. Geburtshilfe Frauenheilkd 46: 450–454

Bloom HJG, Richardson WW (1957) Histological grading and prognosis in breast cancer. Br J Cancer 11: 359–363

Blossey HC, Bartsch HH, Kanne D, Köbberling J, Nagel GA (1982a) The pharmacokinetics of high-dose medroxyprogesterone acetate (MPA) in the therapy of advanced breast cancer. Cancer Chemother Pharmacol 8: 77–81

Blossy HC, Wander HE, Nagel GA, Köbberling J. Kleeberg U (1982b) Medroxyprgesteronazetat in hoher Dosierung beim metastasierenden Mammakarzinom. Vergleichende Klinik, Pharmakokinetik und Pharmakodynamik verschiedener Applikationsformen. Onkologie 5: 13–24

Carroll KK, Gammal EB, Plunkett ER (1968) Dietary fat and mammary cancer. Can Med Assoc J 98: 590–594

Centers for Disease Control Cancer and Steroid Hormone Study (1983) Long-term oral contraceptive use and the risk of breast cancer. JAMA 249: 1591-1595

Chamness GC, McGuire WL (1979) Scatchard plots: common errors in correction and interpretation. Steroids 26: 538–542

Chopra IJ, Chopra SR, Smith SR, Teza M, Salomon DS (1975) Reciprocal changes in serum concentrations of $3,3',5'$,-triiodothryonine (reverse T_3) and $3,3',5$-triiodothyronine (T_3) in systemic illnesses. J Clin Endocrinol Metab 41: 1043–1049

Clark JH, Peck EJ (eds) (1979) Female sex steroids, receptors and function, Morogr Endocrinol 14

De Waard F (1969) The epidemiology of breast cancer. Review and prospects. Int J Cancer 4: 677–586

Fischedick O, Lux H (1977) Zur Epidemiologie des weiblichen Brustkrebses. Gynäkologe 10: 123–128

Grandics P, Puri RK, Toft DO (1982). A new affinity design for purification of non-transformed avian progesterone receptor. Endocrinology 110: 1055–1057

Grill HJ, Manz B, Pollow K (1982) Double-labeling assay system for estrogen and progesterone receptors. Lancet I: 679

Grill HJ, Manz B, Belovsky O, Pollow K (1982) Criteria for the establishment of a double-labeling assay for silmutaneous determination of estrogen and progesterone receptors. Oncology 41: 25–32

Grill HJ, Möbius U, Manz B, Pollow K (1983) 16a-Iodo-3,17β-estradiol: a stable ligand for estrogen receptor determinations in tissues with high 17β-hydroxysteroid dehydrogenase activity. J Steroid Biochem 19: 1687–1688

Grill HJ, Manz B, Belovsky O, Pollow K (1985) Criteria for the establishment of a double-labeling assay for simultaneous determination of estrogen and progesterone receptors. Counting Exchange 1: 1–7

Grill HJ, Heubner A, Manz B, Kreienberg R, Pollow K (1985) Charakterisierung der gestagenen und glucocorticoiden Wirkung von MPA auf der Rezeptorebene. In: Nagel GA, Schulz KD, Kreienberg R, Pollow K (eds) Neue Erkenntnisse über den Wirkungsmechanismus von Medroxyprogesteronazetat. Aktuel Onkologie 30: 15–31

Guthrie D (1982) Treatment of carcinoma of the cervix with bromocriptine. Br J Obstet Gynaec 98: 853–855

Henderson BE, Powell D, Rosario I, Keys C, Hanisch R, Young M, Casagrande J, Gerkins V, Pike MC (1974) An epidemiologic study of breast cancer. J Natl Cancer Inst 53: 609–614

Hesch RD (1981) Das Niedrig–T_3–Syndrom. Dtsch Med Wochenschr 106: 971–972

Heubner A, Manz B, Grill HJ, Pollow K (1984) High-Performance and ion-exchange chromatography and chromatofocusing of the human uterine progesterone receptor: its application to the identification of 21-^{3}H-dehydro Org2058-labelled receptor. J Chromatogr 297: 301–311

Heubner A, Belovsky O, Grill HJ, Pollow K (1985) FPLC-Eine neue Dimension in der Analytik und präparativen Darstellung von Progesteron-Rezeptoren. In: FPLC-Fast Protein Liquid Chromatography. GIT, Darmstadt, pp 89–107

Heubner A, Beck T, Grill HJ, Pollow K (1986) Comparison of immunocytochemical estrogen receptor assay, estrogen receptor enzyme immunoassay, and radioligand-labeled estrogen receptor assay in human breast cancer and uterine tissue. Cancer Res [Suppl] 46: 4281-4285

Hochberg RB (1979) Iodine-25-labeled estradiol: a gamma-emmiting analog of estradiol that binds to the estrogen receptors. Science 205: 1138–1140

Hochberg RB, Rosner W (1980) Interaction of 16a(^{125}I)-β-iodoestradiol with estrogen receptor and other binding proteins. Proc Natl Acad Sci USA 77: 328–332

Izuo M, Lino Y, Tominaga T, Nomura Y, Abe D, Enomoto K, Takatani, O, Kubo K (1982) Hochdosierte orale. Therapie mit Medroxyprogesteron-Azetat beim fortgeschrittenen Brustkrebs: Klinische und endokrinologische Untersuchungen. Med Klin SoNr 2: 23–28

Jensen EV, De Sombre ER (1972) Mechanism of action of the female sex hormones. Annu Rev Biochem 41: 203–230

Jensen EV, Block GE, Smith S (1971) Estrogen receptors and breast cancer response to adrenalectomy. NCI Monogr 34: 55–70

Jonat W, Knapp W, Schumann B, Trapp H, Vanhecke C, Maass H (1984) Orale hochdosierte Gestagntherapie als Versagerschema beim metastasierenden Mammakarzinom. Dtsch Med Wochenschr 109: 46–49

Jonat W, Stegner HE, Maass H (1985) Immunhistochemische Bestimmung von Östrogenrezeptoren im Mammakarzinomgewebe mittels monoklonaler Antikörper-erste klinische Ergebnisse. Geburtshilfe Frauenheilkd 45: 473–476

Judd SJ, Rakoff JS, Yen SSC (1978) Inhibition of gonadotropin and prolactin release by dopamine: effect of endogenous estradiol level. J Clin Endocrinol Metab 47: 494–498

Jungblut PW, Hughes S, Hughes A, Wagner RK (1972) Evaluation of various methods for assay of cytoplasmic estrogen receptors in extracts of calf uteri and human breast cancers. Acta Endocrinol 70: 185–195

Katzenellenbogen BS (1980) Dynamics of steroid hormone receptor action. Annu Rev Physiol 42: 1–357

Ketcham AS, Sindelar WF (1975) Risk factors in breast cancer. Prog Clin Cancer 6: 99–114

King RJB (1976) Intracellular reception of steroid hormones. In: Campbell PN, Aldridge WNA (eds) Essays in biochemistry, vol 12. Academic, London, pp 41–46

Köhler G, Bässler R (1986) Ergebnisse vergleichender immunhistochemischer und biochemischer Untersuchungen zum Östrogen-Rezeptor-Status in Mammakarzinomen. Dtsch Med Wochenschr 111: 1954–1960

Kolodny RC, Jacobs LS, Daughaday WH (1972) Mammary stimulation causes prolactin secretion in non-lactating women. Nature 238: 284–286

Korenman SG, Dukes BA (1970) Specific estrogen binding by the cytoplasm of human breast carcinoma. J Clin Endocrinol Metab 30: 639–645

Kreineberg R, Grill HJ, Melchert F, Pollow K (1985) Hochdosierte MPA-Therapie beim metastasierenden Mammakarzinom: MPA-Serumspiegel und hormonelle Parameter. In: Nagel GA, Schulz KD, Kreienberg R, Pollow K (eds) Neue Erkenntnisse über den Wirkungsmechanismus von Medroxyprogesteronazetat. Aktuel Onkologie 30: 65-77

Kucera H, Smekal G, Spona J (1983) Prolactin level and cervical carcinoma. J Steroid Biochem 19 [suppl]: 144 S

Lessey BA, Alexander PS, Horwitz KB (1983) The subunit structure of human breast cancer progesterone receptors: characterization by chromatography and photoaffinity labeling. Endocrinology 112: 1267–1274

Lewison EF (1976) Role of exogenous Estrogenes. In: Stoll BA (ed) Risk factors in breast cancer. Heinemann, London, p 67

Lilienfeld AM (1963) The epidemiology of breast cancer. Cancer Res 23: 1503–1513

Maass H, Trams G, Sachs H (1970) Das Mammacarcinom. Epidemiologie und Endokrinologie. Gynäkologe 3: 2–6

Maass H, Jonat W (1979) Steroidhormonrezeptoren in Mammakarzinomen. Bericht über ein Consensus-Meeting im National Institute of Health, Bethesda USA. Geburtshilfe Frauenheilkd 39: 761–764

Maass H, Sachs H (1972) Epidemiologie des Mammacarcinoms. Internist (Berlin) 13: 326–331

MacMahon B, Cole P, Brown J (1973) Etiology of human breast cancer: a review. J Natl Cancer Inst 50: 21–42

Mahlke M, Grill HJ, Knapstein P, Wiegand U, Pollow K (1985) Oral high-dose medroxyprogesterone acetate (MPA) treatment: cortisol/MPA serum profiles in relation to breast cancer regression. Oncology 42: 144–149

Malarkey WB, Kennedy M, Allred LE, Milo G (1983) Physiological concentrations of prolactin can promote the growth of human breast tumor cells in culture. J Clin Endocrinol Metab 56: 673–677

McGuire WL (1979) Assays for estrogen and progesterone receptors in human breast cancer tissue. Applications Data, Beckman Instruments, Spinco Division, Palo Alto

McGuire WL, Carbone PP, Vollmer EP (1975) Estrogen receptors in human breast cancer. Raven, New York

Meinhold H (1977) Reverses Trijodthyronin-Neue Aspekte des peripheren Metabolismus der Schilddrüsenhormone. Compact News Nucl Med 4: 55–59

Noel GL, Suh HK, Frantz AG (1974) Prolactin release during nursing and breast stimulation in post-partum and non–post–partum subjects. J Clin Endocrinol Metab 38: 413–423

O'Malley BW, McGuire WL (1968) Studies on the mechanism of action of progesterone in regulation of the synthesis of specific proteins. J Clin Invest 47: 654–664

Pollow K (1983) Die Bedeutung von Hormonrezeptoren für die Behandlung maligner Erkrankungen. Therapiewoche 33: 6809–6825

Pollow K, Kreienberg R, Grill HJ, Melchert F, Knapstein P, Manz B (1984) Hochdosierte Medroxyprogesteronacetat-Therapie beim metastasierten Mamma-Karzinom in Abhängigkeit von der Applikationsform. In: Robustelli Della Cuna G, Nagel GA, Lanius P (eds) Deutsch-Italienisches Onkologisches Symposium. Kehrer, Freiburg, pp 85–100

Possinger K, Willich S, Jaspers L, Langecker P. Schmid L, Wilmanns W (1985) Therapeutische Effektivität einer hochdosierten MPA-Therapie und Wirkung auf das endokrine System. In: Nagel GA, Schulz KD, Kreienberg R, Pollow K (eds) Neue Erkenntnisse über den Wirkungsmechanismus von Medroxyprogesteronazetat. Aktuel Onkologie 30: 15–31

Press MF, Greene GL (1984) Methods in laboratory investigations. An immunocytochemical method for demonstrating estrogen receptor in human uterus using monoclonal antibodies to human estrophilin. Lab Invest 50: 480–486

Raynaud JP (1977) R5020, a tag for the progesterone receptor. In: McGuire WL, Raynaud JP, Baulieu EE (eds) Progesterone receptors in normal and neoplastic tissues. Raven, New York, pp 9–21

Rees LH, Bloomfield GA, Rees GM, Corrin B, Franks LM, Ratcliffe JG (1974) Multiple hormones in a bronchial tumor. J Clin Endcrinol Metab 38: 1090–1097

Reiner A, Reiner G, Spona J, Schemper M, Kolb R, Jakesz R, Holzner JH (1986) Vergleich von immunochemischem und biochemischem Östrogenrezeptor-Nachweis bei Mammakarzinomen und Beziehung zur histochemischen Tumorklassifikation. Verh Dtsch Ges Pathol 70: 243–246

Remmele W, Stegner HE (1987) Immunhistochemischer Nachweis von Östrogenrezeptoren (ER-ICA) im Mammakarzinomgewebe: Vorschlag zur einheitlichen Bewertung des Untersuchungsbefundes. Frauenarzt 28: 41–43

Rose DP, Davis TE (1978) Plasma thyroid-stimulating hormone and thyroxine concentrations in breast cancer. Cancer 41: 666–669

Rose DP, Davis TE (1979) Plasma triiodthyronine concentrations in breast cancer. Cancer 43: 1434–1438

Salimtschik M, Mouridsen HT, Loeber J, Johansson (1980) Comparative pharmacokinetics of medroxyprogesterone acetate administered by oral and intramuscular routes. Cancer Chemother Pharmacol 4: 267–269

Scatchard DG (1949) The attraction of proteins for small molecules and ions. Ann NY Acad Sci 51: 660–672

Schmidt-Matthiesen H (1975) Der Internist und das Genital-und Brustcarcinom der Frau. Die Krebssuche in der internistischen Praxis. Internist 16: 223–231

Schrader WT, Kuhn RW, O'Malley BW (1977) Progesterone-binding components of chick oviduct. Receptor B subunit protein purified to appanent homogeneity from laying hen oviducts. J Biol Chem 252: 299–307

Sherman MR, Tuazon FB, Diaz SC, Miller LK (1976) Multiple forms of oviduct progesterone receptors analyzed by ion exchange filtration and gel electrophoresis. Biochemistry 15: 980–989

Smith RG, D'Istria M, Nguyen TV (1981) Purification of a human progesterone receptor. Biochemistry 20: 5557–5565

Tamassia V (1986) Clinical pharmacokinetics of medroxyprogesterone acetate: relevance for the treatment of breast and endometrial cancer. In: Bolla M, Racinet C, Vrousos C (eds) Endometrial cancers. Karger, Basel, PP 168–176

Thijssen H (1968) Steroid excretion patterns in postmenopausal women. Kanker Jaarboek 18: 171–183

Thomas DB (1984) Do hormones cause breast cancer? Cancer 53 [Suppl]: 3

Toft DO, Gorski JA (1966) A receptor molecule for estrogens: isolation from the rat uterus and preliminary characterization. Proc Natl Acad Sci USA 55: 1574–1581

Turkington RW (1971) Ectopic production of prolactin. N Engl J Med 285: 1455–1458

Vekemans M, Delvoye, L'Hermite M, Robyn C (1977) Serum prolactin levels during the menstrual cycle. J Clin Endocrinol Metab 44: 1222–1225

Von Werder K, Rjosk HK (1979) Menschliches Prolaktin. Klin Wochenschr 57: 1–12

Von Werder K, Fahlbusch R, Rjosk HK (1977) Hyperprolaktinämie. Pathophysiologie, klinische Bedeutung, Therapie. Internist 18: 520–582

Vorherr H (1980) Breast cancer. Urban and Schwarzenberg, Baltimore

Wagner RK, Jungblut PW (1976) Estradiol and dihydrotestosterone receptors in normal and neoplastic mammary tissue. Acta Endocrinol 82: 105–120

Wander HE, Blossey HCh, Köbberling J, Nagel GA (1983) Hochdosiertes MPA beim metastasierten Mammakarzinom. Beziehung zwischen Krankheitsverlauf und Hormonprofilen. Klin Wochenschr 61: 553–560

Waterhouse J, Muir C, Correa P, Powell J (1976) Cancer incidence in five continents. IARC III, Lyon

Wrange Ö, Nordensköld B, Silfverswärd C, Ganberg PO, Gustafsson JA (1976) Isoelectric focusing of estradiol receptor protein from human mammary – a comparison to sucrose gradient analysis. Eur J Cancer 12: 695–700

Wrange Ö, Nordenskjöld B, Gustafsson JA (1978) Cytosol estradiol receptor in human mammary carcinoma: an assay based on isoelectric focusing in polyacrylamide gel. Anal Biochem 85: 461–475

Wynder EL, Bross IJ, Hirayama (1960) A study of the epidemiology of cancer of the breast. Cancer 13: 559–601

New Trends in the Endocrine Treatment of Breast Cancer

H. Maass, W. Jonat, H. Eidtmann, T. Kunz, and G. Kügler

Universitäts-Frauenklinik, Martinistraße 52, 2000 Hamburg 20, FRG

Breast cancer is a hormone-dependent tumor. Procedures for its endocrine treatment were formerly selected on a purely empirical basis. After methods were developed and came into use for measuring hormone receptors, a solid knowledge about the action of steroid hormones in target organs and therefore about the effects of endocrine treatment procedures became available. The following three aspects of the endocrine therapy of breast cancer are discussed here: (a) selection procedures, (b) adjuvant therapy, and (c) new aspects of the endocrine therapy of metastatic breast cancer.

Selection Procedures

The effect of steroid hormones in target organs is connected with the presence of receptor proteins (Jensen 1970; Maass and Jonat 1979).

For the determination of hormone receptors (estrogen and progesterone receptors are usually measured) biochemical and immunohistochemical proecdures are available. The advantage of conventional biochemical methods lies in exact quantification.

The immunohistochemical procedures can be performed in cell suspensions or tissue slices; their disadvantage is the subjectivity of quantification. The progesterone receptor is a reaction product of estrogen action in the target cell, and its presence means an intact reaction chain.

The clinical correlation between estrogen receptors determined by immunohistochemical procedures (ERICA, or estrogen receptor immunocytochemical assay) and the outcome of endocrine therapy shows at least the same level of prediction as the biochemical assay (Table, 1; Jonat and Stegner 1988). Now data on the correlation of the effect of endocrine treatment and the immunohistochemical determination of the progesterone receptor (PRICA) are available (Jonat et al. 1988) Tables 2 and 3 show that the correlation is not as good as that with ERICA. The receptor status is characterized by the hormone dependence of metastases

Recent Results in Cancer Research. Vol. 118
© Springer-Verlag Berlin·Heidelberg 1990

Table 1. ERICA results and response to endocrine therapy in advanced breast cancer and results from conventional assays

Reference	n	ERICA positive	ERICA negative
Pertschuk 1985	43	9/16	2/27
Coombs 1985	56	21/29	1/27
McCarty 1985	23	13/14	1/9
Jonat 1985	20	6/11	1/9
Jonat 1986	10	5/7	1/3
Total	152	54/77 (70%)	6/75 (8%)
Conventional assays	1336	480/852 (56%)	27/484 (6%)

Table 2. PRICA, results and response to endocrine therapy in advanced breast cancer ($n = 79$)

Response	Histoscore positive	
	50–99	100
Complete remission	6 ⎤	3 ⎤
Partial remission	24 ⎦ 49%	22 ⎦ 51%
No change	4	4
Progression	27	20

Table 3. PRICA results and response to the first endocrine treatment step ($n = 38$)

Response	Histoscore positive	
	50–99	100
Complete remission	6 ⎤	3 ⎤
Partial remission	11 ⎦ 57%	9 ⎦ 60%
No change	2	2
Progression	11	6

Table 4. Estrogen (ER) and progesterone receptor (PR) status in asynchronous assays: results of the German Cooperative Receptor Group

Receptor status change	Patients with change recorded			
	n	n	%	% of total
ER $+$ $\rightarrow$ ER $-$	108	44	40.8 ⎤	
				35
ER $-$ $\rightarrow$ ER $+$	109	31	28.4 ⎦	
PR $+$ $\rightarrow$ PR $-$	59	37	62.7	
				29
PR $-$ $\rightarrow$ PR $+$	145	23	15.9	

better than by clinical parameters. J. Allegra (personal communication) observed a comparable remission rate of receptor-positive metastases independent of the site of the metastatic lesion. The receptor status allows prediction for a longer interval between primary treatment and development of metastases. After 5 years the rate of recurrences is equal in the receptor-positive and -negative groups. Receptor status therefore is not a suitable parameter for long-term prognosis, although the time of survival is prolonged (Hähnel et al. 1979).

Hormone receptor status shows time- and therapy-dependent changes. In 25%–30% of all cases we must expect that the receptor status in the primary tumor is not the same as that in later developing metastases. Table 4 shows the results of a cooperative trial in the Federal Republic of Germany (Jonat 1984). If possible, the receptor status should be determined on specimens of metastatic tissue. This can be achieved by immunohistochemical procedures.

Adjuvant Endocrine Therapy

The efficacy of hormone receptor analysis for prediction of the benefit from endocrine treatment in metastatic breast cancer is well established. Additionally, the determination of receptors is of increasing value for the selection of adjuvant treatment procedures.

Analysis of the results of randomized trials make it possible to provide recommendations for the adjuvant treatment of patients with breast cancer. The data of all published randomized trials were analyzed by the Early Breast Cancer Trialist Collaborative group, PETO (1988) and were the basis for treatment recommendations for nodal-positive patients. The original recommendations presented at the Consensus Development Conference at Bethesda, United States, in September 1985 have been modified by Glick in March 1988 (Table 5). These are valid only for patients who are not treated in trials. Premenopausal, nodal-positive patients should be treated by a combination chemotherapy independent of hormone receptor status. Postmenopausal, nonal-positive, and receptor-positive women benefit from tamoxifen therapy. The effect of tamoxifen in combination

Table 5.. Adjuvant treatment of breast cancer. (From Glick 1988)

Receptor status	LN positive Premenopausal	Postmenopausal
Positive	CHT	TAM +/− CHT
Negative	CHT	CHT +/−TAM

LN, lymph node; CHT, chemotherapy; TAM, tamoxifen.

with chemotherapy and/or chemotherapy followed by tamoxifen is not clear compared with that of tamoxifen alone. In postmenopausal, nodal-positive, and hormone–receptor–negative patients chemotherapy should be given. Also for those in this group the value of chemotherapy in combination with tamoxifen or followed by tamoxifen therapy is not certain compared with a chemotherapy alone.

The validity of this recommendations could be confirmed in the cooperative prospective trial in the FRG (Kaufmann et al. 1987) for a risk-adapted subgroup of node-positive patients (hormone receptors positive and one to three involved axillary lymph nodes). CMF chemotherapy was compared with tamoxifen therapy for 2 years. The 6-year results show a clear advantage for chemotherapy in premenopausal patients and for tamoxifen therapy in postmenopausal patients (Fig. 1; Kaufmann et al. 1985). The optimal duration of adjuvant tamoxifen therapy in postmenopausal patients is not yet clear. The comparison of trials summarized in Table 6 shows that at least a 2-year application of 30 mg per day is necessary. Recent trials suggest that an application for 5 years or longer may be reasonable (Scottish Cancer Trial 1987).

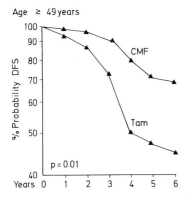 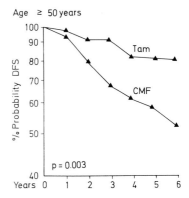

Fig. 1. Probability (percent of patients) of disease-free interval in low-risk breast cancer patients after 6 years. Low risk is defined as one to three lymph nodes involved and estrogen or progesterone receptor positive. *CMF,* cytoxan metothrexat 5-fluoralil; *Tam,* tamoxifen. (From Kaufmann et al. 1985)

Table 6. Tamoxifen dosage and results in randomized adjuvant treatment trials for breast cancer. (From Jonat et al. 1988)

Trial	Maximum exposure (daily dose, duration)	Statistical significance at 5% level	
		Disease-free survival	Total survival
Christie	7.3 g (20 mg, 1 year)	No	No
Danish	10.9 g (30 mg, 1 year)	Yes	No
NATO	14.6 g (20 mg, 2 years)	Yes	Yes
Scottish Cancer	36.5 g (20 mg, 5 years)	Yes	Yes
GABGI			
(Kauf-mann et al. 1985)	21.9 g (30 mg, 2 years)	Yes	No

For nodal-negative patients no standard recommendations can be given at present. Trials are under way to define special risk groups within the group of nodal-negative patients. Risk factors could include morphological factors such as tumor size, tumor cells in bone marrow specimens, grading, and the level of growth factors and molecular biological factors such as hormone receptors, DNA content, oncogene expression, and cell membrane structures. Recently the NIH recommended that all nodal-negative patients be treated by adjuvant procedures with tamoxifen or chemotherapy, depending on receptor status. Most oncologists are of the opinion that an additional selection of risk groups is necessary.

Endocrine Treatment of Metastatic Breast Cancer

The first treatment possibility for metastatic breast tumor was that of endocrine therapy. Ablative therapy with ovarectomy, adrenalectomy, or hypophysectomy is now followed by competition therapy with antiestrogens and inhibitive therapy by aromatase inhibitors and luteining hormone releasing hormone (LH-RH) analogs. The pharmacodynamics of competitive therapy with tamoxifen is based on blockade of the estrogen receptor. Recent investigations by Dickson and Lippman (1987) show that besides the competitive blockade of the estrogen receptor by antiestrogen the induction of the transforming growth factor-β, a growth-inhibiting factor may be the cause of tamoxifen effects, especially in receptor-negative tumors (Erbs et al. 1987). The mechanism of inhibiting drugs such as aromatase inhibitors or LH-RH analogs is based on the blockade of estrogen production in the adrenals, subcutaneous fat tissue, muscles, and possibly the tumor cell itself, or in the case of LH-RH analogs the blockade of the pulsatile LH-RH secretion followed by the absence of the stimulation of the ovarial function. LH-RH analog and aromatase inhibitor therapy therefore means "chemical ovarectomy" and "chemical adrenalectomy."

The average remission rate for all endocrine therapy procedures without selection is 30%, and the duration of remission is approximately 10 months. The

230 H. Maass et al.

advantage of endocrine therapy is the possibility of sequential application of different treatment procedures in the case of remission or no change. Thus long-term remission of patients with metastatic breast cancer can be achieved by a treatment with relatively few side effects. Figure 2 shows the results of an analysis performed on patients at the Department of Gynecology and Internal Medicine of the University of Hamburg by Stolzen bach (1982). Four years after the first appearance of metastases the survival rate of receptor-positive, sequentially treated patients was twice that of receptor-negative patients.

The combination of endocrine procedures shows that occasionally higher remission rates may be observed, but that no significant prolongation of the remission occurs. Possibly, alternating application could be of more success. The theoretical basis for this treatment strategy lies in the fact that the progesterone receptor can be induced by tamoxifen. The administration of tamoxifen alternating with that of progestogens is under study. Selection for endocrine therapy is based on the above-mentioned selection parameters. In premenopausal patients the first step is ovarectomy. In future the application of LH-RH analogs will be the treatment of choice. The first results of trials show comparable remission rates with this kind of treatment as after ovarectomy (Table 7; Thürlimann and Sen 1987). As a second step, after ovarectomy, antiestrogens are given, followed by aromatase inhibitors and high-dose progestogens. It is not yet clear whether the addition of tamoxifen to LH-RH analogs after remission is effective. In postmenopausal patients antiestrogen therapy in hormone-dependent tumors is the treatment of first choice, followed by that of aromatase inhibitors and high-dose progestogens. The results of our own cooperative trial and another trial with a new aromatose inhibitor with fewer side effects than with aminoglutethimide are shown in the Table 8. The remission rates are closely comparable (Table 9). Treatment with anabolic substances at relatively high dose in combination with chemotherapy is performed occasionally in patients with bone metastases. The application of glucocorticosteroids is performed in cases with visceral metastases, especially cerebral metastases and lymphangiosis of the pleura or the lung.

The second and third endocrine treatment steps should be performed only if primary treatment is followed by remission or no change. The probability of a second remission is about 50% if the first treatment was effective and only 12% in patients with progression during the first treatment.

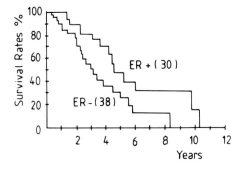

Fig. 2. Percent survival after the first recurrence in estrogen receptor positive and negative patients with metastasized breast cancer following endocrine and cytostatic therapy. Comparison between the two groups, $p < 0.03$. *Parentheses*, number of patients. (From Stolzenbach et al. 1982)

Table 7. LH-RH agonist therapy (goserelin) in advanced breast cancer

Menopausal status	Number of patients/ number of trials	Complete + partial remissions
Premenopausal	231/9	35%
Postmenopausal	93/4	= 10%

Table 8. Side effects[a] of 4-hydroxyandrostene-dione therapy in advanced breast cancer

Trial	Percent of cases
Coombes et al. 1984	35
Jonat 1984	33

[a] Lethargy, rush, nausea.

Table 9. Response to 4-hydroxyandrostenedione therapy in advanced breast cancer among postmenopausal patients

Trial	n	Response duration (months)	Complete + partial remissions
Coombes et al. 1984	100	9	34
Jonat et al. 1988	65	9	30

Endocrine therapy is the most essential part of the interdisciplinary treatment of patients with breast cancer. We are now observing a renaissance in this because of the disappointing results of chemotherapy. Of present endocrine treatment procedures, only tamoxifen is being employed increasingly in the adjuvant situation. A further improvement in this treatment concept can be expected with increased understanding of the biology of breast cancer, the mode of action of the presently available substances, and the development of other effective drugs.

References

Consensus Development Conference (1985) Adjuvant chemotherapy for breast cancer. JAMA 254: 3461–3463

Coombes C, Goss P, Dowsett M, Gazet J-C, Brodie A (1984) 4-Hydroxyandrostendione in treatment of postmenopausal patients with advanced breast cancer. Lancet Dec 1: 1237–1239

Dickson RB, Lippman ME (1987) Estrogenic regulation of growth and polypeptide growth factor secretion in human breast carcinoma. Endocr Rev 82: 29

Early Breast Cancer Trialist Collaborative Group (1988) Effects of adjuvant tamoxifen and of cytotoxic therapy on mortality in early breast cancer: an overview of 61 randomized trials among 28,896 women. N Engl J Med 319: 6181 Peto

Erbs SR, Roberts JV, Baum M (1987) Alternative mechanism of action of "anti-oestrogens' in Breast cancer. Lancet II, Sept 12: 621

Glick J (1988) Adjuvant therapy of primary breast cancer. 3rd International conference, Consensus St Gallen, March 1988.

Hähnel R, Woodlings T, Vivian AB (1979) Prognostic value of estrogen receptors in primary breast cancer. Cancer 44: 671–675

Jensen EV (1970) The pattern of hormone receptor interaction. In: Griffiths K, Pierrepoin CG (eds) Some aspects of aetilogy and biochemistry of prostatic cancer. Alpha Omega Alpha, Cardiff, pp 151–169.

Jonat W, (1984) Experimentelle und klinische Erfahrungen mit Steroidhormonrezeptoren beim Mammakarzinom. Wien Klin Wochenschr 96 (13): 499–508

Jonat W, Stegner HE, Maass H (1985) Immunhistochemische Bestimmung von Östrogenrezeptoren in Mammakarzzinomgeweben mittels monoclonaler Antikörper. Geburtshilfe Frauenheilkd 45: 425–502

Jonat W, Kügler G, von Laffert C, (1988) Biochemische und immunhistochemische Rezeptorbestimmugen. Zuckschwerdt, Munich (in press)

Kaufman M, Jonat W, Caffier H, Hilfrich J, Melchert F, Mahlke M, Abel U, Maass H, Kubli F (1985) Adjuvant chemohormonotherapy selected by axillary node and hormone receptor status in node-positive breast cancer. Rev Endocr Rel Cancer (Suppl) 17: 57–63

Kaufmann M, Jonat W, Caffier H, Kreienberg R, Hilfrich J, Abel Uh Maass H, Kubli F (1987) Adjuvant systemic risk adapted cytotoxic +/− tamoxifen therapy in women with node positive breast cancer. In: Salmon S (ed) Adjuvant therapy of Cancer V. Grune and Stratton, Orlando

Maass H, Jonat W (1979) Steroidrezptoren in Mammakarzinomen. Geburtshilfe Frauenheilkd 39: 761

Scottish Cancer Trial (1987) Adjuvant tamoxifen in the management of operable breast cancer: the Scottish trial. Lancet II: 171–175

Stolzenbach G, Jonat W, Maass H, Strohmeier E, Trams G (1982) Relationship between estrogen receptor values and survival in patients with advanced breast cancer. In: Gergii A (Hrsg) Solide Tumoren und metastasierung. Fisher, Stuttgart (Verhandlgen der Deutschen noelsgesellschaft, Bd III), p 214

Thürlimann B, Senn HJ (1987) LHRH agonists in the treatment of metastatic breast cancer: a review. Tumor Diagn Ther 8: 274–278

Identification of Putative Nonfunctional Steroid Receptors in Breast and Endometrial Cancer

D.S. Colvard, M.L. Graham, N.J. Berg, J.N. Ingle, D.J. Schaid, K.C. Podratz, and T.C. Spelsberg

Departments of Biochemistry and Molecular Biology, Mayo Graduate School of Medicine, Rochester, MN 55905, USA

Introduction

Breast and endometrial carcinomas remain major oncologic problems. Both types of cancer are considered to be responsive to endocrine therapy. This is particularly true in the case of breast cancer whether one considers ablative or additive therapy (Ingle 1984; Ingle et al. 1986). However, tumor responses to steroid therapy vary (Fig. 1). In general, for breast carcinoma, the tumors of about one-half of estrogen receptor (ER)-positive breast cancer patients as assessed by the dextran-coated charcoal assay (DCC assay), respond and one-half do not respond (Edwards et al. 1979; McGuire 1980). Progesterone receptor (PR) status is usually assessed in cases of endometrial cancer, most of which are diagnosed in early clinical stages. Progestational agents are the treatment of choice in cases of advanced disease, yet only 11%–40% of unselected patients respond (Wait 1973); Kohorn 1976; Piver 1980; Podratz 1985). Recent results from a large study indicate that tumors which

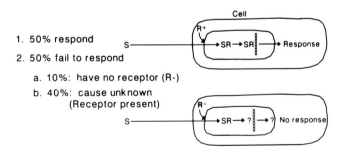

1. 50% respond

2. 50% fail to respond

    a. 10%: have no receptor (R-)

    b. 40%: cause unknown
            (Receptor present)

Fig 1. General tumor responses to steriod therapy. Proposed model for response of tumours from sex steroid target tissues to hormonal therapy includes cells which contain functional receptors and cells which fail to respond for uncertain reasons. *Top panel*, steriod hormone (*S*) freely enters cells from blood and binds to its receptor (*R*) in the nucleus. This complex (*SR*) then binds to acceptor sites on DNA to elicit cellular response(s). *Bottom panel*, the steroid-receptor complex invokes no response. This lack of response could be due to the lack of a functional receptor

contain high levels of PR by the DCC assay show a positive response 60% of the time (Ehrlich 1988).

Although the estrogen (ER) and prosgesterone receptor (PR) assays currently in use clinically have improved the physician's ability to predict a response to hormonal therapy, the DCC assay fails to predict accurately which patients will respond. With the relatively high false-positive rates by the DCC assay and the lack of response by many of these patients, a hormone receptor assay is needed with a substantially higher predictive index. Current methods, such as the DCC assay and immunohistochemical assays, which utilize antireceptor antibodies, identify only the presence of receptor and not any aspect of biological activity of the receptor.

The existence of nonfunctional estrogen receptors (i.e., those able to bind estrogen but unable to become activated and to bind in the nuclear acceptor sites) may explain those breast cancer biopsies which contain ER by the DCC assay but fail to respond to antisteroid therapy (Edwards et al. 1979; McGuire 1980; McGuire et al. 1975). Indeed, the presence of tightly bound nuclear receptors has been reported to correlate with response to endocrine therapy (Leake et al. 1981; MacFarlane et al. 1980). Nonfunctional androgen receptors have also been described in instances of androgen insensitivity in men (Grumbach and Conte 1985). Similarly, some cloned lines of lymphoblastoid cells were found to contain nonfunctional glucocorticoid receptors which, while present, were unable to bind to the nuclear acceptor sites and induce cell responses (Gehring and Tomkins 1974). Thus, a nuclear binding assay was developed by Spelsberg et al. (1987) in an effort to measure the biological activity of steroid receptors in human tumors. The nuclear binding assay, or biopsy nuclear binding assay (BNB assay), which assesses the biological activity of steroid hormone receptors in both animal and human tissues, was then modified to accommodate intact cells from small samples of human tissue such as would be obtained from needle biopsies (Colvard et al. 1988).

The purpose of this study was to identify and quantitate functional steroid receptors in a large series of beast and endometrial carcionmas with use of the BNB assay. These results were then compared to the total cellular binding observed when these cancers were concurrently assayed with the standard DCC assay.

Methods

Tissue Sources. Fresh surgical waste from breast carcinoma was obtained from patients being treated surgically at Mayo Clinic from January 1986 through July 1987. Endometrial carcinoma was obtained from patients treated surgically from February 1984 through June 1986. Tissue for the BNB assay was taken from regions of the biopsy as close to that used for histopathologic evaluation and steroid receptor measurement by a DCC assay (Thibodeau et al. 1981). Tissue samples for nuclear binding assays were placed in MCDB-202 medium for transport to the BNB assay laboratory. Tissue processing was usually begun within 24 h of surgical removal, during which time no measurable loss of nuclear binding was observed.

Nuclear Binding Assay. The steps of the BNB assay are outlined in Fig. 2 and have been described in detail elsewhere (Spelsberg et al. 1987: Colvard et al. 1988). Briefly, fresh surgical specimens are minced in MCDB-202 medium (Irvine Scientific, Santa Ana CA) and digested with type III collagenase (Cooper Biomed, Malvern PA) for 1 h at 37°C. Viable tumor cells are collected by low-speed centrifugation and suspended in medium.

Aliquots of cell suspension were incubated in tubes containing estradiol (17-β-[2,4,6,7-³H]estradiol, S.A. 98 Ci/mmol, New England Nuclear, Boston MA) or promegestone (17-α-methyl-[³H]R5020, 86.2 Ci/mmol, New England Nuclear) in replicate for a final concentration of 10 nM with or without 100-fold excess of the homologous unlabeled steroid for estimation of nonspecific and total binding, respectively, for 1 h at 22°C. After the 1-h incubation, the cell pellets were resuspended in homogenization buffer (50 mM Tris, pH 7.5, 10% glycerol, 10 mM KCl, 0.1% Triton X-100, and 0.1% bovine serum albumin) and gently homogenized in a Teflon pestle glass homogenizer (Thomas type A). The homogenate was layered over 1.4 M sucrose in homogenization buffer and centrifuged for 20 min at 7000 g. Radioactivity was measured in ethanol extracts of the nuclei pellet by liquid scintillation in a LS-5801 liquid scintillation counter (Beckman Instruments, Fullerton CA). DNA was estimated in the nuclear pellet using a modified diphenylamine assay (Burton 1956; Colvard et al. 1988) using a standard curve with calf thymus DNA (Calbiochem, La Jolla CA) treated similarly.

Calcualtions.   The specific nuclear binding in the BNB assay is the mean of the replicate assays for the total binding of [³H]steroid (expressed in disintegrations per minute, DPM, per microgram DNA) minus the corresponding mean of the replicate assays for the nonspecific binding. Specific nuclear binding is then converted to and given as femtomole receptor per milligram DNA. Since a negative calculated vaiue of specific nuclear binding essentially indicates no specific binding, negative values were reset to zero. To calculate receptor molecules bound per cell nucleus from the value for femtomole per milligram DNA, a value of 6 μg DNA per one million cells was used (Sober et al. 1970).

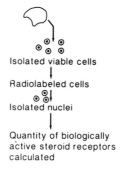

Fig. 2. Steps in the BNB assay. Tumor cells are isolated from fresh biopsies, labeled with tritiated steroid, and the quantity of nuclear-bound receptor is calculated. The procedure is described in more detail in "Methods"

Isolated viable cells
|
Radiolabeled cells
|
Isolated nuclei
|
Quantity of biologically active steroid receptors calculated

Surgical biopsy

Sections rinsed in media, treated with collagenase, filtered

Cells washed and incubated with [³H] steroids, 22°C, 60 min.

Cells disrupted, and nuclei isolated

1. Collection of nuclei on filters
2. Measurement of nuclear bound [³H] steroid
3. DNA quantitated

Total Steroid Receptor Content. Total cellular ER and PR content was assayed by a dual-labeled DCC assay in the Mayo Clinic Medical Laboratories (Thibodeau et al. 1981)

Results and Discussion

Ability of the Biopsy Nuclear Binding Assay to Measure Functional Steroid Receptors.
There are several advantages of the BNB assay over other biochemical assays for steroid receptors. First, the assay measures the number of functional steroid receptors per cell, that is, the number of receptors which can be activated and bound to nuclear acceptors sites. Measurements are made in intact cells rather than homogenized cell cytosol. The BNB assay may be five-to tenfold more sensitive than current immunocytochemical techniques. Lastly, the assay requires substantially less tissue than the DCC assay.

Using the BNB assay, saturable nuclear ER binding has been shown in the avian oviduct and human uterine tissues (Spelsberg et al. 1987; Colvard et al. 1988) as well as human breast carcinoma (Colvard et al. 1988). Only low, nonsaturable binding was found in benign human spleen, a nontarget tissue (Spelsberg et al. 1987; Colvard et al. 1988). The nuclear ER binding was shown to be steroid-specific in breast carcinoma (Fig. 3). Diethylstilbestrol, but not dexamethasone or promegestone (R5020, a synthetic progestin) competed for [³H]estradiol binding. Nuclear [³H]R5020 binding was also shown to be steroid-specific in endometrial carcinoma (Fig. 4). Unlabeled R5020, but not estradiol or cortisol, competed for [³H]R5020 nuclear binding. The above are characteristic of the in vivo nuclear binding of steroid receptors.

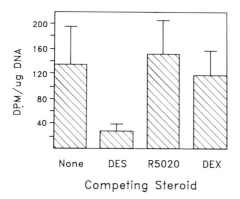

Fig. 3. Steroid specificity of the nuclear binding of [³H]estradiol in breast carcinoma with use of the BNB assay. A fresh breast carcinoma biopsy was digested with collagenase and the cell pellet suspended in MCDB-202. Aliquots of the cell suspension were labeled with 10 n*M* [³H]estradiol alone or with 100-fold excess of either unlabeled diethylstilbestrol (*DES*), promegestone (*R5020*), or dexamethasone (*DEX*). Nuclear binding was determined as described in "Methods". Data presented are the mean ± SD for quadruplicates. (From Colvard et al. 1988)

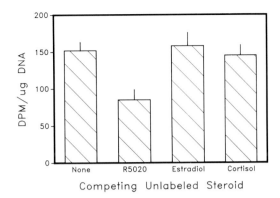

Fig. 4. Steroid specificity of nuclear [³H]R5020 binding in endometrial carcinoma with use of the BNB assay. An endometrial carcinoma biopsy was digested with collagenase and the cell pellet suspended in MCDB-202. Aliquots of the cell suspension were labeled with 10 nM [³H]R5020 alone or with 100-fold excess of either unlabeled R5020, estradiol or cortisol. Nuclear binding was determined as described above. Data presented are the mean ± SEM for triplicates

Correlation of the BNB and DCC Assays in Breast Carcinoma. After the BNB assay was shown to measure specific ER nuclear binding, the BNB assay and the DCC assay were applied to a large set of patients treated surgically for breast cancer, and the results of the two assays were compared. Of the 211 breast cancer patients assayed for ER binding by both the BNB and DCC assays, 140 patients were over 55 years old. This subgroup was chosen for comparative analysis since they are most likely to be postmenopausal.

The BNB values for this set of patients had a range of 0–16 900 fmol nuclear-bound ER per milligram DNA and a median of 840 fmol/mg DNA. The shape of the distribution of the BNB assay values for the patient group under 55 years old was similar. Comparisons were then made between the DCC assay and the BNB assay values for this set of patients. Since only moderate correlation was found (correlation coefficient between the BNB and DCC assays of 0.44) and since the DCC assay has limitations in its predictability of response to hormonal therapy, it was speculated that the BNB assay may provide better or additional, clinically useful information.

As for any new assay, the determination of the lower cutoff value is difficult to determine. Although the cutoff value which would correspond to a "positive" assay result can be answered definitively only when both BNB assay results and the clinical responses to steroid treatment are known for a large set of patients, we have used the clinically observed relationship between DCC assay values and response to hormonal therapy to speculate on a putative cutoff BNB value.

It has been observed clinically that approximately 50% of postmenopausal women who are ER-positive by the DCC assay do not respond to hormonal manipulation. If all of these women fail to respond solely due to lack of functional steroid receptors, then it is speculated that the cutoff of the BNB assay would be

Table 1.   Comparison of BNB and DCC assay values in breast cancer

BNB assay cutoff (fmol ER/ mg DNA)	Assay result[a] BNB	Assay result[a] DCC[b]	n	% of total patients	% of DCC assay positive patients
	−	+	50	36.5	50
1076	+	+	49	35.8	50
	−	−	29	21.2	
	+	−	9	6.6	

The speculated BNB assay cutoff (1076 fmol ER/mg DNA) is based on the observed clinical response of breast cancer patients to hormonal therapy.

[a] The signs + or − denote assay values above or below the cutoff for specific binding, respectively.

[b] The DCC assay cutoff used is 10 fmol ER per milligram protein.

approximately close to the point at which 50% of the DCC assay ER-positive postmenopausal women would have a value less than it. Using a DCC assay cutoff of 10 fmol of estrogen receptor per milligram cytosol protein, the BNB assay results for 99 women who were at least 55 years old and ER positive by the DCC assay were obtained. Among these women, 50% had a BNB assay value less than 1076 fmol/mg DNA. Hence, we speculate that the cutoff corresponding to a positive BNB assay would be approximately 1076 fmol/mg DNA. These results are summarized in Table 1. Using 1076 fmol ER/mg DNA as the BNB assay cutoff, 57% (35.8 + 21.2) of the patients correlated with regards to either positivity and negativity in both assays. Interestingly, 36.5% of the patients displayed positive DCC assay but negative BNB assay values, suggesting the presence of non-functional receptors in those biopsies. Less than 7% of the patients were ER positive by BNB and ER negative by DCC.

If the proportion of DCC assay-positive patients with nonfunctional receptors is less than our assumed proportion of 50%, then the cutoff may be less than our speculated value of 1076 fmol/mg DNA. This would be the case if some patients fail to respond to hormonal therapy for reasons other than having nonfunctional receptors. Based on animal model systems for nuclear receptors needed for gene activation (Spelsberg et al. 1987; Mulvihill and Palmiter 1980; Palmiter et al. 1981), a cutoff of 1000 molecules of nuclear-bound ER per cell was speculated for the BNB assay. Using a putative cutoff of 277 fmol/mg DNA (which is equivalent to approximately 1000 molecules per cell nucleus), 71% of the patients correspond for positivity and negativity (Table 2). Even at this lower cutoff, the BNB assay identifies nonfunctional receptors in 20% of the patients which are ER positive by the DCC assay.

Correlation of the response to hormonal therapy in these patients with the BNB assay is in progress. We hope then to be able to establish the predictive capability of the BNB assay in breast carcinoma.

Table 2. Comparison of BNB and DCC assay values in breast cancer at a lower cutoff

BNB Assay %Cutoff (fmol ER/ mg DNA)	Assay result[a]		n	% of total patients	% of DCC assay positive patients
	BNB	DCC[b]			
	−	+	20	14.6	20.2
277	+	+	79	57.7	79.8
	−	−	19	13.9	
	+	−	19	13.9	

The speculated BNB assay cutoff used (277 fmol ER/mg DNA) corresponds to approximately 1000 molecules nuclear-bound ER per cell nucleus.

[a] The signs + or − denote assay values above or below the cutoff for specific binding, respectively.

[b] The DCC assay cutoff used is 10 fmol ER per milligram protein.

Correlation of the BNB and DCC assays in endometrial carinoma. In this study, 62 endometrial cancer patients were evaluated for total cellular PR using the DCC assay and for nuclear binding using the BNB assay. This group of patients were not separated by stage or grade, although most of the patients were of stage 1 or 2 when surgically treated and assayed for steroid receptor binding. The BNB assay values ranged from 0 to 54 000 molecules PR per cell and had a median of 4805 molecules per cell.

The BNB and DCC assay values were then compared. Only low correlation was observed for the separate points (correlation coefficient of 0.30). PR positivity or negativity was then compared between the two assays. A cutoff of 50 fmol PR per milligram cytosol protein was used for PR positivity with the DCC assay. Again, a cutoff of 1000 molecules of nuclear-bound PR per cell was used for the BNB assay. Using these cutoff values, the correlations between the BNB and DCC assays were determined as summarized in Table 3. Using a cutoff of 1000 molecules per nucleus, both assays correlated for PR positivity or negativity in 63% of the

Table 3. Comparison of BNB and DCC assay values in endometrial cancer

BNB Assay Cutoff (molecules/ nucleus)	Assay result[a]		n	% of total patients	% of DCC assay positive patients
	BNB	DCC[b]			
	−	+	11	17.7	24.4
	+	−	34	54.8	75.6
1000	−	−	5	8.1	
	+	−	12	19.4	

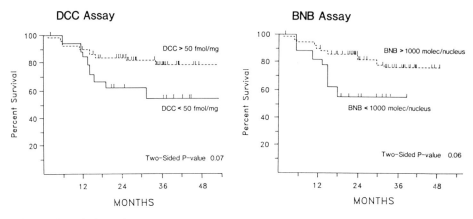

Fig. 5. Correlation of survival in endometrial cancer with the BNB and DCC assays. Clinical disease status was monitored in 62 endometrial cancer patients following surgical treatment and receptor assays. Survival was determined for the patients above and below the assay cutoffs and is shown as Kalpan-Mier plot estimates. Vertical dashes indicate censored cases. *Left*, survival estimates compared with the DCC assay cutoff of 50 fmol PR per milligram cytosol protein ($p = .07$); *right*, survival estimates using the BNB assay cutoff 1000 molecules nuclear-bound PR per cell nucleus ($p = .06$)

patients. Nonfunctional receptors were identified in 24% of the patients with PR-positive DCC assay. Of course, the application of higher BNB assay cutoff values would predict more nonfunctional receptors.

Clinical Correlations in Endometrial Carcinoma. Follow-up data on this set of endometrial patients revealed that patient survival curves, as estimated by the Kaplan-Mier method (Kaplan and Mier 1958), correlated with moderate significance with the BNB assay using a cutoff of 1000 molecules per cell nucleus (two-tailed log-rank significance test (Mantel N 1966), $p = 0.07$; Fig. 5, right). However, the correlation was no better than that with the DCC assay for total cellular PR (two-tailed significance test, $p = 0.06$; Fig. 5, left). Similar analysis of nuclear ER binding and patient survival with the group of breast cancer patients over 55 years old is in progress.

As very few of this group of endometrial carinoma patients were given hormonal therapy, we hope that future studies will reveal whether the BNB assay is predictive of response to steroid therapy in endometrial cancer.

Summary

A nuclear binding assay was developed for the purpose of having available a more predictive assay for hormone responsiveness in human cancers. The BNB assay identified specific and saturable steroid nuclear binding in human target tissues and human carcinomas. When the BNB assay was applied to a large set of breast and endometrial carcinomas, we speculate that nonfunctional receptors were detected in 20%–50% of the patients who were receptor-positive by the DCC assay. Lastly, as responsiveness to hormonal therapy in these cancer patients becomes known, the predictive value of the BNB assay can be established.

References

Burton K (1956) Biochem J 62: 315

Colvard DS, Jankus WR, Berg NJ, Graham ML, Jiang N-S, Ingle JN, Spelsberg TC (1988) Clin Chem 34: 363

Edwards DP, Chamness GC, McGuire WL (1979) Biochem Biophys Acta 560: 457

Ehrlich CE, Young PCM, Stehman FB et al (1988) Am J Obstet Gynecol 158: 796

Gehring U, Tomkins GM (1974) Cell 3: 301

Grumbach MM, Conte FA (1985) Disorders of sexual differentiation. In: Wilson JD, Foster DW (eds) Williams textbook of endocrinology. Saunders, Philadelphia, p 376

Ingle JN (1984) Cancer 53: 766

Ingle JN, Krook JE, Green SJ et al. (1986) J Clin Oncol 4: 178

Kaplan EL, Mier P (1958) J Am Stat Assoc 53: 457

Kohorn EI (1976) Gynecol Oncol 4: 398

Leake RE, Laing L, Calman KC, Macbeth FR, Crawford D, Smith DC (1981) Br J Cancer 43: 59

MacFarlane JK, Fleiszer D, Fazekas AG (1980) Cancer 45: 2998

McGuire WL (1980) An update on estrogen and progesterone receptors in prognosis of primary and advanced breast cancer. In: Jacobelli S (ed) Hormones and Cancer. Raven, New York, pp 337–43

McGuire WL, Carbone PP, Sears ME, Escher GC (1975) Estrogen receptors in human breast cancer: an overview. In: McGuire WL, Carbone PP, Vollmer EP (eds) Estrogen receptor in human breast cancer. Raven, New York, pp 1–7

Momtel N (1966) Cancer Chemother Rep 50: 163

Mulvihill ER, Palmiter RD (1980) J Biol Chem 255: 2085

Palmiter RD, Mulvihill ER, Shepard JH, McKnight GS (1981) J Biol Chem 256: 7910

Piver MS, Barlow JJ, Lurain JR et al. (1980) Cancer 45: 268

Podratz KC, O'Brien PC, Malkasian GD et al. (1985) Obstet Gynecol 66: 106

Spielsberg TC, Graham ML, Berg NJ, Riehl E, Coulam CB, Ingle JN (1987) Endocrinology 121: 631

Thibodeau SN, Freeman L, Jiang N-S (1981) Clin Chem 27: 687

Wait RB (1973) Obstet Gynecol 41: 129

Hormonal Therapy in Endometrial Carcinoma

K.C. Podratz

Department of Obstetrics and Gynecology, Mayo Clinic and Mayo Foundation, Rochester, MN 55905, USA

Introduction

Hormonal therapy began to be used for endometrial carcinoma after Kelley and Baker (1961) reported that endometrial cancer responded to progestational therapy. Multiple empirical trials of progestational agents in the treatment of this disease were reported during the next two decades. Various response rates were recorded, most between 30% and 50% (Bonte et al. 1978; Geisler 1973; Malkasian et al. 1971; Piver et al. 1980; Rozier and Underwood 1974; Smith et al. 1966; Wait 1973). At least part of the variability in these rates undoubtedly reflected differences in how stringently tumor response was defined. Although complete resolution of systemic disease (for example, multiple pulmonary metastatic lesions) for extended periods can occur with hormonal therapy, such responses unfortunately are exceptions to the norm.

During this same period (1960–1980), estrogen and progesterone receptors were identified and characterized, so that our understanding of the molecular mechanism of hormonal action was enhanced. Consequently, attempts to correlate tumor response to hormonal therapy with receptor levels soon were advocated, and success varied. This review highlights the treatment of endometrial cancer with hormonal agents and emphasizes the therapeutic results observed in patients with advanced primary or recurrent endometrial cancer seen at the Mayo Clinic.

Interdependence of Receptors, Pathologic Changes, and Clinical Responses

Correlation of Receptors and Survival

Recent reports correlating survival rates with levels of progesterone receptors in tumor specimens obtained from patients with untreated endometrial carcinoma suggested that progesterone receptor status could be used as a prognostic determinant. Creasman et al. (1985) observed that disease-free survival in patients with

Recent Results in Cancer Research. Vol. 118
© Springer-Verlag Berlin·Heidelberg 1990

endometrial cancer was significantly influenced by the tumor estrogen or progesterone receptors. Similarly, assessing the progesterone-protein interaction in the cytosol of 86 patients with primary endometrial carcinoma, Liao et al. (1986) found that 3-year survival was 80% in patients with tumor-associated progesterone receptor levels above 10 fmol/mg of cytosol protein. In contrast, 5-year survival in patients with negligible tumor receptor levels was 25%. Ehrlich et al. (1988) demonstrated similar results in a larger group of patients; the median survival rate was significantly better in patients with progesterone receptor-positive tumors than in those with progesterone receptor-poor tumors. However, although patients with clinical stage I or II disease and progesterone receptor-rich tumors likewise had a significantly better prognosis, no statistically significant differences were detectable in a similar subset of patients with surgical stage I or II tumors. Recent experience at the Mayo Clinic showed that patients with surgical stage I disease have a significant survival advantage when they have increased levels (> 1000 molecules per nucleus) of nuclear binding of progesterone in endometrial cancer specimens (D. S. Colvard, K. C. Podratz and T. C. Spelsburg; unpublished data). Hence, although a reasonable correlation exists between progesterone receptor levels and survival – suggesting applicability as a prognostic factor – the independence of progesterone receptors from other traditional prognostic factors remains to be proved.

Correlation of Receptors and Tissue Differentiation

Because of the molecular organization required for appropriate steroid-protein interaction to alter cellular control and result in the anticipated hormonal response, changes in the synchronized molecular events might be expected to occur as the degree of tissue differentiation decreases. In summarizing several reports addressing estrogen and progesterone receptor levels according to histologic grade, Kauppila and Friberg (1981) noted that as the grade of endometrial carcinoma increased, the amount of detectable estrogen and progesterone receptors decreased. Most noticeable was the precipitous decrease in measurable progesterone receptors between grade 2 and grade 3 lesions. More recently, Ehrlich et al. (1988) likewise reported that the measurable tumor-associated progesterone receptors were inversely proportional to grade, with again the most marked variance noted between International Federation of Obstetricians and Gynecologists (FIGO) grade 2 and grade 3 lesions. In contrast, no significant correlation existed between estrogen receptors and tissue differentiation. In an assessment of the correlation of nuclear binding of progesterone with tissue histologic findings in 65 patients evaluated at the Mayo Clinic, significant nuclear binding was demonstrable in greater than 85% of grade 1 and grade 2 lesions and in about half of poorly differentiated tumors (D. S Colvard, K. C. Podratz, and T. C. Spelsburg, unpublished data). Hence, evidence continues to accumulate supporting the inverse relationship of tumor-associated progesterone receptors and histologic differentiation.

Correlation of Receptors and Clinical Responses to Hormonal Therapy

Because of the molecular mechanism of hormonal action and the known responsiveness of certain endometrial cancers to hormonal therapy, several investigators attempted to correlate the presence of progesterone receptors in endometrial cancer and the response of these tumors to progestational therapy. In the recent summary by Ehrlich et al. (1988) of seven published series reporting the relationship of tumor progesterone receptors and subsequent responses to hormonal therapy, 34% of the 152 patients had either a partial or a complete response to progestin administration (Benraad et al. 1980; Creasman et al. 1980; Kauppila et al. 1982; Martin et al. 1979; Pollow et al. 1983; Quinn et al. 1985). Of the 52 patients responding to progestational therapy, 79% were designated as harbouring progesterone receptor-rich tumors. The overall response rate was 72% in patients with progesterone receptor-rich tumors but only 12% in patients with progesterone receptor-poor lesions. Although the total number of reported cases of endometrial carcinoma treated with progestational agents having identified progesterone receptor levels is small relative to the frequency with which this therapy is used, the preliminary results, as shown above, are most encouraging.

General Clinical Observations on Hormonal Therapy in Endometrial Cancer

The overall response rate and, more specifically, the long-term survival rate in patients with advanced primary or recurrent endometrial carcinoma treated with progestins have been disappointing at our institution. For patients with stages IA and IB endometrial carcinoma, the 5-year survival rate for the decade before 1962 was not statistically significantly different from that for the decade of 1963 through 1972, when progestational agents were readily available and used for the treatment of advanced primary and recurrent disease (Malkasian et al. 1977, 1980). Furthermore, the 10-year survival rates for clinical stage I grade 3 lesions for the decade before 1962 and the decade after 1963 were 49% and 53%, respectively (not significant). The overall observed response rate for patients subjected to hormonal therapy at our institution has traditionally been substantially below the usually reported response rates of 30%–50%. At least in part, interinstitutional variability undoubtedly reflects the definition of response based on both objective criteria and duration. Often, the assessment of response is influenced by the enthusiasm of the patient and physician because of the notable subjective improvement that frequently accompanies the initiation of hormonal therapy. The disappointing clinical impressions in the treatment of cancer in this normally hormonally responsive organ led to a detailed retrospective assessment of the experience at the Mayo Clinic with progestins and antiestrogens in the treatment of endometrial cancer.

Progestational Therapy

The treatment of advanced primary and recurrent endometrial cancer with multiple progestins at the Mayo Clinic from 1968 through 1980 was assessed by the following stringent response criteria:

1. Complete regression: complete resolution of all lesions for at least 3 months.
2. Partial regression: 50% decrease in the product of lesion diameters lasting at least 3 months without evidence of new lesions during this interval.
3. Progression: 25% increase in the product of the diameters or the appearance of a new lesion.
4. Stabilization: lesions neither regressing nor progressing for at least 3 months.

Objective responses were observed in 16 (11.2%) of 143 patients having clinically measurable disease who were treated for at least 2 months (Podratz et al. 1985). Although four progestational agents were used—17-hydroxyprogesterone caproate, 6-methyl-17-hydroxyprogesterone acetate, 6-methyl-17-acetoxydehydro-progesterone, and 6,17-dimethyl-dehydroprogesterone—there were no statistically significant differences among the various progestins in either objective response or overall 5-year survival.

Objective responses were assessed according to Broders' histologic grade. An inverse relationship was observed as the degree of tissue dedifferentiation increased. Whereas complete or partial responses were detected in 4 of 10 patients (40%) with Broders' grade 1 lesions, only 11 of 71 patients (15%) with grade 2 and 1 of 73 (< 2%) with grade 3 or 4 lesions had objective responses. The sole response in the latter group was recorded as complete for only a minimal 3 months' duration.

Because of the marked disparity of the above-reported response rate of 11.2% and the frequently cited response rates of 30%–50%, the likelihood of excessively rigid response criteria was assessed. For the 16 patients who had partial or complete regression, the 1- and 3-year survival rates were acceptable (88% and 62%, respectively), with a median survival of 57 months. For the 60 patients categorized as stable, a precipitous decline in survival occurred between 1 and 3 years, with a median survival of 13 months. In the 75 patients experiencing progression, an exceedingly rapid decline took place during the first 12 months, with a median survival of only 5 months. Thus, the response criteria noted above resulted in appropriate stratification and furthermore appeared to possess prognostic value when the specific response status was identified after hormonal therapy began.

Despite general acceptance of standard therapy for advanced primary or recurrent endometrial carcinoma for over two decades, the effectiveness of progestational therapy for this disease continues to be recorded predominantly as objective response rather than as overall or progression-free survival rates. In the 155 Mayo patients receiving progestational therapy for more than 2 months, the 1-, 2-, and 5-year survival rates were 40%, 19%, and 8%, respectively (Fig. 1). Furthermore, patients with Broders' grade 3 or 4 tumors had a rapid 12-month attrition rate; no patient with a Broders' grade 4 lesion survived for 24 months, and none with a grade 3 lesion lived for 5 years (Fig. 2). Patients with well- or moderately well-differentiated tumors had a less precipitous attrition rate; nevertheless, the 5-year survival rates associated with grades 1 and 2 lesions were 20% and 19%, respectively. Although occasional striking long-term regressions occurred in patients with well- or moderately well-differentiated tumors, the overall

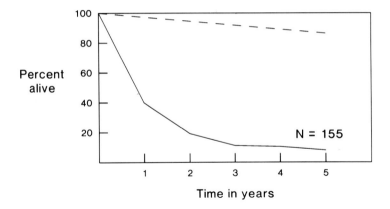

Fig 1. Overall survival after beginning of progestin therapy (*solid line*) and expected survival for age-matched controls (*broken line*). (From Podratz et al. [1985] By permission of the American College of Obstetricians and Gynecologists)

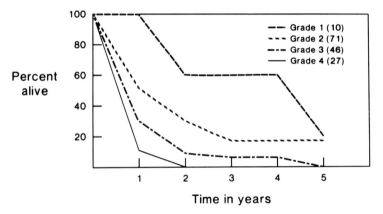

Fig 2. Overall survival by Broders' histologic grade after beginning of progestin therapy. Numbers of patients are shown within parentheses. Grade was unknown in one patient. (From Podratz et al. [1985] By permission of the American College of Obstetricians and Gynecologists)

survival rate of 8% at 5 years, the rapid attrition, and the lack of detectable salvage associated with Broders' early grades 3 and 4 lesions suggest that, at best, progestational agents have a marginal impact on the natural history of this disease.

Assessing survival after hormonal therapy according to tumor volume revealed median survival times of 25, 11, and 5 months, respectively, for patients with residual tumor burdens of under or equal to 10, 11–100, and over 100 cm^3. These observations require cautious interpretation but potentially suggest value in cytoreductive surgery for endometrial cancer before hormonal treatment.

Inasmuch as appreciable levels of progesterone receptors were detected in the vast majority of well- and moderately well-differentiated primary tumors and in a significant number of poorly differentiated primary tumors (D. S. Colvard, K. C. Podratz and T. C. Spelsburg, unpublished data; Ehrlich et al. 1988; Liao et al. 1986), the lack of effective control of advanced primary or recurrent endometrial cancer by progestational therapy shown by the above overall and histologic grade-associated 5-year survival rates appeared to be inconsistent. Plausible explanations include a biased albeit natural selection process in which predominantly patients with progesterone receptor-poor tumors are treated with progestins. Patients with the progesterone receptor-poor primary lesions, which had an unfavourable prognosis, presumably represent most of the patient population that subsequently required treatment for either advanced primary or recurrent disease. With such skewed selection, most of such patients treated with progestational agents would not be expected to have a response. Other suppositions for why tumors non-responsive to hormonal therapy could have evaluable progesterone receptor levels are tissue and tissue versus metastasis heterogeneity, nonfunctional but measurable receptors, altered nuclear acceptors, enhanced hormonal metabolism, and hormonally independent cellular control mechanisms.

Antiestrogen Therapy

Initial reports assessing the efficacy of tamoxifen in the treatment of endometrial cancer suggest objective response rates (33%) similar to those observed with progestins (Swenerton et al. 1984). Likewise, the responses were of minimal medial duration (7 months) and were related to tissue differentiation.

Between 1980 and 1983, a multi-institutional study based at the Mayo Clinic assessed the effectiveness of tamoxifen therapy for 46 patients with advanced endometrial carcinoma. The population consisted of 22 patients with demonstrated refractoriness to progestational therapy and 24 patients not previously exposed to hormonal therapy. After treatment with 10 mg of tamoxifen twice daily, the objective response rate for all patients was 11%; for those without previous progestin therapy, 21%; and for those who had progression with progestational

Table 1. Objective response status to tamoxifen therapy according to prior progestational therapy ($n = 46$)

Response status	Number of patients	
	Refractory to progestin therapy	Did not have progestin therapy
Objective response	0	5
Stabilization (≥ 2 months)	6	11
Progression	16	8
Total	22	24

therapy, 0% (Edmonson et al. 1986; Table 1). Of the objective responses, four were observed in 32 patients harboring well- or moderately well-differentiated tumors, whereas only one was associated among 14 patients with poorly differentiated tumors. Regardless of the response rate, the median progression-free survival interval was only 57 days, and the median overall survival was only 120 days, with 74% of the patient population dead of disease at 1 year. The observations suggest that tamoxifen therapy was not effective in progestin-refractory patients, and further assessment of its potential value as primary adjuvant or salvage therapy for recurrent disease requires additional prospective evaluation.

Combination Antiestrogen-Progestin Therapy

Although the molecular mechanisms controlling the cellular levels of estrogen and progesterone receptors continue to be investigated, the administration of progestational agents is known to cause diminution of the cellular concentration of the progesterone receptor proteins. Therefore, clinicians have expressed concern that the continuous administration of progestins depletes the tumor tissue of these macromolecules and thereby potentially renders the tumor refractory to progestational therapy. In contrast, although antiestrogens cause a decrease in cellular estrogen receptor concentration, they enhance the de novo synthesis of the progesterone-binding proteins. The latter observation led Mortel et al. (1981) to recommend treatment with antiestrogens before or intermittently with administration of the progestational agents.

In 25 patients with endometrial adenocarcinoma, Carlson et al. (1984) evaluated the progesterone receptor concentrations before and immediately after 5 consecutive days of tamoxifen (10 mg twice daily) administration. Before exposure to antiestrogen, 13 of 25 tumors (52%) had detectable levels of progesterone receptors. After tamoxifen pretreatment, there was a significant increase to 21 tumors (84%) having detectable receptor levels. The influence of histologic dedifferentiation again was apparent, because 17 of 17 FIGO grades 1 and 2 lesions were progesterone receptor-rich after tamoxifen therapy in contrast to only 4 of 8 FIGO grade 3 tumors having detectable progesterone receptors. Administering 10 mg of tamoxifen twice daily and 250 mg of medroxyprogesterone acetate intramuscularly weekly, Carlson et al. (1984) observed four responses of 7, 7, 10, and 24 months' duration among 12 patients. Recognizing the limitations of the small number of patients, the authors indicated that the 33% response rate observed with this regimen of combination hormonal therapy approximates the response rates generally reported for progestins alone.

Using an alternative treatment regimen, Bonte et al. (1986) reported an overall response rate of 62% in patients treated in a sequential fashion with tamoxifen (20 mg/day) pretreatment for 1 week followed by medroxyprogesterone acetate (Provera; 150 mg daily) during the following 3-week interval. The 62% response rate exceeded response rates of 51% and 36% reported for medroxyprogesterone acetate and tamoxifen, respectively, given as single agents. Whether these differences constitute a significant increase in tumor response was not addressed by the authors. In contrast, Kline et al. (1987) reported that among 20 patients with recurrent or metastatic poorly differentiated endometrial cancer, only one had a response after sequential treatment with tamoxifen (10 mg twice daily) on days 1–5 and medroxyprogesterone acetate (50 mg twice daily) on days 6–25. On the basis of the presence or absence of both estrogen and progesterone receptors in tumor tissue, Bonte et al. (1986) suggested that combination hormonal therapy be modulated for advanced and recurrent endometrial carcinoma. The authors recommended simultaneous administration of tamoxifen and medroxyprogesterone acetate for "highly hormone-dependent tumors (ER +, PR +)" and sequential tamoxifen and medroxyprogesterone acetate administration for both "strictly hormone-dependent tumors (ER +, PR −) and potentially hormone-dependent tumors (ER −, PR −)."

On the basis of preliminary laboratory (Zaino et al. 1985) and clinical observations, theoretical merit exists for clinical use of simultaneous or sequential antiestrogen-progestin combination hormonal therapy. However, the clinical investigations to date have been predominantly phase II trials, with limited evidence to suggest that combination therapy is superior to single-agent treatment. Again, prospective randomized trials stratified for various risk factors are necessary. Not only rigid response criteria but also progression-free overall survival analyses must be used to compare single-agent therapy with combination therapy.

Summary

Although hormonal agents have been used to treat endometrial cancer for nearly 30 years, response rates have remained essentially unchanged. Furthermore, objective response rates vary considerably from institution to institution, presumably because of differences in accepted response criteria and patient selection. The latter is particularly influenced by the distribution within the treated population of well-differentiated and poorly differentiated tumor histologic types. Nevertheless, the rapid attrition after hormonal therapy begins and the limited long-term salvage in nonselected patients with advanced primary or recurrent disease suggest primary nonresponsiveness or acquired tumor refractoriness to hormonal therapy. The determination of tumor progesterone receptor levels has made it easier to identify patients with sensitivity to such therapy. Recent investigations have shown favourable response rates (72%) after administration of progestational agents in patients with progesterone receptor-rich tumors. Similarly, responses have been reported with antiestrogens and combination progestin-antiestrogen therapy, recent laboratory observations having suggested potential benefit from sequential administration. Although these clinical and laboratory findings are encouraging, the limited duration of objective responses and the poor long-term survival rates continue to temper enthusiasm for routine hormonal therapy. Properly stratified (according to pathologic, biochemical, and clinical criteria), prospective, randomized, double-blind studies with more definitive end points, such as progression-free survival and overall survival, are mandatory to further evaluate the merits of various therapeutic regimens using gonadal hormones.

References

Benraad TJ, Friberg LG, Koenders AJM, Kullander S (1980) Do estrogen and progesterone receptors (E₂R and PR) in metastasizing endometrial cancers predict the response to gestagen therapy? Acta Obstet Gynecol Scand 59: 155

Bonte J, Decoster JM, Ide P, Billiet G (1978) Hormonoprophylaxis and hormonotherapy in the treatment of endometrial adenocarcinoma by means of medroxyprogesterone acetate. Gynecol Oncol 6: 60

Bonte J, Janssens JP, Ide P (1986) Modalities and results of a combined anti-estrogenic therapy by means of tamoxifen and medroxyprogesterone in gynecologic cancerology. Eur J Gynaecol Oncol 7: 45

Carlson JA Jr, Allegra JC, Day TG Jr, Wittliff JL (1984) Tamoxifen and endometrial carcinoma: alterations in estrogen and progesterone receptors in untreated patients and combination hormonal therapy in advanced neoplasia. Am J Obstet Gynecol 149: 149

Creasman WT, McCarty KS Sr, Barton TK, McCarty KS Jr (1980) Clinical correlates of estrogen- and progesterone-binding proteins in human endometrial adenocarcinoma. Obstet Gynecol 55: 363

Creasman WT, Soper JT, McCarty KS Jr, McCarty KS Sr, Hinshaw W, Clarke-Pearson DL (1985) Influence of cytoplasmic steroid receptor content on prognosis of early stage endometrial carcinoma. Am J Obstet Gynecol 151: 922

Edmonson JH, Krook JE, Hilton JF, Long HJ III, Cullinan SA, Everson LK, Malkasian GD (1986) Ineffectiveness of tamoxifen in advanced endometrial carcinoma after failure. of progestin treatment. Cancer Treat Rep 70: 1019

Ehrlich CE, Young PCM, Stehman FB, Sutton GP, Alford WM (1988) Steroid receptors and clinical outcome in patients with adenocarcinoma of the endometrium. Am J Obstet Gynecol 158: 796

Geisler HE (1973) The use of megestrol acetate in the treatment of advanced malignant lesions of the endometrium. Gynecol Oncol 1: 340

Kauppila A, Friberg L-G (1981) Hormonal and cytotoxic chemotherapy for endometrial carcinoma: steroid receptors in the selection of appropriate therapy. Acta Obstet Gynecol Scand [Suppl] 101: 59

Kauppila A, Kujansuu E, Vihko R (1982) Cytosol estrogen and progestin receptors in endometrial carcinoma of patients treated with surgery, radiotherapy, and progestin: clinical correlates. Cancer 50: 2157

Kelley RM, Baker WH (1961) Progestational agents in the treatment of carcinoma of the endometrium. N Engl J Med 264: 216

Kline RC, Freedman RS, Jones LA, Atkinson EN (1987) Treatment of recurrent or metastatic poorly differentiated adenocarcinoma of the endometrium with tamoxifen and medroxyprogesterone acetate. Cancer Treat Rep 71: 327

Liao BS, Twiggs LB, Leung BS, Yu WCY, Potish RA, Prem KA (1986) Cytoplasmic estrogen and progesterone receptors as prognostic parameters in primary endometrial carcinoma. Obstet Gynecol 67: 463

Malkasian GD Jr, Decker DG, Mussey E, Johnson CE (1971) Progestogen treatment of recurrent endometrial carcinoma. Am J Obstet Gynecol 110: 15

Malkasian GD Jr, McDonald TW, Pratt JH (1977) Carcinoma of the endometrium: Mayo Clinic experience. Mayo Clin Proc 52: 175

Malkasian GD Jr, Annegers JF, Fountain KS (1980) Carcinoma of the endometrium: stage I. Am J Obstet Gynecol 136: 872

Martin PM, Rolland PH, Gammerre M, Serment H, Toga M (1979) Estradiol and progesterone receptors in normal and neoplastic endometrium: correlations between receptors, histopathological examinations and clinical responses under progestin therapy. Int J Cancer 23: 321

Mortel R, Levy C, Wolff J-P, Nicolas J-C, Robel P, Baulieu E-E (1981) Female sex steroid receptors in postmenopausal endometrial carcinoma and biochemical response to an antiestrogen. Cancer Res 41: 1140

Piver MS, Barlow JJ, Lurain JR, Blumenson LE (1980) Medroxyprogesterone acetate (Depo-Provera) vs. hydroxyprogesterone caproate (Delalutin) in women with metastatic endometrial adenocarcinoma. Cancer 45: 268

Podratz KC, O'Brien PC, Malkasian GD Jr, Decker DG, Jefferies JA, Edmonson JH (1985) Effects of progestational agents in treatment of endometrial carcinoma. Obstet Gynecol 66: 106

Pollow K, Manz B, Grill H-J (1983) Estrogen and progesterone receptors in endometrial cancer. In: Jasonni VM, Nenci I, Flamigni C (eds) Steroids and endometrial cancer, vol 25. Raven Press, New York, pp 37–60

Quinn MA, Cauchi M, Fortune D (1985) Endometrial carcinoma: steroid receptors and response to medroxyprogesterone acetate. Gynecol Oncol 21: 314

Rozier JC Jr, Underwood PB Jr (1974) Use of progestational agents in endometrial adenocarcinoma. Obstet Gynecol 44: 60

Smith JP, Rutledge F, Soffar SW (1966) Progestins in the treatment of patients with endometrial adenocarcinoma. Am J Obstet Gynecol 94: 977

Swenerton KD, Chrumka K, Paterson AHG, Jackson GC (1984) Efficacy of tamoxifen in endometrial cancer. Prog Cancer Res Ther 31: 417

Wait RB (1973) Megestrol acetate in the management of advanced endometrial carcinoma. Obstet Gynecol 41: 129

Zaino RJ, Satyaswaroop PG, Mortel R (1985) Hormonal therapy of human endometrial adenocarcinoma in a nude mouse model. Cancer Res 45: 539

Hormone-Secreting Ovarian Tumors

A. Pfleiderer

Abteilung für Frauenheikunde und Geburtshilfe II, Universitäts-Frauenklinik,
Albert-Ludwigs-Universität, Hugstetter Straße 55, 7800 Freiburg i. Brsg., FRG

There are three interesting aspects of hormone secreting ovarian tumors: the clinical features of granulosa cell tumors, the effect of testosterone production in ovarian tumors, and hormonogenesis in epithelial tumors of the ovary.

Clinical Features of Granulosa Cell Tumors

Incidence and Age. The granulosa cell tumor is considered to be the prototype of a hormone secreting tumor. According to the literature (Scully 1979; Schulze-Tollert and Pfleiderer 1986), 1%–2% of all ovarian tumors are thought to be granulosa cell tumors. In the years 1980–1986 in our clinic we found 3.8% granulosa cell tumors among all malignant tumors of the ovary. Between 1966 to 1988, 54 women with granulosa cell tumor came to our hospital. Of these, 31 were primarily operated on by us, 17 were referred to us for further therapy, and 6 came because of recurrence (Table 1). Twelve patients were aged between 20 and 49 years, 42 were postmenopausal, and 14 were over 70 years of age. There were no children among our patients.

Table 1. Granulosa cell tumors and age

Age of patient (years)	n
20–29	1
30–39	3
40–49	3
50–59	10
60–69	17
70–79	14

Six patients, aged 27, 27, 28, 31, 36, 55 years, were treated because of recurrence.

Recent Results in Cancer Research. Vol. 118
© Springer-Verlag Berlin·Heidelberg 1990

Table 2. Prognosis in granulosa cell tumors by stage

Stage	Total number of patients 1968–1988	Number of patients 1966–1983	Survival (n)	Death due to tumor
I	21	16	14	1
II	16	14	8	3
III	7	5	1	3
IV	2	2	0	2
Unknown	2	2	1	0

Staging and Cure. Of the 48 cases treated in our hospital, 21 were of stage I, 16 stage II, and 9 stages III or IV (Table 2). The 5-year survival rate, 24 out of 39 verifiable cases (62%), was substantially more favorable than that reported in ovarian carcinoma (Pfleiderer 1984). This, however, is due to the higher percentage of cases in stages I and II; in terms of the respective stages, prognosis of the granulosa cell tumor is comparable to that of epthelial ovarian carcinoma (Pfleiderer et al. 1976).

Para-aortic Metastases. Unlike typical ovarian carcinomas, granulosa cell tumors seem to have a special tendency to form para-aortic lymph node metastases. Three cases may illustrate this.

Case 1: A 55–year–old patient was operated on in 1977 for endometrial carcinoma. During surgery a granulosa cell tumor limited to one ovary was also found. Eight years later a larger upper abdominal tumor 8.5 cm in diameter appeared which was diagnosed as a metastasis of granulosa cell tumor in a para-aortic lymph node. After operation and postoperative irradiation 3 years later the patient experienced recurrence in supraclavicular nodes.

Case 2: Ten months after operation (abdominal hysterectomy with both adnexes, omentum, and pelvic lymphadenectomy) for granulosa cell tumor of stage Ib in a 31–year–old woman, an inoperable upper abdominal tumor 26 × 15 × 15 cm in size was found starting from para-aortic metastases. Chemotherapy with six cycles of cisplatin, vinblastine, and bleomycin brought about a clinical complete remission. After 2 months, however, the patient died from meningiosis carcinomatosa.

Case 3: H. A. Hirsch (personal information) reported a 67–year–old patient with a unilateral granulosa cell tumor. By careful pelvic and para-aortic lymphadenectomy in only one out of 76 examined lymph nodes (at the renal vein) was a tumor metastasis found.

These experiences show that granulosa cell tumors may be treated very well in young women by a fertility-conserving operation if no metastasis is observed beyond the ovary. Operation, however, must include careful pelvic and para-aortic lymphadenectomy.

Table 3. Evidence of estrogen production in granulosa cell tumors

No	5		
Yes	17	77%	81%
Combined with endometrial cancer	5		
Not evaluable	24		

Production of Estrogen in Granulosa Cell Tumors. The granulosa cell tumor is especially active in estrogen production (Pfleiderer 1984; Schulze-Tollert and Pfleiderer 1986; Scully 1979). In infancy granulosa cell tumors are relatively rare. If they occur, there is pseudopubertas praecox. In the reproductive period of life, anomalies of cycle such as amenorrhea or metrorrhagia are found. Postmenopausal bleedings are typical. Occasionally, a painful swelling of the breast may occur. As a morphological substrate of persistent estrogen production, a glandular-cystic hyperplasia of the endometrium is generally to be found. Ovulation is inhibited. The contralateral ovary is smaller than normal – if it is not affected with tumor, which is seen in only about 5% of cases – and does not show any larger follicles. The cortical area is collagenized as in the polycystic ovary syndrome. After removal of the tumor, there occurs within a few days a withdrawal bleeding. The combination with an adenocarcinoma of the endometrium is well known. According to the analyses of Björkholm and Silfverswärd (1980) on 687 granulosa cell tumors, the frequency of subsequent endometrial carcinomas is increased by a factor 4.4. The latency period is 8.9 years on average.

In 24 of the cases of granulosa cell tumor we observed, we could not determine whether there was estrogen production (Table 3). Five were operated on for adenocarcinoma of the endometrium, and granulosa cell tumor was discovered coincidentally. Of the remaining 22 cases, in five cases it was so clear that there was no sign of bleeding. Thus, we found signs of estrogen production in 77% and 81%, respectively. In no case was there a sign of androgen production.

The Importance of Testosterone Formation in Ovarian Tumors

Sertoli and Leydig cell tumors are considerably rarer than those of granulosa or theca cells. Sertoli and Leydig cell tumors probably develop directly from female cell elements of the ovarian stroma or from granulosa cells by transformation; these tumors are characterized by a virilization which is very dramatic for the patient herself (Scully 1979).

As Breckwoldt et al. (1988) showed, removal of a Leydig cell tumor leads to a strong drop in blood testosterone level. At the same time, the cholesterol level declines, although more slowly. A second important aspect of this process is the influence of testosterone on the lipoprotein profile (Breckwoldt et al. 1988). After removal of a Leydig cell tumor in a 65-year-old women, the blood testosterone level dropped from 3.2 to 1.16 ng/ml. Along with the decline in total cholesterol level the beta fraction of lipoproteins dropped. As is well known, from the relationship between low-density (LDL) and high-density (HDL) lipoproteins an arteriosclerosis risk factor can be determined. This risk factor increased to 2.07 and then decreased to 1.29 with the drop in testosterone (M. Breckwoldt 1988, personal information). In a second patient, 74 years old, Breckwoldt and his group made similar observations: preoperative testosterone was measured at 1.42 ng/ml and postoperative testosterone at 0.11 ng/ml. With the drop in testosterone, the beta fraction and total cholesterol dropped as well and again produced a shift in the LDL/HDL quotient. Here, the risk factor decreased from 2.67 to 1.13.

These observations suggest that testosterone substantially influences LDL and very low density lipoprotein fractions. Moreover, they demonstrate the importance of testosterone in the risk of arteriosclerosis.

Formation of Steroid Hormone in Epithelial Ovarian Tumors

Signs of Hormonal Activity. The symptom of genital bleeding with simple ovarian carcinoma is well known yet is seldom explained. In analyzing the material in our hospital from 1957 to 1974 we found vaginal bleeding in 24.9% of all primary ovarian carcinomas. In 17.9% this was not due to carcinoma itself (Table 4). In 1963 cells were first described in connective tissue of typical adenocarcinoma of the ovary which showed a strong reaction to some dehydrogenases, aminopeptidases, and lipids (Pfleiderer 1963; Woodruff et al. 1963). These cells have been termed enzymatically active stromal cells (EASC).

Histochemical Analysis of EASC. The EASC are characterized by a strong NADP-dependent dehydrogenase reaction including NADPH and NADH cytochrome c reductases (Fig. 1). Of the NAD-dependent dehydrogenases, only lactate dehydrogenase activity (in 90%) and malate dehydrogenase activity (in more than 80%) are found. Alkaline phosphatase also seems to occur regularly. In addition, these cells are not uniform. Cytochrome oxidase, butyrate and glycerol phosphate dehydrogenases, galactosidase, aminopeptidases nonspecific esterases, and various lipids were discovered in only some cases. It is especially remarkable that 3β-ol-steroid dehydrogenase, using dehydroepiandrosterone for substrate, presents a

Table 4. Bleeding in epithelial ovarian carcinoma

	n	%
Total no. of patients with ovarian carcinoma	402	
Patients presenting with vaginal bleeding	100	24.9
From cancer of endometrium	16	4.0
From penetration of vagina	12	3.0
Unexplained premenopausal bleeding	22	5.5
Unexplained postmenopausal bleeding	50	12.4

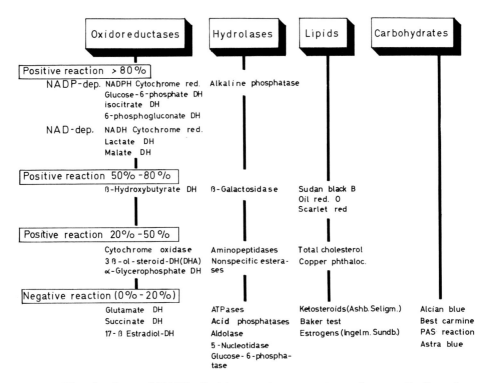

Fig. 1. Histochemistry of EASC. *Positive reaction*, percentage of enzymatically active stromal cells stained. (From Pfleiderer and Teufel 1976)

slight reaction in only about one-third of cases. Glutamate, succinate, and 17β-estradiol dehydrogenases, most of the specific phosphatases, and all carbohydrate reactions are negative in these cells (Pfleiderer and Teufel 1968, 1976). The EASC, which morphologically appear as luteinized theca cells, theca cells, or simple stroma cells, have only a few enzymatic reactions in common and are different in regard to lipids and all other enzymes. Probably, as in the development and regression of follicle and corpus luteum, enzymatically active stromal cells are luteinized and then fall into regression. Possibly the enzymatically active fibrocytes are the first step of theca-like cells which are then luteinized and finally filled with cholestrol (Teufel 1969). Enzyme patterns of the enzymatically active stromal cells and the theca cells are equivalent (Pfleiderer and Teufel 1976).

Incidence of EASC. EASC occur very seldom in young women (Fig. 2). In those below the age of 40 we have noticed such cells only once: this was a case of theca cell tumor in a 16 – year – old girl with hirsutism. On the other hand, EASC occur in a very high percentage of patients after menopause, which suggests extraovarian factors and perhaps the influence of hypophyseal gonadotropins. These cells are found in granulosa and theca cell tumors, but also in multilocular cystomas and carcinomas. They occur almost as a rule in mucinous cystomas and mucinous

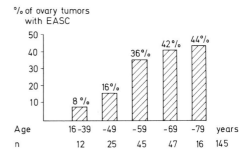

Fig. 2. Occurence of EASC and age.
(From Pfleiderer and Teufel 1976)

Table 5. Type of ovarian tumor and occurrence of EASC. (From Pfleiderer and Teufel 1976)

	n	% containing EASC
Epthelial tumours	113	30
Serous	49	14
Mucinous	21	72
Endometrioid	26	38
Unclassified	17	12
Stromal tumors		
Granulosa cell	9	48
Theca cell	4	100
Fibroma	6	0
Miscellaneous		
Dermoid	1	0
Brenner	1	0
Metastatic carcinoma	9	33

Table 6. EASC and postmenopausal bleeding. (From Pfleiderer and Teufel 1976)

	Ovarian tumors without EASC	Tumors containing EASC
Postmenopausal bleeding ($n = 15$)	6% (4/64)	42% (11/26)
Glandular cystic endometrium ($n = 3$)	0 (0/14)	38% (3/8)
Carcinoma of endometrium ($n = 10$)[a]	4% (4/97)	12% (6/48)

Included are women at least 2 years after menopause and without granulosa or theca cell tumors.
[a] Includes cases with granulosa cell tumors.

Table 7. Proportion of EASC in tumor volume[a] and postmenopausal bleeding. (From Pfleiderer et al. 1973)

	n	EASC % of tumor volume
No bleeding	12	1.6%
Postmenopausal bleeding	5	2.4%
Endometrial carcinoma	5	0.4%

[a] Planimetric measurement.

carcinomas as well as in one-third of all endometrioid and alveolar adenocarcinomas of the ovary (Table 5).

EASC are of major importance in menopausal bleeding (Table 6). In only 6% of 64 women with ovarian tumors without EASC were postmenopausal bleedings observed. On the other hand, postmenopausal bleedings occured in 42% of cases in which enzymatically active stromal cells were present in the ovary. A still clearer correlation was seen in comparison with cystic-glandular hyperplasia of the endometrium. Even in cases of simultaneous carcinoma of the endometrium we more frequently find enzymatically active stromal cells in ovarian tumors (Table 6).

In postmenopausal patients with typical ovarian cancers and EASC in the stroma of these tumors, there is a direct relationship between the proportion of EASC within the tumor and the occurrence of postmenopausal bleeding (Table 7). The higher the proportion of EASC in tissue, the more frequently bleedings occur. The proportion of EASC in ovarian tumor tissue with simultaneous endometrial carcinoma is noticeably low (Pfleiderer et al. 1973).

References

Björkholm E, Silferswärd C (1980) Granulosa- and theca-cell tumors. Incidence and occurrence of second primary tumors. Acta Radiol 19: 161–167

Breckwoldt M, Neulen J, Wieacker P, Geyer H, Wieland H (1988) Wirkung von Sexualsteroiden auf das Lipoproteinprofil. Dtsch. Med Wochenschr 113: 218–220

Pfleiderer A (1963) Histochemische Untersuchungen and Ovarialkarzinomen. Paper presented at the 129th meeting of the Mittelrheinische Gesellschaft für Geburtshilfe und Gynäkologie, Mainz, May 18–19

Pfleiderer A (1984) Das Ovarialkarzinom. In: Döderlein G, Wulf KH (eds) Klinik der Frauenheilkunde und Geburtshilfe, vol VIII. Urban and Schwarzenberg, Munich, pp 714/1–714/174

Pfleiderer A, Teufel G (1968) Incidence and histochemical investigation of enzymatically active cells in stroma of ovarian tumors. Am J Obstet Gynecol 102: 997–1003

Pfleiderer A, Teufel G (1976) Hormone production in ovarian carcinomas. Histochemical approach in stroma reaction. Oesterr Z Onkol 3: 83–90

Pfleiderer A, Karzel M, Morlok KF, Schaal R (1973) Neue Methoden zur Beurteilung der Wirkung von Zytostatika bei Ovarialkarzinomen. II. Planimetrische Vermessung enzymhistochemisch gefärbter Gewebsschnitte. In: König PA, Pfleiderer A, (eds) Neue Aspekte in Diagnose und Therapie des Genitalkarzinoms der Frau. Enke, Stuttgart, pp 75–81

Pfleiderer A, Wipprecht KG, Ritzmann H, Tan TH (1976) Die Potenz der malignen Entartung der Ovarialtumoren. Fortschr Med 94: 81–88

Schulze-Tollert J, Pfleiderer A (1986) Stromatumoren. In: Pfleiderer A (ed) Maligne Tumoren der Ovarian. Enke, Stuttgart, pp 99–110

Scully RE (1979) Tumors of the ovary and maldeveloped gonads. In: Atlas of tumor pathology. Armed Forces Institute of Pathology, Washington (Second series, fascicle 16)

Teufel G (1968) Vorkommen und Bedeutung von Thekaelementen in Ovarialtumoren. Histochemische Untersuchungen. Medical dissertation, University of Tübingen

Woodruff JD, Williams TI, Goldberg B (1963) Hormone activity of the common ovarian neoplasm. Am J Obstet Gynecol 87: 679–698

Ovarian Hormones and Carcinoma of the Uterine Cervix

D.S. Mosny[1] and H.G. Bender[2]

[1] Frauenklinik, Medizinische Einrichtungen der Universität Düsseldorf, Moorenstraße 5,
  4000 Düsseldorf, FRG
[2] Universitäts-Frauenklinik, Theodor-Stern-Kai 7, 6000 Frankfurt/Main 70, FRG

Introduction

The biochemical analysis of steroid receptors is a routine technique in breast cancer, endometrial cancer, and ovarian cancer because the receptor concentration has prognostic value and is also a decisive factor in the choice of further therapy.

Various authors have identified estrogen (ER) and progesterone receptor (PR) protein in squamous cancer of the cervix uteri by means of biochemistry. Nevertheless, antihormonal treatment of cervical cancer usually shows no effect (Hoffmann and Siiteri 1980; Potish et al. 1986). Indeed, primary surgical treatment of premenopausal women is intended to achieve a normal ovarian function (Husseinzadeh et al. 1984). After therapeutically induced or normal arrest of ovarian function in patients with cervical cancer, sexual steroid hormones are substituted without negative side effects on survival time. Several larger studies have shown that the steroid hormone receptor content in cervical carcinoma has no prognostic value, and that there is no significant difference in survival time between receptor-positive and receptor-negative patients (Martin et al. 1986).

These clinical experiences are scarcely reconcilable with the thought that the matrix tissue of the cervical neoplasia – the squamous epithelium of the cervix or vagina – shows clear signs of hormone dependence (Lohe and Baltzer 1984). For example, menstrual cycle diagnosis is based on typical cycle-dependent morphological changes. Typical atrophic changes of the squamous epithelium occur after extinction of ovary function. The atrophic changes of the epithelium are reversible by local or systemic treatment with ovarian hormones.

In the present preliminary study 45 cases of normal or neoplastic cervical tissue were studied immunohistochemically by ER and PR staining to analyze the discrepancy between the hormone dependence of healthy squamous epithelium of the uterine cervix and the independence of cervical neoplasia. (Bolla et al. 1982; Cao et al. 1983; Fenton et al. 1986; Garau et al. 1986; Hunter et al. 1987; Martin et al. 1986; Yajima et al. 1985).

Recent Results in Cancer Research. Vol. 118
© Springer-Verlag Berlin·Heidelberg 1990

Methods

To evaluate immunohistochemical staining in relation to the menstrual cycle 25 specimens were obtained at hysterectomy from patients in Düsseldorf University Hospital. The histology was evaluated to exclude any neoplastic lesion of the squamous epithelium. Eight specimens were obtained at biopsy from suspicious cervical lesions detected by colposcopy. Ten tumor specimens were obtained during Wertheim-Meigs operations or exenterations. All representative samples of the ectocervix uteri were immediately removed from surgical specimens and were deep-frozen at −80°C until further use.

The immunohistochemical staining was performed on frozen sections of 5 μm. The ER protein was detected using the ER immunocytochemical analysis kit (Abbott, Wiesboden, FRG) with primary antibody H 222. The PR protein was detected by means of the monoclonal antibody PR 1808 (Dianova, Hamburg, FRG) at a dilution of 1:300 and overnight incubation at 4°C. Slides were then treated with the Vectastain ABC peroxidase method (Vector Laboratories, Burlingame, California, USA).

The results were analyzed according to a score system, using the parameters of staining intensity (no staining $= 0$, slight $= +$, medium $= + +$, severe $= + + +$) and staining distribution (basal cells, parabasal cells, intermediate cells, superficial cells, stroma cells).

Results

The ER protein concentration depends upon the menstrual cycle. In the early proliferative phase all layers are negative. In the later proliferative phase the basal and parabasal layers of the healthy ectocervix begin to show an immunohistochemical staining reaction. At the end of the proliferative phase and throughout the secretive phase positive cell nuclei can be found in all layers. A weak reaction to ER staining is found only in mild dysplastic lesions of the uterine cervix; severe dysplastic forms and carcinomas are all ER negative. In comparison with the squamous epithelium, the ER concentration of the stroma is more pronounced, but no menstrual cycle dependent changes can be detected. An ER-positive stromal reaction is found in some of the carcinoma cases. In squamous cell tissue no positive PR reaction can be found. In most cases, adjacent stroma and cervical glands show highly positive PR staining, although there are no changes related to the menstrual cycle.

Discussion

The squamous epithelium of the uterine cervix is under the control of steroid hormones, as seen in Papanicolaou smears of the vagina and uterine cervix of mature women (Drill 1976; Fujimoto et al. 1986; Hunter et al. 1987; Soost 1980). Various investigators have identified cytoplasmic ER and PR in neoplastic cervical specimens (Hunter et al. 1987; Potish et al. 1986; Sandborn et al. 1975; Yajima et al. 1985). However, in most reports no precise distinction is made between epithelia and stroma. In some cases the possibility cannot be excluded that a mixture of epithelium and stroma was used for the biochemical investigation of receptor content. Only Bloch 1979 mentions the difficulty of separating the epithelium for the biochemical measurement of ER protein by the dextran-coated charcoal method (DCC). About 35% of his specimens were discarded because insufficient tissue remained after separation of epithelium and stroma.

The biochemical analysis of receptor concentration in normal squamous epithelia of the internal female genitalia produces varying results. In most cases no changes or only very slight, insignificant, menstrual cycle dependent ER changes were detected (Cao et al. 1983; Sanborn et al.1975; Yajima et al. 1985). However, Garau et al. (1986) found significantly higher ER concentrations in the secretive phase compared with the proliferative phase.

Hoffmann et al. (1980) explain the increasing ER concentration during the menstrual cycle by a positive feedback mechanism caused by estrogen hormone. They conclude that the receptor concentration depends not only on the tissue specimen (ER endometrium > ER endocervix > ER cervix-stroma > ER ectocervix) but also on the hormonal influence acting on the tissue. Cyclic hormonal changes modify the degree of cell differentiation in the upper layers of the cervical squamous epithelium (Schellhas 1969). By means of radioautography Schellhas detected the highest turnover rate in the basal and parabasal layers and concluded that the cells of the lower parabasal layers are the main source for cell renewal.

Gould et al. (1983), using the technique of in vitro steroid auto radiography, observed changes in the nuclear ER content in normal human cervix and vagina during the menstrual cycle. In the early phase of proliferation the vaginal epithelium shows nuclear estrogen binding sites in the basal layer only. In the later proliferative and midcycle phases steroid receptors can be clearly identified in the parabasal and intermediate layers. The superficial layer binds estrogen weakly at this stage. In the secretive phase, the stroma and all layers of the vaginal epithelium are decidedly positive in respect to nuclear estrogen binding sites. Nuclear labeling is consistently greater in stromal than in epithelial cells. Labeling intensity in the ectocervix was similar but less pronounced (Gould et al. 1983). There are clear parallels between our findings and the results reported by Gould et al.

The biochemical determination (DCC method) of the ER and PR protein in cytosol of cervical neoplasia produces varying results. The proportion of tumors with positive ER varies between 13% and 71% (Bolla et al. 1982; Ciocca et al. 1986; Ford et al. 1983; Hunter et al. 1957; Martin et al. 1986; Yajima et al. 1985); for those with positive PR it varies between 6% and 40% (Bolla et al. 1982; Hunter et al. 1987). On average, adenocarcinomas of the uterine cervix show higher receptor concentrations than squamous carcinomas (Gaor et al.1983; Martin et al. 1986; Yajima et al. 1985). Other authors (Ford et al. 1983; Yajima et al. 1985) observed a decreasing ER concentration in cervical neoplasia compared with normal tissue.

However, nontumorous stroma and muscle tissue may play an important role in influencing the results of biochemical receptor analyses in tissue homogenates.

Various authors (Cao et al. 1983; Hoffmann et al. 1980; Sanborn et al. 1975; Soutter et al. 1981) have found that the ER concentration is definitely higher in cervical stroma tissue than in the squamous epithelium of the ectocervix. Thus, in the analysis of ER in the cytosol of cell homogenates which are not representative of the neoplastic cells the stroma cells may cause an incorrectly positive result (Farley et al. 1982). Budwit-Novotny et al. (1986) demonstrated this phenomenon in endometrial cancer. Our immunohistochemical analyses also detected ER-positive stroma cells among the tumors.

Our results showed a decrease in or loss of ER in neoplastic cells of the squamous carcinoma of the uterine cervix. The lack of ER in the tumor cell of cervical carcinoma may explain why a continuation of estrogen influence in premenopausal women does not cause a tumor progression (Martin et al. 1986), why the survival time is independent of the biochemical steroid receptor concentration (Martin et al. 1986), and why antihormonal treatment has no appreciable therapeutic success (Ford et al. 1983). Summarizing our results, we conclude that they do not contradict empirical and clinical evaluations.

However, one must remember that the hormonal influenceability of the stroma cells could result in the production of intracellularly active substances; this could lead, for example, to epidermal growth factor or transforming growth factor. Furthermore, we take the view that investigations must be carried out to determine whether the threshold value for ER and PR protein, determinable by means of the immunohistochemical staining method, really corresponds to the hormonally dependent reaction of the cell in vivo. In our opinion these points need further study.

References

Bloch B (1979) Hormone receptors in cervical intraepithelial neoplasia. Obstet Gynecol Surv 34 : 868–869

Bolla M, Chedin M, Chambaz E, Racinet C, Martin PM (1982) Steroid receptors in cancer of the uterine cervix. Bull Cancer 69 : 384

Budwit-Novotny DA, McCarty KS, Cox EB, Soper JT, Mutch DG, Creasman WT, Flowers JL, McCarty KS (1986) Immunohistochemical analyses of estrogen receptor in endometrial adenocarcinoma using a monoclonal antibody. Cancer Res 46 : 5419–5425

Cao Z, Eppenberger U, Roos W, Torhorst J, Almendral A (1983) Cytosol estrogen and progesterone receptor levels measured in normal and pathological tissue of endometrium, endocervical mucosa and cervical vaginal portion. Arch Gynecrl 233 : 109–119

Ciocca DR, Puy LA, Lo Castro G. (1986) Localization of an estrogen-responsive protein in the human cervix during menstrual cycle, pregnancy, and menopause and in abnormal cervical epithelia without atypia. Obstet Gynecol 155 : 1090–1096

Drill VA (1976) Effect of estrogens and progestins on the cervix uteri. J Toxicol Environ Health (Suppl) 1 : 193–204

Farley AL, O'Brien T, Moyer D, Taylor CR (1982) The detection of estrogen receptors in gynecologic tumors using immunoperoxidase and the dextran-coated charcoal assay. Cancer 49 : 2153–2160

Fenton J, Asselain B, Magdelenat H (1986) Dosage des recepteurs d'oestorgene et de progesterone dans les epitheliomas du col uterin (A propos d'une serie de 101 cas). Bull Cancer 73 : 124–126

Ford LC, Berek JS, LaGasse LD, Hacker NF, Heins YL, DeLange RJ (1983) Estrogen and progesterone receptor sites in malignancies of the uterine cervix, vagina and vulva. Gynecol Oncol 15 : 27–31

Fujimoto J, Tamaya T, Watanabe Y, Arahori K, Sato S, Okada H (1986) Steroid receptors in uterine cervical cancers. Acta Obstet Gynecol Jpn 38 : 575–582

Gaor YL, Twiggs LB, Leung BS, Yu WCY, Potish RA, Okagaki T, Adcock LL, Prem KA (1983) Cytoplasmatic estrogen and progesterone receptors in primary cervical carcinoma: clinical and histopathologic correlates. Am J Obstet Gynecol 146 : 299–306

Garau JM, di Paola GR, Charreau EH (1986) Estrogen and progesterone receptor assays on the vulvar epithelium. J Reprod Med 31 : 987–991

Gould SF, Shannon JM, Cunha GR (1983) The autoradiographic demonstration of estrogen binding in normal human cervix and vagina during the menstrual cycle, Pregnancy, and the Menopause. Am J Anat 168 : 229–238

Hoffman PG., Siiteri PK. (1980) Sex steroid receptors in gynecologic cancer. Obstet Gynecol 55: 648–652

Hunter RE, Longcope C: Keough P (1987) Steroid hormone receptors in carcinoma of the cervix. Cancer 60: 392–396

Husseinzadeh N, Nahhas WA, Velkeley DE, Whithney CW, Mortel R (1984) The Preservation of ovarian function in young women undergoing pelvic radiation therapy. Gynecol Oncol 18: 373–379

Lohe KJ, Baltzer J (1984) Malignome der Cervix uteri in Bender H G(ed) Gynäkologische Onkologie. Thieme Stuttgart

Martin JD, Hähnel R, McCartney AJ, De Klerk N. (1986) The influence of estrogen and progesterone receptors on survival in patients with carcinoma of the uterine cervix. Gynecol Oncol 23: 329–335

Potish RA, Twiggs LB, Adcock LL, Prem KA, Savage LE, Leung BS (1986) Prognostic importance of progesterone and estrogen receptors in cancer of the uterine cervix. Cancer 58: 1709–1713

Sanborn BM, Held B, Kuo HS (1975) Specific estrogen binding proteins in human cervix. J Steroid Biochem 6: 1107–1112

Schellhas HF (1969) Cell renewal in the human cervix uteri. Am J Obstet Gynecol 104: 617–632

Soost HJ (1980) Zellen eines normalen Vaginal- und Zervixabstrichs. In: Soost HJ, Baur S (eds) Gynäkologische Zytodiagnostik. Thieme, Stuttgart

Soutter WP, Pegoraro RJ, Green-Thompson RW, Naidoo DV, Joubert SM, Philpott RH (1981) Nuclear and cytoplasmatic oestrogen receptors in squamous carcinoma of the cervix. Br J Cancer 44: 154–159

Yajima A, Yamauchi R, Wade Y, Furuhashi, Toki T, Tase T, Oikawa N, Sato S, Takabayashi T, Ozawa N, (1985) Cytoplasmatic estrogen receptors in carcinoma of the uterine cervic. Gynecol Obstet Invest 20: 103–108

Subject Index